AF361524

SAVORING CARE

Savoring Care

Flourishing with Diabetes Across Cultures

EDITED BY JESSICA HARDIN
AND EMILY MENDENHALL

UNIVERSITY OF TORONTO PRESS
Toronto Buffalo London

ISBN 978-1-4875-6569-5 (CLOTH)   ISBN 978-1-4875-6572-5 (EPUB)
ISBN 978-1-4875-6570-1 (PAPER)   ISBN 978-1-4875-6571-8 (PDF)

Library and Archives Canada Cataloguing in Publication

Title: Savoring care : flourishing with diabetes across cultures / edited by Jessica Hardin and
   Emily Mendenhall.
Names: Hardin, Jessica A., editor | Mendenhall, Emily, 1982– editor
Description: Includes bibliographical references and index.
Identifiers: Canadiana (print) 20250288052 | Canadiana (ebook) 20250288109 | ISBN
   9781487565701 (paper) | ISBN 9781487565695 (cloth) | ISBN 9781487565718 (PDF) |
   ISBN 9781487565725 (EPUB)
Subjects: LCSH: Diabetics—Care—Cross-cultural studies. | LCSH: Type 2 diabetes—Alternative
   treatment—Cross-cultural studies.
Classification: LCC RC662.18 .S28 2025 | DDC 616.4/62406—dc23

Cover design: Will Brown
Cover image: Alice Noir, *Anjali Mudra*, The Noun Project

We welcome comments and suggestions regarding any aspect of our publications – please feel free to contact us at news@utorontopress.com or visit us at utorontopress.com.

Every effort has been made to contact copyright holders; in the event of an error or omission, please notify the publisher.

We wish to acknowledge the land on which the University of Toronto Press operates. This land is the traditional territory of the Wendat, the Anishnaabeg, the Haudenosaunee, the Métis, and the Mississaugas of the Credit First Nation.

University of Toronto Press acknowledges the financial support of the Government of Canada and the Ontario Arts Council, an agency of the Government of Ontario, for its publishing activities.

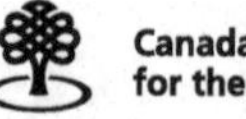

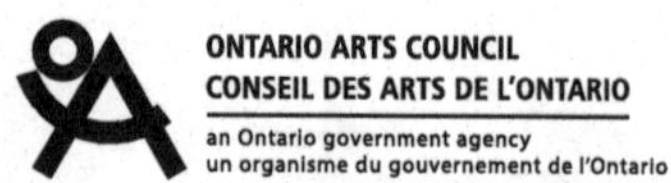

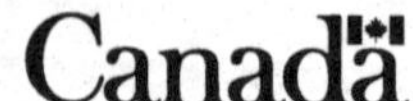

Contents

Introduction: Flourishing with Diabetes ix

EMILY MENDENHALL AND JESSICA HARDIN

1 Complicating Relations: On Research Obligations and Creating Space for Difference 1

JESSICA HARDIN, SAUNIMA'A MA FULU-AIOLUPOTEA, UILA LAIFA LIMA, RAMONA BOODOOSINGH, TAUAITALA POLOIE LEES, TAUSALA AIAVAO, AND FALELUA MAUA

Section One: Diabetes Is *Always* Relational

2 Funeka's Kitchen: Diabetes Healing in Soweto Living Rooms through Prayer and Commensality 19

EMILY MENDENHALL, LINDILE CELE, AND EDNA N. BOSIRE

3 Grace between Wives: Living the Good Life in Senegal 31

EMMA NELSON BUNKLEY, FATOUMATA DIAGNE, AND NDÈYE AMINATA MBAYE

4 Tinkering: Getting By with Diabetes through Creativity and Relational Care in Fiji 43

TARRYN PHILLIPS AND EDWARD NARAIN

5 Ancestral Healing: Interconnected Legacies of Sugar in Brazil   57

   D. BURNETT

Section Two: Diabetes *Always* Reflects Social Structures

6 Friends Can Heal Pain in the Midst of Trauma:
   Manuela's and Alyshia's Story   73

   MANUELA FUENTES AND ALYSHIA GÁLVEZ

7 Socio-Somatic Generativity: A Life Story from Vietnam   88

   TINE M. GAMMELTOFT AND DUNG VŨ

8 Footsteps: How Did We Get Here?   106

   JAMES DOUCET-BATTLE

9 Disruption: Centering Native Youth Voices for Health
   and Healing in Arizona   120

   TOMMEY JODIE, JESSE PABLO, LAUREL BELLANTE, AND
   MEGAN A. CARNEY

Section Three: Diabetes Is about *More than* Diet

10 Iatrochemistry: Recipes that Heal   145

   EMILY YATES-DOERR

11 Connecting Care, Connecting Chronic Illness:
   Community, Rural Health, and Insecurity in Hidalgo,
   Mexico   161

   EMILIA MERCEDES GUEVARA

12 Don Agustín's Crafts: Patience, Skill, and Creativity in
   Weaving the Weft of Life   175

   LAURA MONTESI

Section Four: Diabetes Is *More than* Numbers

13 Embodied Measuring   195

   PALLAVI LAXMIKANTH

14 Thriving while Struggling to Access Care in India   210

LESLEY JO WEAVER

15 Confianza and Collaborative Care: The Value of Patient-
Physician Partnerships   224

JESSICA P. CERDEÑA AND GENESIS SANTOS

Epilogue   237

EMILY MENDENHALL AND JESSICA HARDIN

Author Biographies   241

Index   251

Introduction: Flourishing with Diabetes

Emily Mendenhall and Jessica Hardin

Sneha walked the streets in Old Delhi, searching for a flat residing in a government housing complex. Most people living there had moved from slums scattered throughout the city, and Sneha had spent hours there listening to people's stories about living with diabetes. Before the turn of the century, type 2 diabetes, a condition of insulin resistance, was uncommon or possibly undetected among lower-income Delhiites. Even though this diabetes type was for years expected to emerge among the wealthy, people across income groups in Delhi were developing the condition younger, and it was becoming common among middle and lower-middle class residents, though it sometimes took years to be diagnosed. Sneha found the right flat and softly rapped on the door, noting that the woman she was visiting had young children.

Mona opened the door and nodded her head to Sneha, expecting her. Her gold bangles chimed as Sneha entered the small flat and observed the woman's striking face, her black hair clipped together with a hairclip. Mona's tall frame was covered by a green salwar kameez that had been washed again and again for years. She led Sneha to a room that was locked, where they found a private space for guests that was brightly painted yellow with adorning orange pillars. Although they were somewhat outdated, Sneha observed a sofa, a computer, and a few paintings and posters, too. The house was clean and comforting, and Sneha took a seat on the sofa.

After tea was served, Mona and Sneha slowly moved to conversation about Mona's life. She was married at nineteen and lived with her husband, his mother, father, sister, and his sister's husband. None of them were currently working since her husband left work due to a brain disorder, and his father retired when his heart problems intensified and his type 2 diabetes got worse. "Everyone has a little diabetes," she said when she was talking about both her father-in-law's health condition and her own. Sneha perked up and scribbled something in her notebook. The commonness and acceptance of diabetes was one of the most pervasive themes emerging from her hundreds of interviews. Sneha had worked with two anthropologists who were trying to understand the experience of diabetes in Delhi for the past several years, first Lesley Jo Weaver (2018), and then her friend Emily Mendenhall (2019). Both were curious about why people dismissed diabetes risk and instead seemed to accept or normalize it in India.

Mona's diabetes came on during pregnancy. After the first delivery, her body stabilized, but gestational diabetes came back in her second pregnancy. She was incredibly careful during her pregnancies and was able to control her sugar. After her second baby was born, she wasn't checked again until she became very sick and discovered that her gestational diabetes had progressed to type 2 diabetes.

Mona manages her diabetes on her own, making sure not to mention her own diabetes to her family. Instead, she focuses on her father-in-law's needs and is careful in preparing his foods and managing his medicines. She watches what she eats, too, but rarely discusses her own risk. This is in part because her husband is living with an illness, too. His brain condition makes his behavior erratic and keeps him from working. She is also struggling with the loss of her brother and frequent small conflicts with her mother-in-law. Mona, however, describes how it's important to keep calm and accept one's fate. She sleeps well and feels safe in her neighborhood. She unburdens her stresses in conversations with her sister. They share everything – from parenting her two boys to struggles with their husbands. Having someone to speak with calms her body and helps her through the hardest of times. These are some of the most critical elements for controlling her health and managing her sugar.

Mona is one of some 537 million adults who are currently living with diabetes in the world. This number is predicted to rise to 643 million by

2030 and to more than one billion by 2050. In the United States alone over 11 per cent of Americans live with diabetes. These numbers are staggering.

Yet, we have found that despite the extraordinary risk and burden of this health condition, many people like Mona make do and even thrive. Anthropologist and family physician Jessica Cerdeña (2022, vi) has coined this "imperative resilience." In her work with immigrant women living with diabetes in the northeast United States, she found that women exhibit "daring and devotion" as they navigate precarity, illness, and stress. In this book, we center the relational dynamics around diabetes that Cerdeña suggests fuel an imperative resilience that has long been sidelined, even while recognizing the social hierarchies that make living well in the world difficult. We argue that social support systems involving siblings, spouses, parents, children, neighbors, and friends play an outsized role in people's health and the ingenuity they need to live well with diabetes, particularly when access to reliable and routine medical care proves difficult.

For too long, medical counseling and treatment for diabetes has been framed as the only "commonsense," rational, and moral response to a diabetes diagnosis, centering the need to reconsider how people eat and what people eat. We counter this narrow focus and, as anthropologists often do, offer alternative logics and illuminate other rational responses. Hence, the stories in this book question overly simple public frames for diabetes that focus explicitly on inputs and outputs – a notion that diabetes is a choice for which individuals are utterly responsible.

Scholars have demonstrated for decades now how a focus on individual choices obscures structural conditions. The monetization of health care in places like the United States narrows clinical attention to metrics-based possibilities for interventions because they are both profitable and efficient in terms of time (Closser et al. 2022; Horton et al. 2014). Global health infrastructures that privilege technological solutions to structural problems are also embedded in efficiency logics that reproduce the global inequalities that they seek to redress (Pfeiffer and Chapman 2010). Scientific design, particularly when it comes to obesity and diabetes, reduces environmental complexity to BMI or caloric intake (Valdez 2018; Warin and Gunson 2013). These critiques demonstrate the profound challenges involved in working against enduring structures that privilege capital over health, treatment over social change, and individual responsibility over shared responsibility.

Our approach to diabetes is to decenter medical narratives around diabetes, which are often stigmatizing and suggest that people center illness in their lives above all else. Instead, we have found that people live with diabetes in ways that are profoundly shaped by their families and environments. For these reasons, we take a bit of a different approach than many medical anthropologists working on diabetes, as well as our earlier work on the topic. We consider how people *live well with diabetes* and adopt the construct of flourishing proposed by medical anthropologist Sarah Willen: an "active process of striving to live in keeping with one's defining values, commitments and vision for the future, as individuals and in the context of one's family and the communities to which one belongs" (Willen et al. 2022). As opposed to positive psychologists who consider flourishing an explicitly psychological state, we recognize how flourishing is not an endpoint but rather a pursuit or journey (Willen 2022). We are also inspired by Black feminist anthropologists Ashanté Reese and Hanna Garth, who in writing about diverse Black food cultures explore how people "make a life" within contexts where the state fails to meet community needs (Reese and Garth 2020, 2). Writing about flourishing is inspired by the possibilities that emerge "when we turn to the everyday ways people *make a way outta no way*" to "theorize Black ways of distributing food under structural constraints" (Reese 2020, 31; italics original; see also Hartman 2019).

We reframe diabetes in terms of flourishing to highlight that diabetes is not a metric or choice, but rather a lived experience that is nested within a more robust and complicated social world. We have found that, in various contexts, many people perceive chronic illness as a path through which people journey, adapt, and transform while mitigating the various social, political, and economic structures that shape a life journey (Schmidt-Sane et al. 2023; Cele et al. 2022). As an active pursuit, many people remake a way to find meaning, support, and well-being, despite adversities. The stories we present in this book, then, are meant to provide a window into this otherwise view, a view that makes the idea of individual choice seem strange and aims to stimulate the imagining of more complex approaches to the threshold of body and environment (Paxson 2023; Moran Thomas 2019). Thinking otherwise, as Laura Meek and Julia Alejandra Morales Fontanilla argue, is a core feminist concept, analytic framework, and method – a "political commitment to the insistence of the possible against the pull of the probable" (2022, 274).

SIMPLE STORIES

There is no question that type 2 diabetes has skyrocketed in the past several decades across different kinds of economic contexts. On the surface, the story of why rates of diabetes continue to climb seems simple: people are eating more of the wrong foods, and if we could change people's minds about adopting a healthy diet, then we could be freed of the scourge of diabetes and its associated condition, obesity. This commonsense frame, however, makes invisible all the ways in which changes in how we eat reflect other step-by-step changes in how we move, think, interact, and share in our changing world. Food is not only material but wrapped up in one's identity, family, and culture. As a condition seemingly defined by the dysregulation of insulin, diabetes is in fact defined by the dysregulation of economies and ecologies that have come to shape social contexts (Gálvez 2018).

Anthropologists are experts at observing structures – that is, patterned social interactions, the institutional organizing of resources, and the norms and values that inform how these patterns unfold. When it comes to diabetes, anthropologists have long demonstrated the ways that structural inequalities and violence have shaped who gets sick and who is spared. This biopolitical approach shows how trauma (Mendenhall 2012, 2019), migration (Carney 2015), hunger (Yates-Doerr 2015), food insecurity (Carruth and Mendenhall 2019), trade (Gálvez 2018), race (Doucet-Battle 2021), gender (Weaver 2018), and changes in land relations (Hardin 2021) all shape life changes when it comes to diabetes. As two medical anthropologists who have investigated questions around type 2 diabetes for years in very different contexts – Samoa, India, South Africa, Kenya, and the United States – we have found that rarely does diabetes affect everyone equally.

On the one hand, the epidemiological context in which someone lives profoundly shapes how one experiences diabetes alone and together with other health conditions, from hypertension, heart disease, anxiety, and autoimmune conditions to tuberculosis, fevers, and

HIV. The commonness of diabetes was stark in Mona's story, for example, when she suggested that "everyone has a little diabetes" in Delhi (Mendenhall 2019), thereby actively normalizing the condition. At the same time, Jessica Hardin (2019) has found in her research in Samoa that people frequently situate diabetes within a broader cluster of illness, often saying, "I have all of them," referring to having a combination of metabolic disorders.

On the other hand, from where, when, and how people seek care plays a profound role in how they understand their health condition, manage their disease, and pursue medical care. For instance, people seeking care within a pluralistic health system like India's, where multiple private and public care options exist, may need to strategically navigate multiple access points for medical care at once. These may be public or private, biomedical or spiritual, pharmacological or social. Someone might access routine diabetes care from a public clinic and seek specialized care from a private provider. They might seek medications from a government facility and seek other therapies from a private pharmacy or traditional healer. They might seek the support of a therapist or seek solace from a faith healer. What this looks like differs meaningfully across systems, cultures, and economies of care, and these frames matter when thinking about diabetes.

Recognizing the complexity of illness and care experiences is particularly important for recognizing how diabetes risk is constructed differently from place to place.[1] We know diabetes is not a simple process of calories in, calories out, as is often suggested by the media and medicine through the axiom of choice and the emphasis on individual responsibility.[2] This metrification of health reduces social, cultural, economic, and political complexity in ways that obscure how communities are differentially exposed to risk. Seth Holmes (2013, 17), a medical anthropologist and physician, suggests that

> many experts who study what are called "risk behaviors" in the field of public health might say that these push and pull factors are weighed in the individual's "decisional balance" when such a person chooses whether or not to engage in a risky behavior [like migration or consuming sugary foods]. Such a view assumes a rationally acting individual, maximizing her self-interest and having control over her destiny through choice. Minimized in these

analyses is a focus on the central importance of structural context and the ways in which structural forces constrain and inflect individual choice and direct the options available to people.

There are many limitations to a choice-based model of health, but for our purposes, we want to highlight two. First, choice is an overly simplistic way to understand how people go about feeding themselves and their families. Our everyday lives are not filled with dichotomous choices of healthy options or unhealthy options. Selecting ingredients, snacks, or meals often requires a calculus of exposure: a choice between the vegetables that are pesticide soaked but may offer nutrition to your children or the instant noodles that will fill their bellies and spare them from that toxic exposure (Yates-Doerr 2014). Individual behavioral interventions are predicated on a false choice, based in a simplistic world where opting to avoid unhealthy options is likened to eating a daily diet flush with fruits and vegetables. Second, behavioral approaches do not address the biochemical realities of dysregulated insulin. As a hormone secreted by the pancreas that reduces sugar in the blood, insulin is also closely linked to our environments through stress pathways. Cortisol, a stress hormone, can work on cells to make them insulin resistant. This is one psychophysiological pathway through which social dynamics can afflict and transform the material body.[3] Socially, biologically, and ecologically, focusing diabetes care only on "modifiable behaviors" is an approach constrained by what we imagine is possible, not an approach that reflects scientific complexity. Indeed, anthropological work on diabetes has stood for a distinct departure from medical and public health frames that have long centered individual choice.

DIABETES IN MEDICAL ANTHROPOLOGY

As a condition that clearly demonstrates the porosity of our bodies in our environments, or the ways that our outside environments and our foods shape our internal mechanisms, diabetes has served as a bellwether of global change, emerging at sweeping rates around the world alongside other world-shifting patterns that have changed how we work, play, and eat. Tracking these changes at simultaneous local and global levels has been enormously helpful to anthropologists as they have tried for generations to understand what it means to be human in today's rapidly changing world.

Biological anthropologists have long worked to understand what has come to be thought of as the epidemiological transition – that is, the macro-level theory of why, around the world, patterns of disease have shifted from communicable (like cholera or HIV) to noncommunicable (like diabetes or depression). Stephen McGarvey, an epidemiologist and biological anthropologist, for instance, used obesity and eventually diabetes to explain how and why globalization, framed at that time as modernization, was rapidly transforming human society (McGarvey et al. 1993). Leslie Sue Lieberman (2003), taking an evolutionary perspective, has argued that humans in both developed and developing countries are metabolically maladapted for our current environments, which shape the kinds of foods we eat and the kinds of spaces in which we live and work. In this light, diabetes began to be thought of as a "disease of modernity" or a "disease of civilization."

When anthropologists study diabetes, we are analytically positioning it as indicative. Diabetes has been an incredibly important disease to study because of the ways it has emerged in relation to social change, particularly in response to globalization, "as a force, a process and a set of relations" over the past seventy-five years (Manderson and Smith-Morris 2010, 8). Since World War II, changes in labor, manufacturing, immigration, and supply chain management, and the emergence of neoliberal logics, have made diabetes a fundamental (bio)marker of modernity. Though the earliest anthropological science on this topic fashioned diabetes as a consequence of modernization, it sometimes naturalized population-wide experiences of chronic illness as a logical and inevitable result of modernization. Emily Mendenhall (2019) has argued that this misrecognizes modernity for the poverty that stems from rapid global change. Emily Yeats-Doerr (2022) names it precisely when she writes that theorizing about macro-level change accredited to modernity is "taking place against the backdrop of imperial history" that is often naturalized or erased from analytic attention.

One of the first ethnographies to tackle this problem was Carolyn Smith-Morris's 2008 book, *Diabetes among the Pima: Stories of Survival*. She argues that understanding motherhood, foodways, and identity is as significant to understanding high rates of diabetes as genetic factors. In fact, she argues that the overestimated role of genetics in diabetes risk often makes potential structural changes to redress the harms of settler colonialism difficult to see, never mind implement. The outsized public and scientific attention to genetic risk only reproduces the ways that individuals are blamed for their conditions (Warin et al. 2016). In the years following Smith-Morris's book, a wave of medical anthropologists took to the topic of diabetes and obesity. Interest in the topic reflected the historical moment in which newly trained anthropologists were emerging – a time when panic over obesity was sweeping across the United States and beyond (SturtzSreetharan et al. 2021). By 2020, there were several influential sociological and anthropological books that presented the rise of obesity as a function of global capitalism, and its accompanying moral panic as a form of racialized, gendered, and classed-based blame for systemic, global change.

Feminist anthropologists also took a particular interest in the study of obesity, tracking how ideals about good bodies are naturalized in clinical and global health practices at the expense of the complex science that troubles the use of the neat and tidy BMI metric (Jeske 2021; Warin et al. 2008; Warin 2015). What becomes evident in these ethnographies is the inseparability of studying obesity and studying diabetes, hypertension, kidney disease, and cardiovascular disease. To study one, in many ways, is to study the others. Medical anthropologists demonstrate this and, in doing so, demonstrate the intersecting social experiences that shape how diabetes manifests in bodies and in communities. Diabetes never occurs in isolation: trauma, migration, and hunger also become engines for metabolic change.

And yet, when diabetes sweeps through communities and stays, people around the world make meaningful lives through their faith, friendships, and activism while cultivating resilience (Cerdeña 2023). This is why we elevate stories where people make sense of diabetes in relation to the day-to-day complexities of the lives they live, often finding joy apart from illness, and managing their symptoms, medications, and clinical expectations as best they can. Some might even be labeled "noncompliant" while still striving to manage diabetes in ways that make sense to them (Weaver 2018). While many people have the resources to achieve this by reducing stress and changing their environments, diets, exercise habits, and pharmacological routines, others don't have those resources. Others may have the resources to make these behavioral changes but cannot change the toxicity of their environments, in terms of chemical exposures or the lived realities of everyday racism (Solomon 2016; Doucet-Battle 2021). Regardless of their socioeconomic status and myths of what drives glucose "control," people around the world actively strive to make uncomfortable symptoms subside while crafting livable, and sometimes thriving, worlds.

A GUIDE TO THINKING WITH THIS BOOK

Our sections are organized into four ways of thinking about diabetes from the perspective of medical anthropology. First, it's important to recognize how **diabetes is *always* relational**, meaning that diabetes is socially enacted, embodied, and shared. Living with diabetes is work. It requires careful management, a distinct kind of sensitivity to technologies that translate potentially dangerous embodied experiences into metrics, and a re-evaluation of the meaning of what constitutes good and healthy foods.

From a relational perspective, diabetes isn't simply about managing blood sugar levels; it's about how people live within networks of care, respond to the expectations of family, friends, and health-care providers, and navigate social and cultural norms around food, restriction, and money. Consider, for example, Jessica's ethnography of how Pentecostal Samoans manage their diabetes through salvational logics; that is, how they understand their health as a measure of their faith. In this example, people in Bible study groups or attending sermons forge new interpretations of the meaning of diabetes in relation to their spiritual lives, where the ups and downs of glucose might reflect the ups and downs of emotions like anger, anxiety, or sadness that are managed by turning to spiritual tools. This spiritual focus, however, is not only about an individual relationship with God but also comes about through the intensive work of praying with others, alongside everyday forms of comfort, such as consoling a friend whose husband left her or attending a Zumba class with a pregnant friend who found out they have diabetes. Diabetes is managed in concert with others, through talking, sharing food, or giving people rides to their appointments. In these ways, experiences of diabetes are forged through deeply personal, social, and cultural relationships. The interpersonal dynamism of diabetes reveals how the work we do for our loved ones and friends to cultivate life with dignity and generosity is often central to the diabetes experience.

Second, **diabetes *always* reflects social structures**. The stories in this book illuminate – in different and socially situated ways – how diabetes and other chronic illnesses emerge around the globe in relation to steepening global inequalities that stem from neoliberal economic change. The concept of structural violence is a good starting point. Paul Farmer describes structural violence as "violence exerted systematically – that is, indirectly – by everyone who belongs to a certain social order," a notion that is intended to help us understand "the social machinery of oppression" (2004, 307). In some ways this construct fails to put "gendered and racialized histories of conquest, settler colonization, and dispossession into conversations focused on economics or politics" (Gálvez, Carney, and Yates-Doerr 2020, 640). Some feminist scholars, including those writing for this book, suggest that recognizing these layered histories is imperative to understanding how illness is experienced and embodied differently within and between peoples. At the same time, diabetes is much more complex than simply a marker of insulin resistance. In addition to this layering of social context, diabetes is often experienced alongside other chronic, acute, and social conditions that stem from deeply unequal contexts. Emily has argued, for example, that diabetes is never a disease experienced in isolation but rather is a syndemic condition defined by "synergistically interacting epidemics," such as diabetes *with* depression, domestic violence, emotional distress, social isolation, and infections (Mendenhall et al. 2022, 1359; Mendenhall 2012, 2019).

This focus on syndemics should demonstrate the point clearly that **diabetes is about *more than* diet**. There is a powerful shadow of morality imbued in the obesity and diabetes literature, which propagates a profoundly moral discourse about self-control. This moral discourse attributes a collection of poor individual choices to a lack of virtue or fortitude to resist temptation. This is also a largely Christian ideal, rooted in cultural beliefs suffused with notions of virtuosity, that is closely linked to fat shaming and body image dialogue in Western cultures like the ones we live in (in the United States) (Hardin 2019; Gerber 2012; Griffith 2004). This scholarship suggests that fat is linked to one's inability to control, reflecting a Western and deeply gendered construct of personhood that is rooted in capitalist notions of self (Bordo 1993). In these ways, how big a body is and how elevated one's hemoglobin A1C is deem if someone is a "bad" patient or a "good" patient, who follows nutritional guidelines and clinical protocols for keeping sugars controlled and weight low. Such views certainly compete with other moralities, such as patients' roles as parents, partners, children, friends, religious practitioners, workers, and citizens. How people navigate this morality – within the interstices of good and bad, health and sickness, obedience and deviance – is a central theme we explore.

This focus on diet, food management, and self-control falls short of the emerging science that demonstrates the ways that environmental toxicity shapes our metabolic processes. Environmental toxins, especially the endocrine-disrupting chemicals that infuse all aspects of our lives through the plastics we use, the pesticides we are exposed to, and the industrial products that make life possible at a global scale, are increasingly associated with the development of diabetes – something our interlocuters have been describing for some time. One anthropologist, Harris Solomon (2016), takes this understanding of the porosity of our bodies as a starting point to argue that metabolic living defines our times. He does so through the lens of urban India, where diabetes and obesity emerge through processes of absorption, blurring the lines between environment and body. Throughout this book, contributors introduce the reader to nurses, anthropologists, mothers, and friends who creatively and lovingly navigate the blurry lines between food, medicine, and poison in their unrelenting search for healing.

Finally, this leads up to the important recognition that despite the seeming simplicity of health metrics like glucose or weight, **diabetes is *more than* numbers**. Medical anthropologists have come to see metrics as powerful tools in isolating individuals from environments in scientific studies of disease, clinical care, and interventions, both for chronic illnesses like diabetes and also a host of entangled social and health problems (Adams 2016; Benton 2015; Yates-Doerr 2015; Sangaramoorthy 2014). As with dietary change, when patients fail to lower their metrics, they are blamed: *You have no self-control! Did you take your medication!? What did you eat? How many steps are you walking each day?* In fact, when patients focus on numbers, or experience the stigma of not living up to their target numbers, their health and well-being may be affected negatively (Brewis and Wutich 2014; Brewis 2014). Though for some, focusing on numbers may be a way to gain power and refocus more energy on other meaningful things in life.

For the past fifty years, studies have demonstrated that diet-focused prevention efforts don't work, and metabolic disorders are increasingly linked to environmental exposure. Why do individualized measures and interventions persist in both public health and medicine? Natali Valdez (2022) takes this question head-on in her ethnographic study of obesity in pregnancy in randomized control trials in the United States and the United Kingdom. She argues that when scientific tools isolate individual behavior as data, these techniques then discount the role of social environments in contributing to obesity risk, and in turn the vital impacts of systemic racism are also erased. These forms of systemic racism are therefore not the target of intervention; instead, the individual's eating and exercise habits are targeted for interventions because they are measurable.[4] In light of this, we introduce women who integrate metrics in different ways into their complex lives, where they navigate stress, trauma, and family demands.

In this book, we describe the lives of people in seemingly radically different places, following the ways diabetes is a life, and it is not a life. Through diabetes people make meaning but rarely is diabetes the core of one's identity. For some, diabetes may be a window through which they observe other traumatic experiences in their lives, from interpersonal to medical trauma. Yet, for others, it may be a way through which they deepen relationships with family members, friends, or groups in their community or online, thereby cultivating friendships and support networks that they would not have without the illness. In these ways, we share stories about diabetes that decenter diabetes and place the illness and identity within complex, messy, and full scenarios through which people navigate everyday life.

This book is simultaneously about diabetes and not about diabetes. We bring together scholars, practitioners, patients, and friends to story complexity into global-level explanations for the emergence of diabetes at multiple scales. And while there is particularity to diabetes experiences when it comes to critically and anthropologically understanding how people make meaning and act upon and understand their circumstances, diabetes stands in for disease as an analytic category. Whether we are examining COVID-19, HIV, cancer, or malaria, diseases are socially constructed while also socially constructing. To understand the social construction of disease is to situate meaning alongside material contexts, to keep individuals and communities in focus alongside the systems that they navigate. Experiences of illness are fundamental to human experience across space and time; we bear witness to these experiences in relation to the historical processes that have come to define bioscientific and biomedical modes of managing illness, where knowledge is squarely individualized and technological fixes are imagined to be the magic bullet (Packard 2016). Just as the people we write about across these chapters, we situate diabetes as a prism for understanding the complex interplay of biosocial dynamics that operate at micro and macro levels, from the individual to the community, from microbiome to macrobiome (Benezra 2023; Carney and Gálvez 2019).

ORIENTATION

Our writing about diabetes differs from how diabetes has commonly been written about in anthropology, public health, and medicine. Our stories stand in contrast to a unifying "global" narrative of diabetes that narrows how we might think about the condition. We present stories of living well using an asset-based approach as opposed to a deficient approach to community health. This approach is common in public health and stands in contrast to the historical approach to communities through a deficit lens – where communities are targeted with a top-down approach and external expertise is used to define problems and the shortcomings of communities. The asset approach, in contrast, emphasizes community strengths and capacities, uses collaborative methods, and is community driven.

To illuminate the multiple ways in which people are savoring care, we experiment with storytelling to offer a way of thinking about diabetes that recognizes how health inequities are reproduced within racist and settler colonial systems, and how people flourish despite them. People find joy in their relationships, developing new recipes that celebrate the flavors and textures of their families' foods, or cultivating new routines that are life-giving. We invite you to consider what we might learn from stories that bring into focus the enormous potential of people to make life not only endurable but distinctly meaningful through the prism of illness.

We encourage you to think about building a healthier world by listening to how people create nourishing relationships within contexts of steep inequalities. In doing so, we question universal approaches (eat less, exercise more) to hold at bay our assumptions about how health works and to center the communities and people living with illness as experts themselves (see Hsu et al. 2024). There is potential to think better about diabetes globally by understanding the multiplicity of relations, strategies, and knowledge that people employ to live well despite diabetes.

Our approach reflects what is becoming increasingly common in anthropology – to move beyond critique, to explore "the threshold of possibility" that anthropology has to offer the world (Pandian 2019, 4). This book gathers stories from around the world that imagine a world *with* diabetes where illness is a journey nested within a complex life filled with love, joy, suffering, despair, and commensality. We do not try to "solve" the problem of diabetes, as if there is a singular solution to an illness that reflects complex local biologies around the globe. To bear witness to the stories presented here is to recognize that ecologies matter in ways that Margaret Lock (1993) envisioned when she challenged the assumption that biology is a fixed or purely natural category. Instead, we see that diabetes emerges in a biosocial way, where food, toxic exposure, chronic stress, trauma, and microorganisms differently constitute diabetes "risk." We encourage you to listen to the diverse voices – from New York to Samoa, Brazil to Guatemala, Senegal to Vietnam, Baltimore to Mexico – to reflect on possibilities for solidarity and action that embrace thriving alongside struggling, flourishing despite adversity. To refocus attention on living well, as we do in this book, is not to erase the ways that our worlds are shaped by all sorts of structural inequalities but to question what there is to learn *from* and *with* communities that flourish in these situations.

METHODOLOGICAL EXPERIMENTATION

This book is organized around a collection of composite, personal, and observational stories compiled through ethnographic work. Anthropologists tend to share the idea that stories can be transformative, and we believe that the stories to follow have the potential to change how you think about living with diabetes, not only from a cross-cultural perspective but also through the lens of patients who live complex and full lives. Each author builds on long-term fieldwork and relationships that come from in-depth engagement. In some cases, these chapters are written by cultural anthropologists who have conducted ethnographic fieldwork, participating in and observing the daily lives of a community for up to twenty years.

Traditionally, in anthropology, ethnographers are expected to learn about a community different from their own, to learn a language and strive to understand life and how people make sense of their lives. Today, anthropologists conduct ethnography in their home communities as well. Our field sites are no longer defined by discrete groups or communities but now are often focused on the institutions that shape people's lives, from clinics to policy spaces to classrooms. In more collaborative ethnography, anthropologists partner with interlocutors, community members, or other actors involved in the community in which they work. Many of our authors take this approach, which you will see by the co-authorship among the many collaborative research teams.

Many authors in this book depart from traditional ethnographic writing to engage in a more inventive style of ethnographic fiction, vignette, or creative ethnography. This writing provides more flexibility to convey a scene that may have emerged through interviews, participant observation, and years of learning about how people engage in and around their illness. Putting protagonists in conversation together provides an opportunity to show clearly the complexities and challenges people face while living well with illness. It opens space for new kinds of thinking, revealing the ways people live well together and support one another in shared spaces. This is a kind of dialogue between ethnographers and their counterparts, depicting an intimate reading and understanding of how people grapple with and overcome the challenges of living with complex chronic illness.

Before we jump into our four sections – of thinking of diabetes in terms of relationality and social structures and beyond diets and numbers – we turn to Jessica's research team, which struggled immensely with the project of writing about *living well with diabetes*. In some ways, this was because the research team spent time with people struggling to manage their conditions amid structural barriers that impede medical models for achieving good health. Instead, people more routinely found good health in faith and friends, commensality, and community. In what follows, we illuminate how our collective writing teams have grappled with thinking about how people who live with diabetes enact imperative resilience in their everyday lives, relationships, and communities. We demonstrate how notions of well-being – of living well in the face of adversity – are individually defined, collectively constructed, and contextually understood. We emphasize here, and throughout the stories in this book, how the relationships of people and their communities, as the writers who have come together to construct these stories, are central to how we think about illness, well-being, and the project of medical anthropology itself.

NOTES

1 For more on how obesity and diabetes research flattens differences within African American and Black communities see Doucet-Battle (2016) and McClure (2016).
2 For more on the history of metabolic thinking see Landecker (2013).
3 This dynamic relationship has been described through various frameworks, such as syndemics, chronicity, local biology, the theory of fundamental causes, and ecosocial theory (see Mendenhall and Weaver 2018).
4 Moreover, this scientific research often relies on the invisibility of Black labor in cardiometabolic research more broadly – something James Doucet-Battle (2021) argues in his book *Sweetness in the Blood* as he draws attention to the double bind of racializing risk. As Black communities are the focus of interventions and scientific communities aim to diversify their subject pool, African American communities are targeted to participate in research that has served to create world-changing diabetes drugs–drugs that are not always equally accessible by all communities.

REFERENCES

Adams, Vincanne. 2016. *Metrics: What Counts in Global Health*. Durham: Duke University Press.

Benezra, Amber. 2023. *Gut Anthro: An Experiment in Thinking with Microbes*. Minneapolis: University of Minnesota Press.

Benton, Adia. 2015. *HIV Exceptionalism: Development through Disease in Sierra Leone*. 3rd ed. Minneapolis: University of Minnesota Press.

Bordo, Susan. 1993. *Unbearable Weight: Feminism, Western Culture, and the Body*. Berkeley: University of California Press.

Brewis, Alexandra A. 2014. "Stigma and the Perpetuation of Obesity." *Social Science & Medicine* 118 (October): 152–58.

Brewis, Alexandra A., and Amber Wutich. 2014. "A World of Suffering? Biocultural Approaches to Fat Stigma in the Global Contexts of the Obesity Epidemic." *Annals of Anthropological Practice* 38, no. 2: 269–83.

———. 2019. *Lazy, Crazy, and Disgusting: Stigma and the Undoing of Global Health*. Baltimore: Johns Hopkins University Press.

Carney, Megan. 2015. *The Unending Hunger: Tracing Women and Food Insecurity Across Borders*. Berkeley: University of California Press.

Carruth, Lauren, and Emily Mendenhall. 2019. "'Wasting Away': Diabetes, Food Insecurity, and Medical Insecurity in the Somali Region of Ethiopia." *Social Science & Medicine* 228: 155–63.

Cele, Lindile, Sarah S. Willen, Maydha Dhanuka, and Emily Mendenhall. 2021. "Ukuphumelela: Flourishing and the Pursuit of a Good Life, and Good Health, in Soweto, South Africa." *SSM – Mental Health,* 1: 100022.

Cerdeña, Jessica P. 2023. *Pressing Onward: The Imperative Resilience of Latina Migrant Mothers*. Berkeley: University of California Press.

Doucet-Battle, James. 2016. "Sweet Salvation: One Black Church, Diabetes Outreach, and Trust." *Transforming Anthropology* 24 (2): 125–35.

Gálvez, Alyshia. 2018. *Eating NAFTA: Trade, Food Policies, and the Destruction of Mexico*. 1st ed. Oakland: University of California Press.

Gálvez, Alyshia, Megan Carney, and Emily Yates-Doerr. 2020. "Chronic Disaster: Reimagining Noncommunicable Chronic Disease." *American Anthropologist* 122 (3): 639–40.

Gerber, Lynne. 2012. *Seeking the Straight and Narrow: Weight Loss and Sexual Reorientation in Evangelical America*. Chicago: University of Chicago Press.

Griffith, R. Marie. 2004. *Born Again Bodies: Flesh and Spirit in American Christianity*. Berkeley: University of California Press.

Hardin, Jessica. 2019. *Faith and the Pursuit of Health: Cardiometabolic Disorders in Samoa*. New Brunswick, NJ: Rutgers University Press.

Hartman, Saidiya. 2019. *Wayward Lives, Beautiful Experiments: Intimate Histories of Social Upheaval*. New York: W. W. Norton & Company.

Hsu Vox Jo, Moodie Megan, Abigail A. Dumes, Emily Lim Rogers, Chelsey Carter, Emma Broder, Daisy Couture, Ilana Löwy, and Emily Mendenhall. 2024. "Patients as Knowledge Partners in the Context of Complex Chronic Conditions." *Medical Humanities*: medhum-2024-012957. https://doi .org/10.1136/medhum-2024-012957.

Jeske, Melanie. 2021. "Constructing Complexity: Collective Action Framing and the Rise of Obesity Research." *BioSocieties* 16 (1): 116–41.

Landecker, Hannah. 2013. "Postindustrial Metabolism: Fat Knowledge." *Public Culture* 25 (3): 495–522.

Lieberman, Leslie Sue. 2003. "Dietary, Evolutionary, and Modernizing Influences on the Prevalence of Type 2 Diabetes." *Annual Review of Nutrition* 23 (1): 345–77.

Lock, Margaret. 1993. "Encounters with Aging: Mythologies of Menopause in Japan and North America." In *Aging and the Life Course,* xiv–xliv. Berkeley: University of California Press.

Manderson, Lenore, and Carolyn Smith-Morris. 2010. *Chronic Conditions, Fluid States: Chronicity and the Anthropology of Illness*. New Brunswick, NJ: Rutgers University Press.

McClure, Stephanie. 2016. "Symbolic Body Capital of an 'Other' Kind: African American Females as a Bracketed Subunit in Female Body Valuation." In *Fat Planet: Obesity, Culture, and Symbolic Body Capital*, edited by Eileen P. Anderson-Fye and Alexandra Brewis. Albuquerque: University of New Mexico Press.

McGarvey, Stephen T., Paul D. Levinson, Linda Bausser-Man, Daniel J. Galanis, and Conrad A. Hornick. 1993. "Population Change in Adult Obesity and Blood Lipids in American Samoa from 1976–1978 to 1990." *American Journal of Human Biology* 5 (1): 17–30.

Meek, Laura A., and Julia Alejandra Morales Fontanilla. 2022. "Otherwise." *Feminist Anthropology* 3 (2): 274–83.

Mendenhall, Emily. 2012. *Syndemic Suffering: Social Distress, Depression, and Diabetes among Mexican Immigrant Women*. Walnut Creek, CA: Left Coast Press.

———. 2019. *Rethinking Diabetes: Entanglements with Trauma, Poverty, and HIV*. Ithaca, NY: Cornell University Press.

Mendenhall, Emily, and Lesley Jo Weaver. 2018. "Diabetes." In *The International Encyclopedia of Anthropology*, edited by Hilary Callan, 1–6. Oxford: John Wiley & Sons, Ltd.

———. 2019. "Socially Determined? Frameworks for Thinking about Health Equity and Wellness." In *Well-Being as a Multidimensional Concept: Understanding Connections between Culture, Community, and Health*, edited by Janet Page-Reeves, 1–6. Lanham, MD: Lexington Books of Rowman & Littlefield.

Moran-Thomas, Amy. 2019. *Traveling with Sugar: Chronicles of a Global Epidemic*. Oakland: University of California Press.

Packard, Randall. 2016. *A History of Global Health: Intervention into the Lives of Other People*. Baltimore: Johns Hopkins University Press.

Paxson, Heather, ed. 2023. *Eating beside Ourselves: Thresholds of Foods and Bodies*. Durham: Duke University Press.

Pandian, Anand. 2019. *A Possible Anthropology: Methods for Uneasy Times*. Durham: Duke University Press.

Reese, Ashanté M., and Hanna Garth, eds. 2020. *Black Food Matters: Racial Justice in the Wake of Food Justice*. Minneapolis: University of Minnesota Press.

Sangaramoorthy, Thurka. 2012. "Enumeration, Identity, and Health." *Medical Anthropology* 31 (4): 287–91.

Schmidt-Sane, Megan, Lindile Cele, Edna N. Bosire, Alexander C Tsai, and Emily Mendenhall. 2023. "Flourishing with Chronic Illness (es) and Everyday Stress: Experiences from Soweto, South Africa." *Wellbeing, Space, and Society* 4 : 100144.

Solomon, Harris. 2016. *Metabolic Living: Food, Fat, and the Absorption of Illness in India*. Durham: Duke University Press.

SturtzSreetharan, Cindi, Alexandra Brewis, Jessica Hardin, Sarah Trainer, and Amber Wutich. 2021. *Fat in Four Cultures: A Global Ethnography of Weight*. Toronto: University of Toronto Press.

Trainer, Sarah, Cindi SturtzSreetharan, Amber Wutich, Alexandra Brewis, and Jessica Hardin. 2022. "Fat Is All My Fault: Globalized Metathemes of Body Self-Blame." *Medical Anthropology Quarterly* 36 (1): 5–26.

Valdez, Natali. 2022. *Weighing the Future: Race, Science, and Pregnancy Trials in the Postgenomic Era.* 1st ed. Oakland: University of California Press.

Warin, Megan. 2015. "Material Feminism, Obesity Science and the Limits of Discursive Critique." *Body & Society* 21 (4): 48–76.

Warin, Megan, Karen Turner, Vivienne Moore, and Michael Davies. 2008. "Bodies, Mothers and Identities: Rethinking Obesity and the BMI." *Sociology of Health & Illness* 30 (1).

Willen, Sarah S., Abigail Fisher Williamson, Colleen C. Walsh, Mikayla Hyman, and William Tootle. 2022. "Rethinking flourishing: Critical insights and qualitative perspectives from the U.S. Midwest." *SSM – Mental Health* 2: 100057.

CHAPTER ONE

Complicating Relations: On Research Obligations and Creating Space for Difference

Jessica Hardin, Saunima'a Ma Fulu-Aiolupotea, Uila Laifa Lima, Ramona Boodoosingh, Tauaitala Poloie Lees, Tausala Aiavao, and Falelua Maua

Your way
Objective
Analytic Always
doubting
The truth
Until proof comes
Slowly
Quietly
And it hurts

My way
Subjective
Gut-feeling like
Always sure
Of the truth
The proof
Is there
Waiting
And it hurts   – Konai Helu Thaman

When Jessica brought the prompt to the team during our Zoom meeting – *What does it mean to thrive with diabetes? What does it mean to live well with diabetes?* – the Zoom room fell silent. The question seemed to linger in the air, heavy and unanswered.

Crickets.

Ma was the first to break the stillness. With a quiet nod, she unmuted herself. "There is no living well," she said, her voice firm, tinged with the weariness of too many years of seeing her patients and family members arrive early at the end of life. "They just don't come until it's too late." Ma has been a community nurse since 1971. Her hands have cared for generations, and she has prayed over those generations as well. Her words carried the authority that only experience – and disappointment – could bear. She is our team leader not only because of her standing in the community but because of her clarity of thought; Ma's words cut right to the heart of our collective work.

Let's step back for a moment.

We are a team of researchers: There's Jessica, a white anthropologist, alongside Ma, Tausala, Falelua, and Tala, all Samoan nursing faculty. We're joined by Uila, a Samoan physician, and Ramona, a scholar of Indo-Caribbean descent with a focus on development studies. For the past four years, we've been immersed in studying the ravages of diabetes complications, mostly having to do with slow-healing wounds, infections, and eventual lower-limb amputation. We have documented the slow, insidious damage done by years of dysregulated glucose. We have focused on how individuals and their families manage a rapidly changing set of symptoms, as their lives become embroiled with the daily work of managing a small cut that becomes a life-threatening wound within weeks or months.

The prompt about *thriving* – living well with diabetes – had quickly spiraled into something much darker, a reflection on why so many people end up in the hospital with no choice but amputation. The question seemed almost naive against the backdrop of this shared struggle.

"What else can we do for these people?" Ma asked, bewildered. Her voice rose just slightly, more in exasperation than anger. "I don't know what else to do to make them listen, to make them follow through. They never listen. Not until it's too late, and then they act like they knew nothing."

Her frustration was palpable; decades of watching diabetes swell into a tidal wave of suffering had taken its toll. And as a woman in her seventies who managed her own diet, taking medications daily for her own health, Ma felt the sting of watching her advice go ignored. Whether she spoke to her family, her church, or her patients, the refrain was always the same: "Change your food, change your life." But they didn't. They couldn't. "They go right back," she said, throwing up her hands.

After a few minutes of silence, Jessica asked a question she felt she had been asking for decades: "Why? Why is it so hard to change?"

We talked about what the critical literature would say – dietary change isn't a simple matter of willpower. Structural conditions of eating, shaped over the twentieth and twenty-first centuries in Samoa and elsewhere, make it nearly impossible to change what one eats. The flow of cheap, calorie-dense, salt- and sugar-laden foods into a fledgling cash economy has fundamentally altered how people feed themselves and their families (Gewertz and Errington 2010; Cassels 2006; Singer 2014). We also know that it's not just diet that shapes who gets sick and who doesn't; it's the chronic stress of living under these conditions of change, of never seeming to have enough of what one needs to be healthy, and the varying degrees of toxicity that we all manage in our foods, water, and ecologies (Langwick 2018; Roberts 2017; Mendenhall et al. 2012; Nading 2020). Public health scholars might point to cultural norms, to the significance of feasting, to the fabric of Samoan life itself (Elstad et al. 2008; Rosen, DePue, and McGarvey 2008). But none of that felt satisfying, not to Ma, not to any of us sitting in that Zoom room.

Some of the team shrugged, shaking their heads. Others softly interjected: Maybe pride? Laziness? Faith? No one seemed to have the answer. Ma's frustration grew. "I want you guys from overseas to really look at what's happening here in Samoa. Diabetes is increasing. Is it enough, what we're doing?"

Uila's face flickered onto the screen. She was in the middle of her clinical rotation at a rural hospital on Savai'i. The walls behind her were bare, the fluorescent lighting harsh. She began quietly, acknowledging Ma's frustrations with respect. "We have some primary care," she said, her voice steady but thick with emotion. "But people don't come early enough."

Her voice cracked. She paused, blinking away the tears that gathered in her eyes. "When we diagnose them, they start counting the years – until amputation, until death."

A photo appeared in the chat – a man's foot, blackened, the flesh necrotic and sunken, chunks of it missing. Uila had been treating him earlier that day. The others on the Zoom didn't react, accustomed to these kinds of images. But Jessica winced, instinctively minimizing the image.

"We have a systemic problem," Uila continued, her words measured but full of urgency. "Our health care is built so people are supposed to use the rural clinics. But they don't. And by the time they come to the hospital, it's too late."

Tala jumped in. "It's not just diet and exercise. They need to know the signs, the symptoms of complications. They don't see it coming." Falelua added, "Self-care, I think we need to teach about the importance of self-care." Tausala noted, "The change needs to come from being a child, as they grow to become an adult, serving family."

"But," Ma interjected, her voice as steady as ever, "behavior doesn't change unless they come to the end. And then it's too late."

We left this meeting frustrated. Theories that make sense in our academic work were coming up short. The structural conditions – the environments that allow diabetic wounds to persist, glucose to become chronically dysregulated – are real; they are felt and understood by the people navigating them. But what were we to do with these critiques in our meeting as we bore witness to the ravages of dysregulated glucose on the body and on the family?

Here's the thing about this work: we are in it as witnesses to the profound inequalities that shape our worlds, that shape who gets sick and who doesn't. To observe structural conditions is inescapable; Samoans and anyone experiencing structural violences will be critical analysts of the conditions through which they expertly navigate (Biehl and Petryna 2013; Pigg 2013). But analyses that end with a critique of structural inequalities can fall flat, as they did in our meeting. Thinking about thriving despite these conditions is one way to make space for the extraordinary efforts of individuals, their families, and their communities to support, love, and just be with people as they navigate deeply unfair and unequal worlds. But, as we were in the thick of our analysis, thriving seemed to brush aside the profoundness of the experiences of people who shared their stories with us.

We can, of course, tell stories of that support, love, and being-with. Falelua shared a Samoan proverb, which the group agreed was a fitting metaphor to explain the importance of relationality in everyday life:[1] "A lavea lou vaematua, e logo atoa lou tino uma." (When your big toe is hurt, your whole body feels it.) Here the whole body represents the aiga, which is translated as *family* but means quite a bit more – the family is the organizing unit of people's lives; most people live in multigenerational settings, where lineages are defining features of everyday experience, and while the family is a source of obligation, it is also a source of support (Efi 2018; Suaalii-Sauni et al. 2014). Another proverb that speaks to the ways that families provide a gravitational grounding in everyday life is "O le tagata ma lona aiga, o le tagata ma lona fa'asinomaga" (Every person belongs to a family, and every family belongs to a person) (Mew et al. 2024). This characterizes the gentle balance of individualization and collective orientation, the mutual obligation of individual to collective and vice versa. Samoan theologian Therese Lautua writes, "While each human being is their own person, everyone is understood in relation to their family, wider community and the land to which they belong" (2023, 75). When the toe hurts, or becomes infected, the whole family feels it.

We share two brief stories below that reflect what we heard in countless interviews and personal conversations; namely, the importance of faith and family cannot be overstated. These stories also demonstrate the core of Ma's frustration – both Tupua and Levi understood the risks involved in their diets prior to amputation. And there are reasons behind this that we could explain, having to do with gendered hierarchies and the importance of food as an expression of respect, alongside the realities of being a professional in Samoa today and not being able to afford fresh fruits and vegetables. Instead, we'd like you to hear their stories without an analytic agenda, a simple being with them in regret, humor, and hope.

TUPUA: "I'M JUST LIKE A MAN WITH TWO LEGS"

Diagnosed in 2002, Tupua reflects somberly during our interview about the pivotal decisions he made – or failed to make – that led to the amputation of his leg. As we sit in his large fale Samoa – a circular, thatched home with no walls – the dry-season sun filters through the open sides of the structure, casting gentle shadows across the Chinese-made plastic woven mats on the floor. Tupua, in his fifties, wears a T-shirt with the logo long since faded and a lavalava, his graying hair neatly trimmed. His eyes carry the weight of years of regret and resilience.

When we ask him why he initially avoided taking his diabetes medication, his response is steeped in a blend of faith and self-reproach. "To be honest," he says, "because I'm a pastor." He explains that his deep faith in God led him to prioritize spiritual healing over medical intervention, a choice he now deeply regrets. "My faith in God was strong, but my carelessness had its impact," he adds, a note of sadness in his voice. Despite his regret, his faith remains steadfast, directing him to view his eventual acceptance of medical treatment not as a contradiction but as an extension of divine grace.

Following the amputation, Tupua's approach to health transformed. He now takes insulin and regards his doctors and nurses as "gifts from God." He continues to believe in divine miracles but recognizes that medical treatment is a crucial part of the healing process, a kind of miracle in itself. His faith has evolved; rather than diminishing, it now encompasses the support of medical professionals.

Tupua attributes the onset of his diabetes to the unhealthy imported foods he consumed while working in American Samoa. Tupua served as a pastor, living in a substantial multistory home that was built by the church community, adjacent to the church. As pastor, he and his family were fed by the church. He didn't work the land as he wasn't from this village and didn't have access to land. His work was pastoral, and in return, the congregation's obligation was to care for him (Latai 2015; Muaiava 2015). Coming from Samoa, the independent nation, to American Samoa was a shock to him in the beginning. The foods he was accustomed to eating, such as taro and banana, were replaced with rice and instant noodles. Most of his congregation worked in the formal economy, working in education, for the government, or in the fisheries. They fed him and his family via their earnings, buying foods from the shops. When he reflects back on this time, he thinks it was these foods that caused his diabetes.

Where we sit now, behind Tupua is a small vegetable garden with leafy greens, cucumbers, and tomatoes growing. These are the "clean" foods he eats now, from his own family land. He has come to embrace this change, but it wasn't without sacrifice. With Tupua's prolonged sickness and eventual amputation, he felt he couldn't serve as pastor any longer.

Moving from the pastor's house, a kind of home known to demonstrate a level of conspicuous consumption as it reflects the wealth of the community, to a modest wooden fale is not a choice that many would make. But for Tupua, he felt his family land called to him; he wanted to return to the gardens he had worked as a young man before leaving for theological college. Despite the challenge of working with crutches, Tupua feels enlivened by the opportunity to experience the peace of living this life, of working his gardens (see also Hardin 2021). More important, though, is his ability to continue to serve in his role as a family leader, father, and pastor. Though he is not a pastor in his current church, he is an elder and continues his pastoral calling with this new congregation. "I'm just like a man with two legs," he says with a touch of pride, "and I thank God for my children; they support me every step of the way."

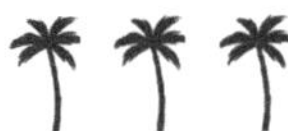

LEVI AND PO: "NOW, HE HAS THE CHANCE TO LIVE"

Palm trees flap above our heads one afternoon in Apia, the capital city, as we gather with Levi and Po at a restaurant popular with politicians and professionals. Levi, a radio celebrity, receives nods and handshakes from passersby. His wife joins us, having taken time off from her job at the bank. Their youngest child, three years old, plays quietly nearby as we order lunch – fried spring rolls, poke, and fish fingers. Levi is positive, speaking with confidence, though it is clear his wife has carried much of the burden.

"My blood sugar was very high, and I lost a lot of weight – that's how I knew it was dangerous," Levi begins, explaining how a swelling in his foot had led to the amputation of his leg. "Before this, they recommended insulin, but I never wanted to take it. When I saw the private doctor, they said it was my fault, because of my carelessness."

His wife raises an eyebrow and smiles. "At that time, the doctors advised him to exercise and control his diet, but he loves his meat and beer. Now, he's improved – he takes his injections, doesn't drink, doesn't party, and eats what we cook for him."

Levi, a little embarrassed, describes how exhausting it was to go through the fifteen operations required to amputate both of his legs and how challenging it was to manage the financial pressure of not being able to work for the full year it took to recover. But now, back on the radio, he shares his experience to help others. "I tell people with diabetes they need to eat right, take their medications, and go for regular checkups. Don't wait until it's too late."

His wife reflects quietly, "We thank God he is able to work again. We fasted as a family for this because we thought he would be bedridden." As the conversation slows, we turn to our food, picking at the pupus.

She continues, her voice soft but steady, "It was hard for me. In the past, Levi wasn't focused on being a father or taking care of himself. He just ignored me. But during the surgeries, I told him, 'I'm putting everything into this because I love our kids. How can we take care of them if we can't take care of ourselves?' Finally, he understood."

Levi, trying to lighten the moment, adds, "I was a tough case." With a laugh, he continues, "But now, I'm really looking at our children, so they don't end up like me. When they eat too much, I say, 'Hey, no, no.' I remind them they'll have to do more chores to burn off the fat." His wife smiles and nods, adding, "The kids were scared at first, but now we're all learning to take care of our health. It's hard, sometimes expensive, to eat right, but we saw what happens if we don't. We could've lost him. Now, he has the chance to live."

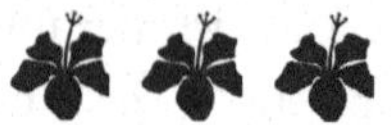

These are stories that demonstrate how people live well with diabetes. Among our interviews, however, these stories are matched by those whose outcomes haven't been so positive. Through our years working on this project, we witnessed people die under similar circumstances or nurse wounds for years that wouldn't heal (see also Moran-Thomas 2019a). We struggled to write a chapter about thriving because we witness both kinds of stories all the time. We see the people we have come to know in our communities and in our clinical work encounter near death or die. We see them experience hopelessness and fear as individuals while their families support them with dignity, generosity, and love. But this is what it means to live and work in a community, in Samoan communities in particular, and to understand the work that is needed to ensure that everyone is cared for.

We approached this chapter cautiously, hoping to make clear that clinical medical practice and public health policies that emphasize individual behavioral change alone (diet, exercise, etc.) are insufficient. For one, they don't work (Hardin, McLennan, and Brewis 2018). As Ma frustratingly shared, information about how to prevent diabetes is abundant in Samoa (and around the world); Tupua and Levi "knew" how to prevent diabetes, and yet they didn't. This is where a structural critique is useful, as encouraging individuals to eat differently does nothing to confront those structural conditions, including the availability of unhealthy, imported foods, chronic stress, and a lack of health-care access. Encouraging individuals to eat differently also doesn't acknowledge that shifting how an individual eats is also about shifting how a household eats, how they procure their food, and how they prepare those foods. Eating together is an everyday social achievement, a part of cultivating alimentary dignity, which is not always easily changed because of a single individual (Garth 2020).

Our stories highlight what chapters across this volume do so brilliantly – that people like Tupua, Levi, and Po rely on their faith and families to endure and redefine what it means to live well, even after devastating complications. In some cases, as with Tupua and Levi, people do manage to change their lives, but it is not through individual will alone. Family members like Po and her children, the land that Tupua was entitled to return to, the support of his church in his retirement, all of these aspects of their lives made changing their circumstances possible. Anthropologists have been pointing to the "slow care" required for individuals to navigate the barrage of symptoms that people living with diabetes deal with (Moran-Thomas 2019). And yet the norms of clinical practice, medical science, and public health intervention continue to focus on the individual.

As with other chapters throughout this book, we approach flourishing with special attention to our own relations as collaborators, working to nourish our connections through the way we write. Our research relationships are inspired by Pacific-based critiques of the ways that research has been historically used as a colonial tool of domination (see George and Gibson 2018; Thaman 2009). In her landmark book, *Decolonizing Methodologies,* Māori scholar Linda Tuhiwai Smith writes, "The ways in which scientific research is implicated in the worst excesses of colonialism remains a powerful remembered history for many of the world's colonized peoples. It is a history that offends the deepest sense of our humanity" (1999, 1). Inspired by that book, across the Pacific there has been a flourishing of decolonial research and writing focused on challenging Western knowledge production. Tonga scholar Konai Helu Thaman, the author whose poem opens this chapter, is a leader in decolonizing Pacific studies who calls for integrating Pacific ways of knowing into higher education and research in Oceania more broadly as "an inclusive and holistic way of thinking" that "champions stewarding nature, participating in community, and valuing interpersonal relationships" (Thaman 2003, 12).

The flourishing field of Pacific research methodologies that has developed over the past forty years is embedded in "an era of (anticolonial, antiimperialist, antiracist, antisexist) questioning of approaches to knowledge that were based on normalized (colonial, capitalist, imperialist, patriarchal) projects and world views" (Leenen-Young and Uperesa 2023, 10). Ultimately, these research methodologies "provide paradigms for ethical community-centered research with Pacific peoples framed within priorities of relationality, reciprocity and responsibility" (18). From the perspective of Pacific studies, collaboration isn't an inherently transformative or positive thing, particularly in the context of broader research trends that make collaboration essential (Rosenberg 2010). In fact, collaboration has come to mean so many things that it has become almost an empty term (Benezra 2023). It's notable that in the Pacific research methodologies literature there is very little discussion of collaboration. Instead, research is understood as relational and, as a result, also reciprocal (Aini et al. 2023; West 2023).

We are not claiming that we are decolonizing our research, but we are taking fundamentals in the movement to decolonize research as a starting point in our relationships with each other. Our team aims to organize ourselves by prioritizing relatedness and reciprocity as an explicit way of challenging typical power arrangements on international research teams where funding flows from the Global North to collaborators in the Global South, and research outputs may flow from South to North (Hardin et al. 2023; Enari and Matapo 2021). For our team, this means ongoing, slow trust building through our regular Zoom meetings, where we aim for transparency around workload, we discuss our individual professional and personal needs for the research, and we sometimes disagree and have to repair trust as a result. The description of the meeting that opens this chapter reflects a core tension in our team as we confronted our different goals for the research and the limits of academic critique. Our work, however, is incomplete.

While Jessica and Ramona felt it important to share with global audiences the limitations in primary care in Samoa and the broader failures of prevention efforts, Ma felt strongly that there is primary care available and people do have the knowledge they need to change their behaviors. To call out these structural inadequacies was, in a way, criticizing Ma's life's work, the team's colleagues, and the work to which they have dedicated their careers. Still others on the team felt differently–Uila a bit in-between, recognizing that there is some opportunity for primary care, but as it is designed now, people don't use it. Tala felt people do have prevention knowledge but not complications knowledge, and Falelua thought people needed to think about diabetes in terms of self-care. Tausala felt the family needed to be at the center of any effort. As an academic, Jessica has spent her career critiquing an individual behavioral approach to addressing diabetes and, as a nurse, Ma has spent her career trying to help people make changes to their behavior. We were left at an impasse. Our views, seemingly irreconcilable.

Understanding research as relational doesn't require everyone to have the same goals, motivations, and interpretations. But it does require what Emily Yates-Doerr calls "careful equivocation": "a research technique attuned to unsettling binaries that does not result in sameness or unity" (2019, 297). At the impasse of understanding individual behavior as constrained by structures and the loving wish that people would make changes in their lives, we as a team continue to work together, organized by our mutual commitments and curiosities, breathing space into our differences as a way of doing research differently, writing about research differently.

In reflecting on our work, it is clear that the search for a single truth about thriving with diabetes is elusive and fraught with the weight of structural conditions and individual choices. Nor is it possible to produce a single truth about collaboration; as Eve Tuck and K. Wayne Yang write, "Solidarity is an uneasy, reserved, and unsettled matter that neither reconciles present grievances nor forecloses future conflict" (2012, 3). However, what our work does reveal is the lived experience of diabetes complications, and it points to an absence of empirical and theoretical attention to those complications. Scholars have yet to carefully think beyond diet and exercise, our critiques so sharp that they don't often extend to the "natural history" of diabetes, a term that epidemiologists use to describe the course of a disease if un-intervened upon. We bore witness to this "natural history." Across the chapters in this book, we see stories of blurry vision, frequent urination, weight loss, mood changes, skin problems, and amputation that result from not only the structural conditions that shape unequal health environments but also the weakness of a prevention-and-control-only approach to diabetes.

But for Ma, and many health providers on the ground in Samoa, there is access to enough for people to manage some kind of change. The stories of Tupua, Levi, and Po are reminders that amid these structural violences, people continue to find ways to live, resist, and redefine thriving – in Ma's terms, find ways to make changes in their behaviors. Importantly, it is not through individual will alone, but through the support of families, faith communities, and the land itself. As critical scholars, we must remain vigilant, recognizing the limits of our analyses while also holding space for the extraordinary efforts of those we study – efforts that challenge the very conditions we seek to critique. For students, scholars, and practitioners, we want to hold open the space for incommensurability to ask what kind of meso-level thinking and revision to clinical practice and policy design can move our analysis beyond the individual, beyond the structural?

Tupua, Levi, and Po live between the analytic ends of "individual" and "structural," begging us as a team to ask, what kind of compromises must we all face in order to do anti-colonial, just science that has the potential to improve people's worlds? There is no single solution, no way to "solve" the problem of diabetes; to do so would be to reduce diabetes to a single issue, and there are no single-issue illnesses (Lorde and Clarke 2007). The complexities we face demand that we go beyond pointing out structural problems, and beyond honoring the resilience, love, and care that sustain people in profoundly unjust worlds. We must work with clinicians, community workers, policy writers, and medical researchers to identify interstitial spaces where it's possible to hold these multiple truths in focus, to measure, interpret, and theorize them in new ways. From our places in the world, from where we write in Rochester, New York City, and Samoa, working together allows us to bring these multiple truths into focus, helping us imagine different futures.

NOTE

1 Samoan words are not italicized to address linguistic hierarchies where non-English languages are marked as "other" through the practice of italicizing (Smith 1999; Somerville 2022).

REFERENCES

Aini, John, Paige West, Yolarnie Amepou, Michael Ladi Piskaut, Cornelius Gasot, Rachel S. James, Jason Steadman Roberts, Patrick Nason, and Anna Elyse Brachey. 2023. "Reimagining Conservation Practice: Indigenous Self-Determination and Collaboration in Papua New Guinea." *Oryx* (March), 1–10.

Beliso-De Jesús, Aisha M., Jemima Pierre, and Junaid Rana. 2023. "White Supremacy and the Making of Anthropology." *Annual Review of Anthropology* 52 (1): 417–35.

Benezra, Amber. 2023. *Gut Anthro: An Experiment in Thinking with Microbes.* Minneapolis: University of Minnesota Press.

Biehl, Joao, and Adriana Petryna. 2013. *When People Come First: Critical Studies in Global Health.* Princeton: Princeton University Press.

Cassels, Susan. 2006. "Overweight in the Pacific: Links between Foreign Dependence, Global Food Trade, and Obesity in the Federated States of Micronesia." *Globalization and Health* 2 (July):10. https://doi.org/10.1186/1744-8603-2-10.

Efi, Tui Atua Tupua Tamasese Ta'isi. 2018. *Su'esu'e Manogi: In Search of Fragrance: Tui Atua Tupua Tamasese Ta'isi and the Samoan Indigenous Reference.* Huia Publishers.

Elstad, Emily, Tusiofo Corabelle, Rochelle K. Rosen, and Stephen McGarvey. 2008. "Living with Ma'i Suka: Individual, Familial, Cultural, and Environmental Stress Among Patients with Type 2 Diabetes Mellitus and Their Caregivers in American Samoa." *Preventing Chronic Disease* 5 (3): 1–10.

Enari, Dion, and Jacoba Matapo. 2021. "Negotiating the Relational vā in the University." *Journal of Global Indigeneity* 5 (1): 1–19.

Garth, Hanna. 2020. *Food in Cuba: The Pursuit of a Decent Meal.* Stanford University Press.

George, Lily, and Lorena Gibson. 2018. "Mahi Tahi: Māori and Anthropology in Aotearoa/New Zealand." Association of Social Anthropologists of Aotearoa New Zealand.

Gewertz, Deborah, and Frederick Errington. 2010. *Cheap Meat: Flap Food Nations in the Pacific Islands.* Berkeley: University of California Press.

Hardin, Jessica. 2021. "Life before Vegetables: Nutrition, Cash and Subjunctive Health in Samoa." *Cultural Anthropology* 36 (3): 428–57.

Hardin, Jessica, Dion Enari, Tarryn Phillips, Tausala Aiavao, Ramona Boodoosingh, Saunima'a Ma Fulu Aiolupotea, Pakilau Manase Lua, et al.

2023. "Developing Trust in Collaborative Research: Utilizing Indigenous Pacific Methodologies to Create Dialogue within Research Teams." *Asia Pacific Journal of Public Health* 35 (8): 529–31.

Hardin, Jessica, Amy K. McLennan, and Alexandra Brewis. 2018. "Body Size, Body Norms and Some Unintended Consequences of Obesity Intervention in the Pacific Islands." *Annals of Human Biology* 45 (3): 285–94.

Horton, Sarah, Cesar Abadía, Jessica Mulligan, and Jennifer Jo Thompson. 2014. "Critical Anthropology of Global Health 'Takes a Stand' Statement: A Critical Medical Anthropological Approach to the U.S.'s Affordable Care Act." *Medical Anthropology Quarterly* 28 (1): 1–22.

Langwick, Stacey Ann. 2018. "A Politics of Habitability: Plants, Healing, and Sovereignty in a Toxic World." *Cultural Anthropology* 33 (3): 415–43.

Latai, Latu. 2015. "Changing Covenants in Samoa? From Brothers and Sisters to Husbands and Wives?" *Oceania* 85 (1): 92–104.

Lautua, Therese. 2023. "A Pacific Qualitative Methodology for the Intersection of Images of God, Cultural Identity and Mental Wellbeing." *Journal of Pastoral Theology* 33 (3): 171–88.

Leenen-Young, Marcia, and Lisa Uperesa. 2023. "Re-Visioning Pacific Research Method/Ologies." *Waka Kuaka* 132 (1 & 2): 9–39.

Lorde, Audre, and Cheryl Clarke. 2007. *Sister Outsider: Essays and Speeches.* New York: Crossing Press.

Maile, Arvin. 2019. *Possessing Polynesians: The Science of Settler Colonial Whiteness in Hawai'i and Oceania.* Durham: Duke University Press.

Mendenhall, Emily, Roopa Shivashankar, Nikhil Tandon, Mohammed K. Ali, K. M. Venkat Narayan, and Dorairaj Prabhakaran. 2012. "Stress and Diabetes in Socioeconomic Context: A Qualitative Study of Urban Indians." *Social Science & Medicine* 75 (12): 2522–29.

Mew, Emma J., Leiema Hunt, Robert L.M. Toelupe, Vanessa Blas, Julia Winschel, Joshua Naseri, Si'itia Soliai-Lemusu, et al. 2024. "O Le Tagata Ma Lona Aiga, o Le Tagata Ma Lona Fa'asinomaga (Every Person Belongs to a Family and Every Family Belongs to a Person): Development of a Parenting Framework for Adolescent Mental Wellbeing in American Samoa." *Children and Youth Services Review* 160 (May):107502.

Moran-Thomas, Amy. 2019a. *Traveling with Sugar: Chronicles of a Global Epidemic.* Oakland, CA: University of California Press.

Muaiava, Sadat. 2015. "The Samoan Parsonage Family: The Concepts of Feagaiga and Tagata'ese." *Journal of New Zealand & Pacific Studies* 3 (1): 73–83.

Nading, Alex M. 2020. "Living in a Toxic World." *Annual Review of Anthropology* 49: 209–24.

Pfeiffer, James, and Rachel Chapman. 2010. "Anthropological Perspectives on Structural Adjustment and Public Health." *Annual Review of Anthropology* 39:149–65.

Pigg, Stacy Leigh. 2013. "On Sitting and Doing: Ethnography as Action in Global Health." *Social Science & Medicine* 99:127–34.

Roberts, Elizabeth F. S. 2017. "What Gets Inside: Violent Entanglements and Toxic Boundaries in Mexico City." *Cultural Anthropology* 32 (4): 592–619.

Rosen, Rochelle K., Judith DePue, and Stephen McGarvey. 2008. "Overweight and Diabetes in American Samoa: The Cultural Translation of Research into Health Care Practice." *Medicine and Health/Rhode Island* 91 (12): 372–77.

Rosenberg, Mark L. 2010. *Real Collaboration: What It Takes for Global Health to Succeed.* University of California Press.

Simpson, Audra. 2007. "On Ethnographic Refusal: Indigeneity, 'Voice' and Colonial Citizenship." *Junctures: The Journal for Thematic Dialogue*, no. 9, 67–80.

———. 2018. "Why White People Love Franz Boas; or, The Grammar of Indigenous Dispossession." In *Indigenous Visions: Rediscovering the World of Franz Boas*, edited by Ned Blackhawk and Isaiah Lorado Wilner, 166–82. Yale University Press.

Singer, Merrill. 2014. "Following the Turkey Tails: Neoliberal Globalization and the Political Ecology of Health." *Journal of Political Ecology* 21:436–51.

Smith, Linda Tuhiwai. 1999. *Decolonizing Methodologies: Researching and Indigenous Peoples.* London: Zed Books Ltd.

Suaalii-Sauni, Tamasailau M., Maualaivao Albert Wendt, Naomi Fuamatu, Upolu Luma Va'ai, Reina Whaitiri, and Stephen L. Filipo. 2014. *Whispers and Vanities: Samoan Indigenous Knowledge and Religion.* Huia Publishers.

Thaman, Konai Helu. 2003. "Decolonizing Pacific Studies: Indigenous Perspectives, Knowledge, and Wisdom in Higher Education." *The Contemporary Pacific* 15 (1): 1–17.

———. 2009. "Nurturing Relationships and Honouring Responsibilities: A Pacific Perspective." In *Living Together: Education and Intercultural Dialogue*, edited by Suzanne Majhanovich, Christine Fox, and Adila Pašalić Kreso, 173–87. Dordrecht: Springer Netherlands.

Tuck, Eve, and K. Wayne Yang. 2012. "Decolonization Is Not a Metaphor." *Decolonization: Indigeneity, Education & Society* 1 (1): 1–40.

West, Paige. 2023. "Conservation as Homogenisation?: Socio-Spiritual-Ecological Futures and Collaborative Relations." *Kritisk Etnografi: Swedish Journal of Anthropology* 6 (1): 49–56.

Yates-Doerr, Emily. 2019. "Whose Global, Which Health? Unsettling Collaboration with Careful Equivocation." *American Anthropologist* 121 (2): 297–310.

Diabetes Is *Always* Relational

Anathi *finds strength in her friendship with Funeka and their prayer group, providing vital emotional support while managing diabetes and HIV.*

Sirah *uses her infectious humor to navigate the challenges of her husband's unstable job and her own health issues, embodying resilience in daily life.*

Koumba, *though not clinically diagnosed with diabetes, shares profound emotional bonds with her co-wives, reflecting their interconnected experiences of illness.*

Penda *transforms her initial isolation due to diabetes into resilience, drawing strength from the unwavering support of her family and co-wives.*

Avinesh *proudly maintains his aging taxi as he navigates Suva's streets, striving to improve his family's life while caring for his mother after her amputation.*

Mari, *newly diagnosed with diabetes, seeks guidance from her spiritual godmother, Mãe Canela, and experiences a dream with her ancestor Isabella that inspires her healing journey.*

Diabetes is profoundly shaped by interactions between individuals, their communities, and broader social, cultural, and environmental factors. Throughout these chapters, we explore everyday spaces where diabetes manifests, shedding light on how daily and historical stresses influence sugar levels. Medical anthropologists emphasize that illness is more than a biological condition; it is intertwined with family dynamics, health-care access, and societal norms. Factors such as access to care, cultural beliefs, and social inequalities profoundly impact how diabetes is experienced and treated, highlighting its deep connection to one's environment and social networks.

This section delves into the relational aspects of diabetes, illustrating how support networks – whether of friends, family, or caregivers – play crucial roles. It explores themes of social suffering, where illness affects entire networks, not just individuals. This perspective challenges simplistic views of health determinants by emphasizing how societal structures shape personal experiences. Medical anthropology's contribution lies in recognizing that while biomedicine treats individuals clinically, illness reverberates through communities. This approach also highlights the complexities of care, obligation, and striving within unequal environments that predispose some to illness more than others, often along gendered and racial lines. It challenges us to move beyond mere structural critiques and explore how relationships and societal norms frame health experiences. In reflecting on these narratives, consider: How can we shift clinical practices to better incorporate the relational and social factors that shape health outcomes, especially in marginalized communities? How can support networks be more effectively integrated into health-care systems to improve diabetes care and management?

CHAPTER TWO

Funeka's Kitchen: Diabetes Healing in Soweto Living Rooms through Prayer and Commensality

Emily Mendenhall, Lindile Cele, and Edna N. Bosire

Anathi arrived at Funeka's threshold twenty minutes before the other members of the prayer group. The taxi had come early, and she had scrambled into the crowded minibus. She found the last seat, right next to a young man, glued to his phone, with long braids and a soft smile pursed upon his lips. Anathi was pleased to squeeze next to him – to feel his calm amid a chaotic day. She'd just left her shift cleaning at Jabulani Mall, working hard all day with a short break for tea and a sandwich she had packed early in the morning. The young man didn't say a word, but the older woman seated to Anathi's right side was muttering under her breath. Anathi smiled at her and nodded, turning toward the younger man, who was texting. She looked over his shoulder, reading, "What r u doing?" She smiled, closing her eyes and rubbing her temples, remembering the joy of dating in the early days, so many years ago. Her shoulders rubbed hard against the older woman, causing her to shift and make space for Anathi. She opened her eyes and stared again over his shoulder at his phone. "C u soon xx," she saw him text. She smiled and felt her stomach grumble. Anathi had been thinking about Funeka's warm bread since she arrived for her shift in the morning.

Anathi's stop came while she was rubbing her hands together, moving the fingers of her right hand deeply into the crevices of her left hand to relax her arthritis. She shimmied out of the bus and put her feet on the dusty street as she saw Funeka's house only fifty meters from the stop. She slowly walked toward her old friend's home, a Wednesday routine that has become part of her survival since she started attending the prayer group more than a decade before. She remembered how she had felt distant from her husband and frustration with her children a decade ago – holding so much anxiety in her body that she could barely function. Slowly, week after week, and year after year, she learned to let go and change her frame of mind. When she was diagnosed with hypertension and later type 2 diabetes, she came to the group for support. It was the women in her prayer group who helped her heal. The window to the house was open, and Anathi could hear soft music playing in Funeka's kitchen. The chilly July wind wisped through her light jacket.

Funeka opened the door before Anathi was able to knock. "Mngani," she said as she pulled her friend's hands into her hands and smiled widely. Anathi's shoulders relaxed as she walked through the door, blocking the wind.

Arriving before the others had become part of their routine – Funeka would have water boiling for tea so they could put out the food together and catch up on gossip. Anathi put down her small bag near the door, feeling relief from letting go of that heavy burden. She immediately collapsed on the couch and leaned back. Funeka heard the water boil.

"You work too hard, my friend," Funeka said without looking up. She was slowly pouring the water into a cup with a rooibos teabag for Anathi. It smelled like Wednesday.

"Phela, I need to pay the bills. The babies have babies."

Funeka scoffed. "Sit. Drink," she instructed.

Anathi breathed in the wafts of tea and started to unwind. Funeka busied herself in the kitchen.

"Have you eaten today, Anathi?" Funeka asked her friend, seeing her close her eyes and settle in for a rest.

Without opening her eyes, she said, "Ridaq, metformin, insulin injections." She rubbed her belly as her tummy grumbled. "All I do is eat pills – I can even smell them in my urine." Funeka clucked her tongue, and Anathi shook her head and laughed lightly to herself. "I drank water all day and ate a small sandwich. I'm okay." Her eyes stayed closed; she tried to relax.

Funeka put a plate of food next to her. She took her soft hands and placed them on Anathi's leg. "Eat now, before they all arrive. We need you today."

As Anathi opened her eyes, the room looked blurry. She took a sip of rooibos and swallowed slowly, feeling the warm water calm her body. The room righted. She took a piece of the buttered bread her friend had prepared for her and bit into it. They didn't always have butter at home – Anathi was the only one regularly working among the four adults in their household. They often didn't have enough food for her two children, her son's wife, and her seven grandchildren. She was hopeful, though, because her son was picking up shifts with a welder on the other side of town.

Symptoms like blurry vision would happen when she didn't eat enough during the day and her sugar became imbalanced. Anathi found it difficult to buy the foods the nutritionist recommended that she prepare for herself. How could she when the grandkids needed shoes and her children had such a difficult time keeping a job? She rarely bought the fish and only bought the cheapest vegetables the nutritionist told her to eat. She'd been "educated" about her diet when she was diagnosed with diabetes a decade ago – but the good foods served in the hospital were not always possible to prepare in her real life.

Anathi was diagnosed with HIV in her mid-thirties. She was frightened at first – in part because her husband had died so suddenly. When he got sick, his health deteriorated fast because he refused to get tested – drugs were just becoming available, and he didn't trust them. "Why would I get tested for something I'd die from anyway without treatment?" Anathi never forgave him for his stubbornness.

When he was dying, she tested positive and started antiretroviral therapy while she nursed him in the last several months of his life. Watching him die caused Anathi great pain, and she constantly grappled with yet another layer of forgiving him. They hadn't always gotten along – but he was *hers*. Every time she knew he was unfaithful, she would turn the other cheek because he would never leave her. His salary was stable, and when he was there, he was loving. "I practice acceptance and move on," she would laugh to her sister. She knew they had built something together – something worth fighting for.

After he passed away, she anticipated feeling anger and fear about her own HIV status. She felt these emotions at first, but she soon learned how to manage her illness. Anathi never missed a checkup and always took her antiretroviral medication – usually getting the medication at the Diepkloof clinic but sometimes going to Baragwanath Hospital for checkups. She knew they were lucky to live in the large, expanded township of Soweto, where there were more jobs, clinics, and middle-class homes than in many of Johannesburg's townships that had more people passing through and living in less secure, shorter-term conditions. Although Baragwanath Hospital in Soweto was painful to visit because it took an entire day to get through her appointments, she knew the care was reliable and the pharmacy was usually stocked.

Anathi learned how the antiretroviral therapy kept the HIV at bay. It was a decade later, when she was diagnosed with diabetes, that her health radically changed her life. This was in part because her treatment now was meant to involve her family. Without the income from her husband, and her children's inconsistent employment, buying preferred foods wasn't a consistent practice for her. And keeping up with her medication while trying to maintain a healthy, balanced diet had become an exhausting part of her everyday life. Sometimes the pharmacy didn't have metformin – the pill she was supposed to take for diabetes – and her illness got worse. This illness wasn't something she could manage on her own. Anathi felt her blurry vision clear.

"The bread is fresh; it tastes nice. Thank you."

"Pleasure," Funeka replied, putting more snacks on the table for their friends and lining up the extra teacups she had for her guests. The teacups were Funeka's most prized possession – she had received them from her mother as a wedding gift, and her mother had written a note to her about how important it was to welcome other mothers into her home, especially after her babies came. Her mother had hosted a prayer group in their home ever since they joined the Zionist church in Diepkloof, after moving to Soweto from KwaZulu-Natal when she was eight.

Funeka went to the fridge and brought out a plastic bottle that was three-quarters full. She had prepared it earlier that morning when she started cooking for the day. All of the grandmothers in her prayer group had diabetes, so she liked to serve *imbiza* when they all gathered on Wednesday evenings. It was a tonic she made from vegetable water – she would ferment vegetables in water, and they would drink the liquid to control their sugar. It had become a weekly habit that they did to acknowledge their shared illness and demonstrate caring for themselves, for each other.

This vignette illustrates how spiritual and social care interweave with biomedical treatment in Soweto. Many people like Funeka and Anathi in Soweto develop multiple chronic illnesses that they manage concurrently. One in five people are HIV positive in Soweto, so it's not uncommon to have to navigate a condition alongside HIV, though the virus has become a chronic illness as opposed to a death sentence like it was when people first started getting sick in the eighties. Today Anathi finds diabetes to be more disruptive than HIV because managing her diet differently from her family is a nearly impossible task.

Yet, she rarely talks about the physical discomforts of her HIV or her diabetes with her family members. Funeka also doesn't talk about her diabetes much beyond their prayer group, in part because she fears people will think she is HIV positive. For years, public health messaging, in an attempt to destigmatize HIV, would assert, "HIV is just like diabetes and cancer!" This made many people with diabetes feel shame and hide their diagnoses, thereby avoiding changing their diets or behaviors, against public health and medical recommendations.

Funeka started the prayer group for women living with diabetes so they could come together to share their stories, struggles with treatments, and emotional burdens. When women joined the group, they often described how they were thinking too much about certain problems in their lives: a child's troubles, a loved one's future, a marriage, their safety. Funeka found it was important to create a space where women could come together to share their struggles and unburden themselves with people who they knew could understand them.

Anathi was the first one to join the group, and their friendship had grown exponentially through their commensality. It was Anathi who showed up during holidays or when the group numbers dwindled during the pandemic. When they weren't forced to stay in their homes for lockdown, Anathi was at Funeka's threshold. When they were in lockdown, they were on WhatsApp, texting and comforting each other. Often they connected through their faith in Jesus, praying over each other and lifting each other up to feel well. Anathi knew that at Funeka's prayer group she often left feeling emotionally unburdened and physically more relaxed.

The door opened, and Tabitha stuck her head in. "Hello?" Funeka clucked her tongue. "I'm coming from church." She paused as she passed over the threshold and started taking off her scarf from around her neck. "I saw Pastor Vusi," Tabitha said as she nodded toward Anathi, who was polishing off the rest of the bread and feeling sturdier. "There is something about the church water that makes me feel calm. It's the best medicine."

Anathi and Tabitha went to the same Zionist church in Diepkloof as Funeka, although they don't remember how they first met. Tabitha went with her parents as a young girl – her parents had been born in Soweto, and she had never lived anywhere else. Anathi had joined as a young mother, soon after her husband died. She sat in the back, absorbing the powerful gospel music and messages. It was several years before she met Funeka.

They met at a bring and share one Sunday afternoon after eating Boerewors rolls a congregation member had prepared for them. They quickly took to each other, and it was in part Anathi's friendship that inspired the group. They soon expanded their circle when Tabitha confided in them about her diabetes one afternoon after the service went late into the day. They met three days later in Funeka's living room and did so every week since. Every session would start with snacks before creating space to hear about each other's weekly struggles and successes not only managing their diabetes but also in all parts of their lives, from emotional well-being to managing money and grandchildren.

Funeka took six plastic cups from her cupboard and put them on the table. Tabitha sat down on the couch and stretched her legs, watching Funeka work. She poured *imbiza* into each glass so they were each half full and smiled as she thought about how important this habit had become: taking in their tonic together to demonstrate their mutual illness and healing.

"I need to see Pastor Vusi tomorrow; I start work at noon, so I should have time to stop by the church. I also need to pick up my medications – they say they are ready by eight in the morning, but I can't know how long I will have to wait. I'm not too worried though – I have plenty of metformin left. I don't always take it," Anathi admitted as she polished off her rooibos.

"He will have already prayed over the water by the time you arrive there, should be plenty of time. I should be there half past eight," Funeka said as she finished pouring *imbiza*. She stopped by the church in the morning to receive the church water and sometimes went in the afternoon, too. She stopped by to see others at the church, but mostly she wanted the healing powers of the church water that Pastor Vusi had prayed over. The routine had become even more important to her since she was diagnosed with diabetes and hypertension. While the hypertension was a bother and required her to take another pill, the diabetes had been something for which she needed Pastor Vusi's support.

For many months after her diagnosis, she felt stress and fear about her diabetes, struggling to modify her diet in a way that was affordable and her cooking in a way her family would accept. Once she started regularly taking church water – visiting Pastor Vusi every morning – she started to feel calm. The other women in her prayer group felt the same way – the church was a sanctuary and space for healing. Yet, Funeka's group had become even more important for Anathi, who could rarely squeeze in an extra trip to church during the week because of her work schedule. Nevertheless, she would wake early to bathe and dress on Sundays in anticipation of spending the day with her friends and staying late into the afternoon.

"It is the water that will heal us," Tabitha said, taking a teacup and eyeing the teapot of rooibos. Anathi sighed and nodded in partial agreement.

"It is our friendship that keeps us going," Funeka said, turning toward Tabitha with a smile. She put her hand on her friend's back, and they both laughed softly together. Anathi crossed her hands on her stomach and leaned back into her chair.

The other three women arrived to Funeka's living room over the next thirty minutes. When Sibongile finally arrived, the six women sat together and drank their *imbiza*. It was the routine they did around their shared diabetes status that would officially start the meeting: drinking together something they believed would lower their sugars and improve their health. Then, the rest of the time together was spent sharing about their week, reading Scripture, singing together, holding hands and sharing in a prayer circle, and supporting each other.

Throughout our decade-long research on chronic illness in Soweto, group meetings in homes of friends and close confidants were described as powerful contexts of healing for people with diabetes and other chronic illnesses. Among eighty-eight people we interviewed recently about living with diabetes and other chronic conditions, we found that more than half ($n = 58$) described different religious practices such as going to church, reading the Bible, and prayer – including self-prayer and being prayed for by others – as key in fostering strength, hope, and meaning in life amid chronic diseases. For instance, one woman said, "It's prayers that keep me strong; it gives me strength to push on." Like Funeka and Anathi, many women emphasized how church and trusting God was a collective source of healing both physically and mentally. As exemplified by one woman: "I don't even feel like I'm sick. The church is healing me, and I feel okay in my body [physical] and mind."

Mashau (2016) reported that an emphasis on prayers and faith healing by the church resulted in medical treatment being rejected in some churches. One woman we spoke to said, "The only thing that is helping me now is church; when I leave the church service, I feel that I have offloaded some stress." Praying together with others in the church and other communal church activities were crucial in providing psychosocial support: "I go to church to be with others. We pray to God together and support each other." Attending church also provided a form of communalism, and people, including the ill, interacted and comforted each other: "The church helps a lot because at church you will hear other people talking about this illness, and I will realize that I am not the only one suffering from these illnesses." Ultimately, many believed in being prayed for by others to improve their health: "I'm a believer, so there's a church that I go to where I pray and ask to be prayed for, and after that, I feel better."

Clinical studies suggest that people's trust in religious practices and beliefs has led to individuals neglecting biomedical care for chronic diseases such as HIV/AIDS (Mattes 2014; Tocco 2014) and cases where parents refused to have their children vaccinated or treated at the hospital (O'Mathúna and Lang 2008). Indeed, seeking care from alternative providers, especially among people living with chronic diseases, is a common practice in South Africa (Mokgobi 2014; Moshabela et al. 2016), although it is unclear what people's long-term health experiences are once they abandon biomedicine altogether (Nyamongo 2002).

This is not surprising since all of the participants shared the common belief that God determines what happens to people's lives. A common sentiment was expressed by one man: "I believe that everything that happens in your life is the will of God; he is the one that takes away sickness from your life so that you can live a good life." Trusting in God's healing power was one way that people accepted their diabetes (or any chronic illness) and moved toward living well with their condition. God was also described as a supreme being and one who had control over people's lives: "God is the Almighty; he knows my life better, just like the chef knows his pots. So I accept what I have and leave it to God." In this context, individuals understood the chronic issues that they had, and perceived that they needed to develop a reciprocal relationship with God by surrendering all their troubles to God in order to attain healing. Many participants without comorbidity viewed their good health as God's favor on their life, while those with comorbidities believed that their healing could only come from God as he is the one who created them.

Many of our participants' strong beliefs that they were healed or would become healed were essential for their ability to cope with and heal amid chronic illnesses (see also Hardin 2019). In other words, finding psychological and spiritual balance amid metabolic or material chaos can serve to improve chronic physical illnesses (Roger and Hatala 2018; Unantenne et al. 2013). For example, people described how having a constant relationship with God through prayer, confiding all their fears and worries to God, helped them feel heard. This was significant in part because very few people felt heard or valued within the biomedical system.

Harris et al. (2016) have demonstrated that patients are happier and more successful in medical treatments – including behavior changes – when they feel heard and valued in decision-making pertaining to their health. Yet patients too often feel silenced, ignored, and misunderstood in biomedical systems of care (Bosire 2020). We have found over several years and hundreds of interviews that biomedicine rarely facilitated trust or a deep sense of healing. In contrast, healing was definite to those who believed and trusted in God's healing powers and were committed to religious practices, such as praying. This is similar to what Jessica Hardin found among Samoan Pentecostals: "Healing is an everyday activity for many evangelical Samoans; it requires striving for divine interdependence as a way to change health behaviors and called for continual attention" (2016, 107). Joel Robbins also argues that Christian rituals "both in their symbolism and their processual design are shaped by the goal of helping those who practice them to overcome the difficulties of ethical self-formation" (2004, 255). In this way, God was conceived as one who was trustworthy and reliable, while medical care was somewhat unreliable and stressful.

Many participants in this study attended the Zion Christian Church (ZCC), one of the fastest growing African Independent Churches in South Africa. Like the women in this story, many people commonly described drinking "church water" – a liquid mixture served at church or prepared for participants to take at home – as a source of healing. Many interlocutors referred to it as "holy water" or "tea" (which was locally called *indayelo*). One woman said it directly, "It's *indayelo* that heals me." Participants reported that church water was prepared by mixing water, oil, tea, and some herbs and then prayed on by a church minister, pastor or *omama bomthandazo*, who are mothers/women of prayer. These women not only prayed for the water in the church but also visited and prayed for church community members in their homes.

Drinking church or holy water is an old and common practice among ZCC members, as well as many other Christians in Soweto. West's (1972) studies on African Independent Churches in Soweto describe the use of holy water among Zionist church members for healing: "Holy water may be given to members of a congregation to heal them of something specific, or else it may be drunk to purify and protect against illness and misfortune" (185). He adds that "The importance of holy water in healing can be seen by the fact that it was given to patients in 79 % of consultations" (213). Recently, based on his interviews with undisclosed ZCC members in Soweto, Mashabela reported that tea and coffee were the old forms of healing: "In the African spirituality worldview, it is critically important to use coffee and tea as they are not invented memories but practically and historically lived memories within the ZCC spirituality" (2017, 6). In other words, tea and coffee were old forms of spiritual healing and have been used since the inception of the ZCC.

In an attempt to investigate our ethnographic findings on a larger scale, we built two surveys about stress and coping that drew from findings from our ethnographic research (Mendenhall et al. 2022). Based on data from 957 people, we found that those who reported less stress, despite living with two or more chronic illnesses, were more likely to have a better quality of life. It was an important finding in part because it revealed how chronic illnesses – alone or combined with one or two other co-occurring conditions – are not what drives quality of life.

Instead, our larger study reveals how crucial the social dynamics and stresses people experience are in driving a good life – with or without diagnosed conditions.

These large survey findings bolster the story from Funeka's kitchen. Putting trust in pastors, friendships, family, and others who can carry a burden forward is a crucial part of healing for many people facing illness in Soweto. When we interviewed thirty of these original eighty-eight Sowetans for a follow-up study on flourishing, we found that flourishing with or without illness was a collective endeavor (as opposed to an individual one, as it often is framed in medicine) (Cele et al. 2021). Flourishing required support from those who helped one come up, often with divine input or influence and in constant dialogue – or even tension – with moral expectations and obligations to one's family or broader community. In this way, the concept of flourishing in Soweto reveals both individual and collective dimensions. Some aspects of the universal definitions hold up (such as individually oriented determination), while, in other aspects (such as *ubuntu*, or caring for others), flourishing in Soweto is highly particular. Moreover, our findings emphasize how upstream factors can fuel a flourishing future, especially when material and financial needs are met.

REFERENCES

Bosire, E. N. 2020. "Patients' Experiences of Comorbid HIV/AIDS and Diabetes Care and Management in Soweto, South Africa." *Qualitative Health Research* 31 (2): 373–84.

Bosire, E. N., L. Cele, X. Potelwa, A. Cho, and E. Mendenhall. 2022. "God, Church Water and Spirituality: Perspectives on Health and Healing in Soweto, South Africa." *Global Public Health,* 17 (7): 1172–1185.

Bosire, E. N., Emily Mendenhall, Shane A. Norris, and Jenni Goudge. 2020. "Patient-Centred Care for Patients with Diabetes and HIV at a Public Tertiary Hospital in South Africa: An Ethnographic Study." *International Journal of Health Policy and Management:* 1–12.

Cele, L., Sarah S. Willen, Maydha Dhanuka, and Emily Mendenhall. 2021. "Ukuphumelela: Flourishing and the Pursuit of a Good Life, and Good Health, in Soweto, South Africa." *SSM – Mental Health,* 1: 100022.

Hardin, Jessica. 2016. "'Healing is a Done Deal': Temporality and Metabolic Healing among Evangelical Christians in Samoa." *Medical Anthropology: Cross-Cultural Studies in Health and Illness* 35 (2): 105–18.

Hardin, Jessica. 2019. *Faith and the Pursuit of Health: Cardiometabolic Disorders in Samoa.* New Brunswick, NJ: Rutgers University Press.

Harris, Bronwyn, John Eyles, and Jenni Goudge. 2016. "Ways of Doing: Restorative Practices, Governmentality, and Provider Conduct in Post-Apartheid Health Care." *Medical Anthropology: Cross-Cultural Studies in Health and Illness* 35 (6): 572–87.

Mashabela, J. K. 2017. "Healing in a Cultural Context: The Role of Healing as a Defining Character in the Growth and Popular Faith of the Zion Christian Church." *Studia Historiae Ecclesiasticae* 43 (3): 1–14.

Mashau, Thinandavha D. 2016. "Moving to Different Streams of Healing Praxis: A Reformed Missionary Approach of Healing in the African Context." *Verbum et Ecclesia* 37 (1): 1508.

Mattes, Dominik. 2014. "The Blood of Jesus and CD4 Counts: Dreaming, Developing and Navigating Therapeutic Options for Curing HIV/AIDS in Tanzania." In *Religion and the Challenges of AIDS Treatment in Africa: Saving Souls, Prolonging Lives,* edited by Rijk van Dijk, Hansjörg Dilger, Marian Burchardt, and Thera Rasing, 169–93. Farnham: Ashgate.

Mendenhall, Emily, Andrew W. Kim, Anthony Panasci, Lindile Cele, Feziwe Mpondo, Edna N. Bosire, Shane A. Norris, and Alexander C. Tsai. 2022. "A Mixed-Methods, Population-Based Study of a Syndemic in Soweto, South Africa." *Nature Human Behaviour.* 6 (1): 64–73.

Mokgobi, Maboe G. 2014. "Understanding Traditional African Healing." Supplement, *African Journal for Physical Health Education, Recreation, and Dance* 20, no. S2: 24–34.

Moshabela, Mosa, Thubelihle Zuma, and Bernhard Gaede. 2016. "Bridging the Gap between Biomedical and Traditional Health Practitioners in South Africa." *South African Health Review.* 83–92.

Nyamongo, Isaac K. 2002. "Health Care Switching Behaviour of Malaria Patients in a Kenyan Rural Community." *Social Science & Medicine* 54 (3): 377–86.

O'Mathúna, Dónal P., and Kelly Lang. 2008. "Medicine vs. Prayer: The Case of Kara Neumann." *Pediatric Nursing* 34 (5): 413–16.

Robbins, Joel. 2004. *Becoming Sinners: Christianity and Moral Torment in a Papua New Guinea Society.* Berkeley: University of California Press.

Roger, Kerstin S., and Andrew Hatala. 2018. "Religion, Spirituality & Chronic Illness: A Scoping Review and Implications for Health Care Practitioners." *Journal of Religion and Spirituality in Social Work* 37 (1): 24–44.

Tocco, Jennifer U. 2014. "Prophetic Medicine, Antiretrovirals, and the Therapeutic Economy of HIV in Northern Nigeria." In *Religion and the Challenges of AIDS Treatment in Africa: Saving Souls, Prolonging Lives,* edited by Rijk van Dijk, Hansjörg Dilger, Marian Burchardt, and Thera Rasing, 119–45. Farnham, UK: Ashgate.

Unantenne, Nimmi, Natasha Warren, Renata Canaway, and Lenore Manderson. 2013. "The Strength to Cope: Spirituality and Faith in Chronic Disease." *Journal of Religion and Health* 52 (4): 1147–61.

West, Martin E. 1972. *African Independent Churches in Soweto.* PhD diss., University of Cape Town.

CHAPTER THREE

Grace between Wives: Living the Good Life in Senegal

Emma Nelson Bunkley, Fatoumata Diagne, and Ndèye Aminata Mbaye

Sirah, Koumba, and Penda, co-wives and diabetics, waited patiently for free glucometers during a community event at the Catholic charity Yoonu Njub, which in Wolof means "way of righteousness." It was a beautiful afternoon, not a cloud in the sky, and the weather was on the cusp of almost too hot and too windy. This is not uncommon in the Sahel, where Saint-Louis, Senegal, is located: the heat remains thick and humid. About thirty of us sat on brown metal folding chairs in Yoonu Njub's largest room, anticipating the event's opening activity. The windows were open to the heat, and a breeze blew in from outside. Sirah fanned herself with a long edge of fabric from her skirt. We, Emma, Fatoumata, and Aminata, were also there – Emma was conducting ethnographic research alongside Fatoumata and Aminata, her research partners.

The organizers of the event, a German family of three – mother, father, and son – had arrived and were presenting to the crowd about a promise of building a gym so that people would have a place to exercise, an idea they had come up with along with the German Lutheran church they represented. Western medicine emphasizes the relationship between exercise, obesity, and diabetes, which informed how the German family thought about health and healing. This was why they believed providing gym equipment would help people living with obesity and diabetes in Saint-Louis. Yet, Sirah, Koumba, Penda, and others listening to their words were not impressed; every day many people in

Saint-Louis walk and labor for hours. For them, gym equipment was foreign and unfamiliar as opposed to comfortable and enabling. In this case, people did not imagine they would exercise themselves away from diabetes; instead, there might be a different relationship between diabetes, exercise, and nutrition that people found essential for their well-being, one not documented by Western biomedicine (Carruth and Mendenhall 2018; Bunkley 2021). Sirah and her co-wives would not be using the gym equipment, but they listened respectfully to the foreigners sharing their project.

When people gathered close, the son of the older German couple pulled up the left sleeve of his green button-down shirt to reveal a white bulge covered in shiny plastic tape. Everyone peered closely at his upper arm to see the technology placed in a curious position. It was a glucometer, installed permanently in his flesh, which, he would go on to explain, helped him monitor his glucose. Fatoumata was called upon to translate from French to Wolof for the young man, which she graciously agreed to do. She rapidly translated for the crowd as people watched him pull out his smartphone from his back pocket and hold it against the machine in his arm. Fatoumata repeated for him the readings that appeared instantaneously on his phone – a sugar range well within normal. "The glucometer reads 75," Fatoumata translated. "This is a good, normal fasting blood glucose. You can see how easily it is for me to monitor," she repeated for the young German man. Collectively, the crowd oohed and ahhed.

There was a brief pause in women fanning themselves as people turned to each other to affirm that what they saw was true. A man in a pressed and glossy bright blue *bubu* (a flowing wide-sleeved robe) raised his hand and asked, "How can I get one of those?" It was the first time many onlookers had imagined that constant surveillance of one's blood sugar was possible. The young German man looked down at his arm and appeared somewhat confused. He glanced, curious, at his parents, seeming to realize that the technology he had installed in his body, the ease of surveillance, was not yet available here. In this moment, he might have realized that his demonstration may not translate well to the people in the crowd if the technology was not something affordable or available for purchase in Saint-Louis. "I don't know," Fatoumata translated for him, "but maybe someday they will have it here." Sirah, Koumba, and Penda, who had traveled from a village a few hours away, fanned themselves and listened as Fatoumata translated. They too had come to the event because of the promise of free glucometers and free medication, which could otherwise be quite costly.

Sitting through this meeting was a demonstration in grace, as participants sat and fanned themselves while the German visitor presented technology unfamiliar and inaccessible to those in the audience–they oohed and ahhed, providing positive feedback to the presenter. They were not quick to anger because the technology was unavailable, but instead were generous in their reception. Grace is something we came to think about while studying disordered metabolisms in Senegal. Beyond this meeting, what does grace offer diabetic women, and what does it ask women to give?

GRACE

Grace, from the Latin root *gratus*, meaning pleasing or thankful, is a character in this story: it is a theoretical concept for understanding social relations among those who are living with a chronic illness. Grace is a gift (Vidal 2014): it is something given, received, and reciprocated. We give grace, in the form of patience, kindness, understanding, and care, to those in our lives who are struggling. We accept grace from others when we ourselves are struggling. For example, Senegalese women trade childcare with each other or cook food for each other, without expectation of return, if someone is sick. This idea of the gift is a key part of how social groups are able to function, through beneficence, through reception, and through reciprocity (Mauss 1925). Metabolic disorders, like diabetes, lay bare the need for grace, for pleasantness and thankfulness, and for gift giving, receiving, and reciprocation in Senegalese women's lives. Sirah, Koumba, and Penda were part of an intricate web of social networks, and as a threesome were their own social network. These networks supported them and allowed them to navigate the complexities of their diseases while maintaining agency and independence. These networks offered them grace – they were given care, time, food, and financial support. Sometimes they were able to reciprocate these gifts, sometimes they were not, but these gifts were offered, nonetheless.

Though the concept of grace predates Abrahamic religions, it is still often thought of in these specific religious terms. In Christianity, theologians talk about the divine grace of God, salvation being the ultimate gift from God. Judaic scholars discuss the relationship between divine grace and divine mercy, often using the Hebrew word *chesed*, love between people or kindness, or the word *chen*, favor or charm. In Islam, grace is thought of as *barakah*, blessings or bounty from Allah. "Surely Grace is in the hand of Allah; He brings it to whomever He decides" (Quran 3:73). At its root, *grace* is gratitude or gratuity (Pitt-Rivers 2011). Grace is something given between people that is extra, that does not always require reciprocity but invites the possibility of return. It is inherently social and often shared, something existing between people and between people and institutions (religious, bureaucratic, medical). Grace allows there to be gratitude, forgiveness, and mercy between people and in their everyday interactions, even amid difficult situations, including diabetes.

This idea of grace being a gift appears in the allegory of the Three Graces, who are often represented as mirth, beauty, and youth. The Three Graces is an old story, with representations of them first appearing in ancient Greek texts and continuing through the Roman Empire to medieval and Renaissance Europe; however, the story is not always the same and is often adapted for temporal and contextual relevance. Yet, the Three Graces are always represented as women: carved as marble statues or appearing in paintings and frescoes. The Three Graces have been written about as representations of the gift – one giving, one receiving, one returning (Pitt-Rivers 2011). Just like in Christianity, Judaism, or Islam, the Three Graces offer a story to us about the significance and importance of giving and receiving.

We offer a Senegalese version of the Three Graces in the context of diabetes – namely, humor, interembodiment, and support – and we tell their tales through Sirah, Koumba, and Penda. Through these three stories, we highlight the importance of grace and of gift giving, receiving, and reciprocating. These acts allow women living with diabetes to find solace, care, and even joy throughout their diabetes experience. These aspects of grace allow us to understand the sociality of metabolic disorders and the ways social support eases the illness experience. Grace allows us to understand the "social work of healing" (Hardin 2020, 651) and the ways in which Senegalese women live well with diabetes.

Diabetes is a universal condition that is mediated by culture, biology, epidemiology, and history to present differently both biologically and emotionally across contexts (Mendenhall 2019). Diabetes refracts the effects the rapidly modernizing and globalizing world has on human bodies and what modernization and globalization look like in different places and in differently placed bodies (Niewöhner and Lock 2018). People perceive diabetes illness and healing through the prism of the possible, and this is a central reason for their divergent perceptions, particularly when it comes to technology like the glucometer the young German man had implanted in his arm. The German family's decision to "educate" the local Senegalese with diabetes about this technology and to promote a gym for the Saint-Louis residents tells us more about German diabetes than Senegalese diabetes. The glucose monitor installed on the young man's arm allows us to peek into technology that isn't "cost effective" or accessible in a place like Senegal as well as the Germans' lack of understanding of the experience of patients tending their diabetes in Saint-Louis (see Moran-Thomas 2019). Germans in Senegal speaking French at a Catholic charity called Yoonu Njub provide a tableau for thinking about the complicated interrelatedness of global health.

The Three Graces of Sirah, Koumba, and Penda offer a lens for thinking about the world around us and the ways our bodies move through that world. Through their stories we see how people in Senegal live well with chronic disease and are not compressed into two-dimensional versions of themselves as suffering subjects (Robbins 2013). In Senegal, technology may not be the most impactful intervention (as it is a source of self-care), and instead reciprocity may be a more powerful conduit of well-being (as it is a source of communal caring).

SIRAH, THE FIRST GRACE, WAS HUMOR

The three women lived in a compound of grey concrete-block houses with zinc roofing. The courtyard of their compound was communal, with shared cooking fires, and chickens, cats, and children all roaming around the freshly swept sandy area. Sirah had invited us to come over while she cooked lunch. The women took turns cooking lunch for each other's families. The children would be home from school to eat before returning for the second half of the day. Opening a large, squeaking gate, Fatoumata and Emma let themselves into the family compound and found Sirah sitting next to a green propane tank with a pan balanced on the top, sautéing onions and garlic, surrounded by uncooked rice, fresh vegetables, fresh fish, and different spices.

Her smile was mischievous as she slit the belly of the glittering silver fish she was preparing for the lunch's *thieboudienne*. "Come help me cook," she taunted, the hot pan sizzling. Emma looked in horror at Fatoumata. Emma didn't even cook in her own home – there was no way she could help cook. Fatoumata laughed and said, "Will you go help her cook?" Fear in her eyes, Emma replied, "Absolutely not. I can't!" Everyone laughed at Emma's incompetence at such a simple act. Fatoumata and Emma sat on worn wooden stools next to a black-and-white cat lounging in the sun.

They asked Sirah, "What work does your husband have?" Looking at Fatoumata and Emma over her shoulder, Sirah deftly finished cleaning the fish's body and commanded, "Find a better job for my husband." The three women laughed again. Her husband, an electrician, didn't have steady work. Even though he was an electrician, he would try and pick up work as a mason or do other odd jobs for which people needed a handyman. Anything to pull in money for the family.

Fatoumata and Emma asked, "Did you go to French or Quranic school?" – a demographic question asked to everyone in the study. Sirah laughed as she began cutting a green bell pepper and responded, "Only primary school because I was a nut." She explained that she had been too wild, couldn't sit still, was always distracting the other children, and did not want to continue with school. The three women laughed together. Sirah's playfulness caught Fatoumata and Emma off guard.

Normally women being interviewed were serious or quiet. Sirah was full of a jovial spirit. A few years prior to our interview, Sirah had experienced a seizure due to uncontrolled high blood pressure. She had been taken to the hospital and had stayed there while the doctors figured out her diagnosis and worked to get her blood pressure under control. Despite the seriousness of her ongoing metabolic illness, she retained an infectious sense of humor. After the interview, Fatoumata and Emma discussed Sirah's convivial nature, her humor, her ability to turn questions back on the interviewers and, in doing so, reclaim her agency and her narrative.

Humor was critical for women navigating their daily experiences, often constrained by their metabolic disorders. Humor was a release, a mitigation of severity, a way to get through. It was also a way "to acknowledge the utter absurdity of misfortune" (Livingston 2012, 147). Through humor, Senegalese women found care (Robertson 2024). Humor allowed women to persist with grace – through chronic treatments, chronic shortages, chronic not knowing. Using humor, Sirah reasserted agency, reclaimed her narrative, turned assumptions on their head. The gift of humor helped women navigate the uncertainty of their metabolic disorders. Humor gave women opportunities for levity in landscapes of gravity.

KOUMBA, THE SECOND GRACE, WAS INTEREMBODIMENT

The women shared a deep empathy with each other that manifested at the biological level through interembodiment. Interembodiment, as Emma has described it, is "the sharing of embodied experiences across and among biological bodies" (2022, 258). Koumba did not have a clinical diagnosis of diabetes, but rather had begun to exhibit classic diabetic symptoms in what we believed to be an interembodied experience with Sirah's and Penda's clinical diagnoses. Koumba was the youngest of the co-wives. She was also the quietest of the three, with bright brown eyes that were always attentive and observing. She had an easy smile. Often, she was laughing with and at Sirah and her jokes. Koumba accompanied Sirah and Penda for glucose checks at the Diabetes Association, and though her sugar would be normal, she complained of headaches, lightheadedness, and frequent urination. Embodiment doesn't end at the boundaries of the skin. Interembodiment refuses the biomedically defined body as bounded and "normal." While clinically she did not have diabetes, she was sharing an interembodied experience of diabetes with Sirah and Penda.

The three women cooked meals and ate together. Women in Senegal are often taught by people affiliated with the biomedical establishment that food is a culprit for diabetes, but when everyone eats the same meal, it becomes difficult to understand why some people manifest diabetes and others do not. It also creates a situation where shared food is suddenly viewed as simultaneously toxic and unavoidable. Common biomedical advice is to cook separate meals for diabetic individuals, which ignores the cultural practice of eating together. Collective eating, diet, and disease management become complicated navigations for Senegalese women (see also Yates-Doerr 2015; Carney 2015; Mendenhall 2019; Weaver 2019; Poleykett 2021).

Koumba was making *akkara*[1] for us when we arrived for a visit one evening. A visiting uncle had started to make *attaya*[2] in the courtyard, and the smell of cooking sugar filled the air. We sat on the corner of Koumba's wooden bed, hovering over her a bit as she sat on the same low wooden stool Fatoumata had used when we visited Sirah a few days before. Koumba shaped the wet, mashed chickpeas into perfect balls and dropped them into boiling oil. She then used a slotted spoon to pull out the fried *akkara* and placed them into a purple plastic tub. "This is too much!" Fatoumata exclaimed. Emma eyed the *akkara* hungrily, and Aminata smiled. Koumba also smiled and told us to eat up. Her uncle arrived with three glasses of *attaya* on a silver tray. We each took a glass, sipping and finishing the delicious and sugary tea before returning the glass to the tray to wait for a second and then third cup. "I can't eat this or drink that," Koumba said, gesturing with her shoulder first to the fried *akkara* and then to the empty *attaya* glasses. "Why not?" Aminata inquired. Koumba replied, "I have to be careful of my diet; it is not good to eat sugar or oil." Emma asked, "Do you have diabetes or hypertension?" Koumba continued to form balls, her palm shiny with oil, and to scoop out the fried and ready pieces, and then replied, "I do not feel well. They say I do not have diabetes, but I know that I do. I have the headaches, and my body aches. Sirah and Penda have diabetes, and I know that I feel like them."

Even absent a clinical diagnosis, Koumba felt the same way as her co-wives. Biologically and emotionally, she had embodied their states of being. This deep empathy, perhaps counterintuitive because it left her weak and feeling poorly, connected her with Sirah and Penda. She deeply empathized with their pain and their experiences. Her interembodiment of their disease experiences brought the three women closer together. It was a form of emotional support. Interembodiment unsettles taken-for-granted ideas about "wellness" – namely the assumption that being well is being individually and independently healthy. Interembodiment surfaces the importance of connection (social and biological) and shows how connection is fundamental to living a life well with others.

PENDA, THE THIRD GRACE, WAS SUPPORT

Winding our way through the sandy lanes to the three women's compound, we passed brightly colored laundry drying on lines strung between buildings, people mending fishing nets, children chasing each other, chickens roaming freely alongside us. We found Penda stitching fuchsia thread into bright blue fabric, forming geometric floral patterns. She sat near the open door, welcoming in the light to aid her in her sewing project. The bed across from Penda was covered in a thick forest-green blanket with a golden lion's face. We sat next to each other on the edge of the bed and watched Penda work.

As she stitched fuchsia and blue together, her shoulders golden from the bright light, Penda told us about how much support she had from her family and the importance of this support in navigating her disease experience. "Yes, my support, my husband, my children always telling me, 'This is nothing; this is only a disease like the others. It's nothing. Do not surrender. Go back to your activities.' My husband and my children supported me until I returned to my normal activities." Penda had originally been diagnosed with diabetes when she began to rapidly lose weight. Fearful of the rumors that would circulate about her and her family because of this weight loss,[3] she hid herself away inside the compound, refusing to go out, do her normal activities, or meet with friends (Bunkley, 2025). The first of the co-wives to be diagnosed, Penda was initially living through the experience without many people to confide in. Her isolation was self-imposed, and her family and co-wives rallied around her, encouraging her not to be afraid.

Women often shared with us that support was critical for making and keeping doctor's appointments, finding financial aid for chronic care, and maintaining a positive and hopeful attitude. More often than not, we were told this in the context of women not having support, making Penda's story somewhat unique. Many women with whom we talked described loneliness, isolation, and a loss of networks able to be relied upon for financial help or help around the house or with children. Some women's husbands left or divorced them because of their diagnosis. Many women had moved into the homes of relatives, finding themselves reliant on brothers and brothers-in-law. The stark contrast of those experiences with those of Sirah, Koumba, and Penda helped us think through what women need to live well with diabetes and the importance of reciprocity through the gift of grace.

In addition to support from her husband and children, Penda and her co-wives supported each other. Co-wives can often experience strife, competition for resources, and jealousy. But Sirah, Koumba, and Penda had a kind, gentle, and generous relationship. Social support allowed women to share resources – time, money, childcare, pharmaceuticals – with each other (see Hardin 2023). Rather than facing the experience singularly, they collectively approached and navigated their metabolic disorders. Social support is the essence of the gift and of grace. It is something given, received, and reciprocated. It is the foundation for relationships, kin structures, and social networks.

CONCLUSION

Grace as a gift, as a reception, as a reciprocity, allows women in Senegal to live well with diabetes. Sirah (humor), Koumba (interembodiment), and Penda (support), the Three Graces, teach us to see the ways women use humor as a form of care, deeply empathize with each other, and support and uplift each other during their illness experiences. This is crucial for a condition like diabetes, which is a chronic disease with acute flareups. Women might feel okay one day and terrible the next. Unpredictable in its timing, diabetes robs people of dependable routines and requires interdependence among their loved ones. The chronicity of diabetes also requires a flexibility of diabetics and those around them. The endless schedule of doctor's appointments, lab visits, strikes at the hospital, the lack of money to go to doctor's appointments and buy pharmaceuticals, the chronicity, the acuteness, the pain, the waiting, all these experiences call for grace to live well with diabetes.

The event at Yoonu Njub puts in stark contrast conceptions of care within global health – Germans arriving in Senegal, Senegalese people as recipients – and the ways people in Saint-Louis perceive and embody care. The German family not only highlighted who had resources and who seemingly did not, but also revealed the ways a disease like diabetes is approached and embodied by different people. The German family conceived of their son's diabetes as largely clinical and isolated, requiring a personal glucometer that is accurate and usable whenever needed for individualized care. And in Senegal, the disease is approached communally, as we can see through the Three Graces. Both methods reveal much about the social nature of disease and the social nature of care.

As the event at Yoonu Njub wrapped up, the locals with diabetes gathered the pieces of diabetic equipment they had been given. The young man rolled down his sleeve to cover up his glucometer implant and buttoned it away. As we observed these actions, of the Senegalese people and the visitors, we thought about the ways diabetes existed in the global health imaginary, the ways in which it was defined, the ways diabetes traveled as a concept from a place like Germany to a place like Senegal. And we also considered Sirah, Koumba, and Penda, co-wives, living with diabetes in Senegal. Three women who had found ways to live well with their chronic disease. Although the young man also found his own way to live well with diabetes (by constantly monitoring it), the communal ways in which the women worked together on food, chores, and the mundane realities of living together demonstrated a different way of living well. When we parted paths at Yoonu Njub that day in April 2019, the Three Graces were giggling with each other – comparing their new glucometers, complete with boxes of test strips, gossiping, at ease and ready to begin their journey home. Together, the Three Graces were navigating the Senegalese diabetic landscape, one filled with uncertainty and scarcity. In each other they found ways to not only survive their disease but flourish with it, charting a new path that was situated within their immediate context, resources, and community (Willen et al. 2021).

NOTES

1 *Akkara* are smashed chickpeas mixed with water and seasoning and then fried as small balls.
2 *Attaya* is the traditional green tea of Senegal and is often made for guests when they visit.
3 Because people might think the weight loss was caused by HIV/AIDS or tuberculosis or a husband who could no longer financially support his family.

REFERENCES

Bunkley, Emma Nelson. 2025. "The Weight of Rumor." *American Anthropologist* 127: 244–54. https://doi.org/10.1111/aman.28053.
Bunkley, Emma Nelson. 2022. "Interembodiment, Inheritance, Intergenerational Health." *Medical Anthropology Quarterly* 36 (2): 256–71.

Bunkley, Emma Nelson. 2021. "Diagnosing Diabetes, Diagnosing Colonialism: An Ethnography of the Classification and Counting of a Senegalese Metabolic Disease." *Medicine Anthropology Theory* 8 (2): 1–26.

Carney, Megan A. 2015. *The Unending Hunger: Tracing Women and Food Insecurity Across Borders.* Oakland: University of California Press.

Carruth, Lauren, and Emily Mendenhall. 2018. "Social Aetiologies of Type 2 Diabetes." *The British Medical Journal* 361: 1–2.

Hardin, Jessica. "Ceaseless Healing and Never-Natural Disasters." *American Anthropologist Vital Topics Forum Chronic Disaster: Reimaging Noncommunicable Chronic Disease* 122, (3): 650–51.

Livingston, Julie. 2012. *Improvising Medicine: An African Oncology Ward in an Emerging Cancer Epidemic.* Durham: Duke University Press.

Mauss, Marcel. 1990. *The Gift: The Form and Reason for Exchange in Archaic Societies.* Translated by W. D. Halls. London: Routledge.

Mendenhall, Emily. 2019. *Rethinking Diabetes: Entanglements with Trauma, Poverty, and HIV.* Ithaca: Cornell University Press.

Niewöhner, Jörg, and Margaret Lock. 2018. "Situating Local Biologies: Anthropological Perspectives on Environment/Human Entanglements." *BioSocieties* 13: 681–97.

Pitts-Rivers, Julian. 2011. "The Place of Grace in Anthropology." *HAU: Journal of Ethnographic Theory* 1 (1): 423–50.

Poleykett, Branwyn. 2021. "Collective Eating and the Management of Chronic Disease in Dakar: Translating and Enacting Dietary Advice." *Critical Public Health.*

Robertson, William James. 2024. "The Butt of the Joke: Humour and Queer Care at an Anal Dysplasia Clinic." *Medicine Anthropology Theory.*

Robbins, Joel. 2013. "Beyond the Suffering Subject: Toward an Anthropology of the Good." *The Journal of the Royal Anthropological Institute* 19 (3): 447–62.

Vidal, Denis. 2014. "The Three Graces, or the Allegory of the Gift: A Contribution to the History of an Idea in Anthropology." *HAU: Journal of Ethnographic Theory* 4 (2): 339–68.

Weaver, Lesley Jo. 2019. *Sugar and Tension: Diabetes and Gender in Modern India.* New Brunswick, NJ: Rutgers University Press.

Willen, Sarah S., Abigail Fisher Williamson, Colleen C. Walsh, Mikayla Hyman, and William Tootle Jr. 2021. "Rethinking Flourishing: Critical Insights and Qualitative Perspectives from the U.S. Midwest." *Social Science and Medicine – Mental Health.*

Yates-Doerr, Emily. 2015. *The Weight of Obesity: Hunger and Global Health in Postwar Guatemala.* Oakland: University of California Press.

CHAPTER FOUR

Tinkering: Getting By with Diabetes through Creativity and Relational Care in Fiji

Tarryn Phillips and Edward Narain

Avinesh feels a little sparkle of pride each time he slips into his taxi. It's a used car shipped over from Japan and eventually purchased third-hand by Avinesh's boss. If he's being honest, the once smooth purr of the electric car has long since become a rattle, betraying its age and constant use. The seat belts no longer retract or clip in, and the cracks in the vinyl seat covers are increasingly oozing a yellow foam. He lovingly fixes its holes and rust and cracks with whatever he can find, and in return for his tinkering, it continues to drive with an endless stoicism that Avinesh appreciates. He proudly distributes business cards he just got printed that say: *Luxury Taxeez. 24 hour call!* The *z* was his oldest daughter Preeti's idea.

As the sun begins to rise, Avinesh has already left the small house that he shares with his mother and two daughters on the outskirts of Suva, Fiji. He pulls his taxi out onto the main road, merging with the bumper-to-bumper line of traffic crawling toward the city. He winds the window down and lets the light, warm breeze sift through his hair. Despite the belching fumes from the buses ahead, he can occasionally still catch a waft of the sweet vanilla from the frangipanni trees. As if in a dance with the cars in front of him, he rhythmically stops, starts, and then rolls again. He drives past all the billboards for the upcoming election, past the wood yards and all the places of worship in a row. A smorgasbord of spiritual options: the Seventh-day Adventist church, the Calvary Temple, the mosque.

To pass time on the road, Avinesh lets his mind wander to what his daughters are doing back home. Now they will be packing leftovers from last night's dal and rice into their metal lunch boxes. They will hand his mother – their *aji* – her medications, just like he has shown them. They will place half a papaya beside her as she lies on her mattress on the ground. (He watches her in his mind: she will swallow the pills, but barely acknowledge the food.) They will walk through the settlement along the muddy path to school, and Preeti will tell Shivashna to hurry up. A weight of sadness bears down on him: his mother is alone in the house. He tries to push the thought away – a neighbor will check in at some stage, and her sister will drop by as always. She won't be alone for long.

The traffic loosens up, and Avinesh shifts into third gear and then fourth, cruising down the hill toward the harbor, where the sun is glinting on the water. Early morning joggers pass each other at the sea wall, street dogs ambling behind them. The beauty of the scene makes him feel a glimmer of possibility. He takes a quick glance at the sun-faded plastic figurine of Hanuman, the Hindu monkey god, swinging from his rearview mirror. The *pundit* says that if we put good karma out into the world, then it will come back to us, if not in this life, then the next. And Avinesh has been working overtime, doing his very best. Things must surely fall into place soon.

Avinesh's taxi rank is just up the street from the Old Victoria Hotel, where the tourists and local elites go for sunset drinks and buffet breakfasts. It's here, Avinesh feels sure, that he is likely to meet the person who is going to solve his problem. He parks across the road from the hotel behind Goundar's and Mota's cars (both his friends are having a nap on retracted seats). He has timed it well today. It is only a couple of minutes before the hotel concierge steps out onto the footpath to flag a taxi with a quick, sharp kissing sound. Goundar jolts up at the noise, starts his engine, and peels off. Mota soon does the same. Eventually the concierge gains eye contact with Avinesh, meaning it's his turn.

He brings the taxi to a stop outside the lush, white-column foyer. The hotel guests waiting for him on the marble steps are a couple that look to be in their forties. They are of South Asian descent like him and yet are immediately recognizable as not-from-around-here. It's their casual but expensive-looking ripped jeans, cotton T-shirts, and Birkenstocks. The concierge opens the door for them, bowing slightly.

"Thanks, mate," the man says in a surprisingly broad Australian accent. Or maybe it is a New Zealand accent. Avinesh can't tell the difference.

They slip into his back seat, and he bobs his head in welcome. The passengers are still weighing out different options of what to do for the day, and he waits patiently for them to decide. He hopes they might be adventurous and seek a more intrepid day trip to the inland or a visit to Sigatoka several hours away. This has happened once or twice and can be a wonderful midweek bonus. Eventually, though, they settle on the markets, only a short drive away.

As they drive down the palm tree-lined street, Avinesh looks at them in the rearview mirror.

He begins the usual way. "Where you from? Australia? New Zealand?"

"Auckland." The man smiles at him from the back seat.

"Ahhhh. You are escaping the coldness, isn't it?"

"Yup!"

"Enjoying your holiday?"

"It's not so much a holiday. My father was from Fiji. He migrated to New Zealand after the '87 coup."

Avinesh chuckles. "Welcome back, *bhai*. We are brothers!"

"Ha ha, yeah, thanks. It's pretty cool," the man continues as he watches Suva whirl past, "to see my roots."

The woman points something out to her husband, and he laughs, turning to watch something whiz past. He turns back around to Avinesh. "Dad started with nothing. Then he went on to build a big IT empire. It's international now. Two hundred employees."

Avinesh nods, impressed. He also knows a thing or two about having nothing. His own parents thought about leaving during the 1987 unrest, too, when Indo-Fijians felt especially unwelcome here. He remembers whispered conversations, and the sound of soft crying from his parents' mattress at night. They couldn't raise the funds in the end and stuck around, eking out enough to keep their kids in school. What a different life they might have led.

The man is still talking. "Dad's always wanted to give back to Fiji, though. He started a charitable foundation last year in his name. To help the needy."

"*Acha, acha.*" Avinesh bobs his head in admiration. "Has a good heart, *haana?*"

"Exactly," the man says.

The woman is now looking at Avinesh with interest.

"What's it like," she asks, "driving taxis in Suva?"

Avinesh has been waiting for this question. He knows how he must answer. "Oooh, it's very, very hard," he says. "Too many taxis, not enough business." He glances at her in the mirror. "I work every day and every night, but still, not enough." He takes a poetic pause. "I can't even buy my mother the wheelchair she needs."

He leaves it there, feeling he has been subtle but heartfelt. There are, of course, untold details to this story. They are too raw, and he is not quite ready to package them up and deliver them to his passengers. He does not tell them, for example, how the doctors cut off his mother's leg early one morning to save her life. How his active, funny, full-of-life mother, who used to rib him constantly, has retreated into herself. No longer able to bathe herself, visit the neighbors, or see her sister on the other side of the village whenever she wants. She is deeply, irrepressibly sad. Not even her granddaughters can make her laugh anymore, no matter how much they try. He notices how Shivashna hams up her playfulness. Preeti talks extra loudly about the things she knows her *aji* likes to hear about – her grades at school, her plans for careers and marriage and children. But still they haven't been able to raise a smile. His heart breaks each time he sees their sweet empathetic faces, soldiering on.

"Nawww," the woman replies from the back seat. "I'm sorry to hear about your mum."

Tomorrow is the girls' end-of-year awards ceremony. It will be the first one *ever* that his mother hasn't attended. He has a feeling that if only they could get her there, it would make a world of difference. He has even considered carrying her over his shoulder – fireman style – to where he parks the taxi outside the settlement. But that is too undignified for her. He really needs that wheelchair. He's been trying to get one for months, by any means possible. The closest he came was when someone told him there was an abandoned wheelchair frame outside MaxValu supermarket (or "min value" as he always jokes to his passengers). Avinesh went to inspect it, but the vinyl seat was completely ripped, the wheels were rusted and immobile. Even for him, it was a little too broken.

"Oh my God!" The man exclaims, surprising Avinesh with his delayed reaction. But he is pointing at a boy vendor outside the cinemas. "How good do those pineapples look? So much *yellower* than the Auckland ones."

Avinesh wends the taxi past the shipping yards with the containers stacked on top of each other, past the bustling bus station, toward the markets. The passengers look awestruck, craning their necks to see the colorful chaos in front of them. He pulls in beside the footpath, ignoring the honk of impatient traffic behind him. As he switches off the engine, Avinesh lands the punchline crisply and clearly. With quiet sincerity, he says, "If you have anything to spare for the wheelchair, this would be very much helpful."

The woman looks at him apologetically. "Sorry," she says, with a pained look on her face, "we give in other ways." Avinesh smiles in understanding.

The price on the reader is $3.20, and the man hands over a fifty note. Avinesh pulls a small wad of notes from his pocket – his float for the day – and rifles through it, giving the man the first twenty note of change. He deliberately takes his time finding the second note, hoping that at some point the passenger might tell him to keep the rest. The man waits for Avinesh to count it out to the cent.

"Dhanyawad," the man says, trying *thank you* in Hindi with his strong Kiwi accent.

Avinesh nods. "Have a blessed day!" He opens the dash compartment to pull out a business card. "If you need a –" but the man has closed the door now, and the couple disappear into the throng of market-goers.

After he leaves the markets, Avinesh does several more fares in a row. He is flagged down by a barefooted and friendly iTaukei man, who he takes to his friend's house at a nearby settlement, and then finds two earnest-looking Americans wanting to go to the Pacific Theological College. Neither of them is any more fruitful than the strict cost of their fares.

He is grateful when ten o'clock rolls around, marking the agreed-upon time to go to the arcade. Through the open windows of the food court, he can see his taxi driver friends Mota and Goundar have already commandeered the usual table. They wave him over, and he gestures that he is coming.

"Coffee please, Aunty," he says to the woman at the stall on the left, who has been there for decades and surely is about ninety years old by now.

"Huh?" The older woman says, leaning one ear over the counter.

"COFFEE PLEASE, AUNTY! NO SUGAR!" He places a dollar fifty on the counter, and she nods and turns toward the urn.

This no-sugar thing is new for him. He refrains from looking at the cabinet full of brightly colored sweets – the milky *barfi*, the syrupy *gulab jamun*, and the fluorescent *jalebi*. Lately, Avinesh has started to feel that diabetes is coming for him, too. He has begun to question all the undetected signs he missed in his mother – the regular trips to the toilet, the uncharacteristic grumpiness, the little wounds that just wouldn't get better. So Avinesh now looks more closely at the food he eats, at an almost granular level – each crumb is potentially the last straw.

Aunty hands him his boiling hot instant coffee with milk powder. At the table with his motley crew of friends, Goundar is cackling at something Mota just said. Mota looks up. "Story, *bhai*?"

"Nothing much." Avinesh sits down, sipping his hot, watery coffee. They debrief about this morning's business. "Made contract, yet?" Avinesh quips.

Goundar sniggers. "Ha, not even close!" It usually takes them most of the day to pay the taxi owner's cut and break even. Mota bites into a warm roti parcel. The smell of the salty potato curry wrapped in the flatbread immediately makes Avinesh want one, too. He takes a deep breath and lets the craving pass.

"Okay, okay, okay." Goundar brings order to the session. "Moment of truth, eh?" He pulls out his cheap, cracked smartphone, and they all huddle around it. He clicks on the familiar icon for the We'veGotThis! app – little hands pressed together in a thank-you gesture.

It was Goundar's idea to set up a crowdfunding campaign. You can't do it from Fiji, so he asked his cousin-brother living in Sydney to do it. They had crafted the message a month ago:

> *Help Ashni get a wheelchair!*
>
> *Pliz help! Urgent! Ashni is a very good woman all her life. She is loving mother and grandmother. She did not know she has diabetes until doctor says amputation. Now she is a handicap! We only need $300AUD to buy a wheelchair. See attached medical report for proof. Pliz help Ashni.*

The last time they looked, the campaign had already raised forty dollars. Two anonymous people – probably friends of Goundar's cousin-brother – had both pledged twenty dollars each. Avinesh was so touched. Even forty dollars would go a long way to help. But Goundar explained that he probably wouldn't see that money unless they reached the target.

There have been no new donations. The guys are all silent for a moment. Goundar refreshes the page once and then twice, as if donations might come in as they speak. Avinesh had hoped that it might – what's that word Preeti uses? – "go viral" like that one they'd seen about the cute American kid, but it won't happen for tomorrow.

Mota mentions the new batch of wheelchairs that the Australian embassy is apparently donating. (It was in the news.) No one knows yet how it's going to work – apparently it will go through a charity, and there will be a waitlist – but he says he will keep trying to find out. His friend's brother-in-law's cousin works at the place where the Australian funds get distributed, so Mota will lean on him when the time comes.

"Acha," Avinesh says, getting up from his chair, signaling to his friends that he will be okay and that they can all leave for their next shift.

"That's it, *bhai,*" Mota says encouragingly. "If we keep a clean heart, it'll happen."

After a long day of driving, Avinesh is barely able to keep his eyelids open in the dusky Suva light. Needing something to revive him for the long drive ahead, he decides to pull into MaxValu. His resolve slips away as he walks past the tantalizing refrigerator full of fizzy, caffeinated drinks. Caving, he buys a bottle of cola and takes the first refreshing sip, bubbles pleasantly burning the back of his throat. It is *exactly* what he needed.

In the carpark, Avinesh can't help but have another look at the abandoned wheelchair frame. It's still there, sitting unloved in the darkness behind the bins. He turns it upside down and creaks it forward. He wonders if he could just dribble some oil onto the axle, whether the wheels might lubricate through their rust and begin to roll. He then tugs at the ripped vinyl seat. It pulls away from the chair altogether, completely disintegrated by the weather. It occurs to him that if he could just secure two or three planks of wood onto the frame, then he could tie a pillow down with some string for a kind of seat. It is a long shot, but he is running out of options. He makes a split decision. He clunks and clanks the frame into the back seat of his taxi and begins the drive home.

When the taxi is safely parked next to the settlement, he trudges through the mud, awkwardly carrying the unwieldy wheelchair frame toward his one-bedroom house. His back aches when he finally sets the metal structure down outside the shack. A waft of pumpkin curry greets him at the door – Preeti has been cooking – and he feels a sudden, beautiful wash of relief to be home.

Inside, the girls have fallen asleep. Still in their school uniforms, they are draped over their grandmother on the armchair, the dulcet tones of the Filipino soap opera they all follow religiously still bubbling away from the small television in the corner. His mother, covered in a blanket and surrounded by her granddaughters, looks almost peaceful.

After a few bites of curry, Avinesh pulls up his sleeves and sits down beside the wheelchair frame, feeling a burst of energy to fix it tonight.

He has a warm, glowing thought. *This will do.*

♿ ♿ ♿

Although Avinesh and his family are fictional characters, they are composites of many people we have met through our combined lived experience growing up and working in Suva (Edward) and conducting long-term ethnographic research on poverty and type 2 diabetes in Fiji (Tarryn). This small Pacific Island nation has a rich and complicated history with sugar, which in turn provides a unique foundation from which to examine the country's contemporary battle against diabetes.

Avinesh's family, like Edward's, is descended from Indians who in the late 1800s and early 1900s were forced or tricked by the British colonial administration into migrating to Fiji and other outposts of the empire. Referred to locally as *girmitiya* (an Indian mispronunciation of the English word *agreement*), they were indentured to work on the sugar cane plantations in brutal conditions of exploitation, abuse, and starvation not dissimilar to slavery (Lal 1998). After the indenture system was abolished in 1916, many indentured laborers remained in Fiji, and some continued to farm sugar. Ethnic tensions have sometimes bubbled over between Indo-Fijians and Indigenous Fijians (iTaukei), and the country has had four military coups since 1987. After these periods of unrest, many of those Indians who had sufficient capital migrated overseas to Australia, New Zealand, Canada, and beyond, as did the passengers in the story above. Those that have stayed in Fiji, however, have both a strong connection to Indian culture and a loyal, if complicated, patriotism for their adopted island home (Narain and Phillips 2024; Trnka 2005).

Nearly a third of all Fijians are officially diagnosed with diabetes, although that is likely an underestimate. The country has the highest documented per-capita rate of premature death from diabetes-related complications in the world. Wealthier people with diabetes and those who have access to the diaspora are often able to manage their condition by engaging in regular health-care checkups, seeking nutritional advice, and being able to afford insulin-measuring technologies. Yet for poorer Fijians, this is not always possible. In addition to high rates of stroke and blindness, at least three Fijians a day are having limbs amputated due to diabetes-related complications. Many of these people, like Avinesh and his family, come from peri-urban informal settlements, where there is typically poor water and sanitation, limited access to fresh, nutritious food, and worse health outcomes (Phillips and Narayan 2017).

Despite these metrics and financial limitations, many family members work creatively and collaboratively to care for their diabetic loved ones in these challenging circumstances. We have followed Avinesh, his daughters, and his friends in their entrepreneurial attempts to raise funds for a wheelchair for his mother, Ashni. A recent amputee, Ashni experiences the comorbidities of poverty, depression, and diabetes common among women in the Global South (Mendenhall et al. 2016; Weaver 2017). While we do not want to gloss over the suffering and deprivation that often comes with amputation in impoverished settings, we do want to foreground the simultaneous moments of playfulness, good humor, spiritual strength, resourcefulness, and communitarian efforts to uphold the dignity of people living with diabetes. We used the metaphor of tinkering as a way of highlighting this humanity.

To tinker, like Avinesh does with his aging taxi, is an ongoing process of making do with what one has in order to mend any problems that arise with practical, creative, and thrifty solutions. Anne-Marie Mol (2008) and her colleagues (Mol et al. 2015) developed the metaphor of "tinkering care" to examine how people do their best to care for others despite "the complex ambivalence and shifting tensions of care" (2015, 14). While biomedical definitions of what "good" care should look like are often rather narrow, this everyday ethic of care moves away from a singular moralized narrative of "good," toward the possibility for multiple, context-dependent "goods" (Mol 2008). We like this approach because it sheds a different light on *failure* in contexts of care. Rather than a "reason for moral blame, a negative verdict" (13), failure can instead be framed as an opportunity to "try again, try something a bit different, be attentive" (14). It is important to mention here that Mol and colleagues were writing about care in mostly Western, industrialized settings. More recently, Supuni Liyanagunawardena (2023) argued that in resource-limited settings such as her field site of Sri Lanka (and in this case, Fiji), *tinkering* may downplay the immense effort required to care for a loved one against the odds, and that *wrangling* may be a more effective metaphor. We agree with Liyanagunawardena's point that mobilizing resourceful care and maintaining optimism in the face of repeated setbacks can be a much heavier task in low-income contexts. And yet, we still feel that tinkering has conceptual value. For us, wrangling implies an adversarial struggle to regain control over one's destiny. Tinkering, on the other hand, is a more subtle, ongoing process of getting by. The tinker is often aware that their solutions are likely to be incomplete and temporary. In this way, those who tinker to provide good care are not always consciously fighting the system or reflecting on injustice when they do so. Tinkering can emerge through – and alongside – faith, love, creativity, playfulness, and pride. It thus encapsulates the dignified strength that we witnessed time and again among people living with diabetes and their caregivers in Fiji.

For Ashni, Avinesh's mother, her prior independence and ability to fulfil her culturally defined gender roles as Indian mother and grandmother (see also Weaver 2019) are severely hampered by her amputation. Avinesh feels certain that improving her mobility will address these needs, both at a practical and symbolic level. And yet a wheelchair is expensive and seemingly beyond his reach. He thus tinkers with what he has available – economically, socially, and spiritually – to somehow secure the resources.

One tool he has available to him is taxi driving – a gendered and racialized affordance. Driving taxis has long been viewed by lower-income South Asian men across the globe as one of limited ways to achieve upward social mobility, which both leads to and stems from structural racism (Hussain 2019; Sarkar 2019). In Fiji, the realities of the overcrowded taxi sector and sometimes exploitative relationships between owners and drivers make profits very difficult to come by. In our research and experience, many Indo-Fijian drivers supplement the fares themselves by seeking alternative and informal ways of making money as a driver, such as crafting narratives of suffering and hardship – stories that are often just as genuine as they are performative – in order to evoke a sympathetic monetary offering from passengers, or brokering other services for visitors including phone repair, tourism guidance, and organizing access to recreational drugs. In public discourse, this practice is often cast as manipulative and nefarious. We instead sought to reframe it as a creative solution to inequality, often motivated by a desire to provide better care for loved ones.

A second avenue Avinesh and his friends lean into is crowdfunding, through the fictional app We'veGotThis! A 2022 article in *The Guardian* reported that Fijians who were suffering from diabetes-related complications were turning to crowdfunding to source funds for life-saving medical interventions (Panepasa 2022). Private hospitals and the Ministry of Health in Fiji had even explicitly offered to help patients set up crowdfunding campaigns by providing them with a detailed medical report to prove the legitimacy of their claims. The headline of the article was "Fundraise or Die."

To elicit a philanthropic response, campaign organizers – like Goundar's cousin-brother in the story – must become "sympathy entrepreneurs," crafting a marketable narrative of worthiness (Wade 2023; see also Clark 1997). However, the odds are stacked against campaigns for people like Ashni. Sufferers of chronic conditions are at a disadvantage on these platforms, rarely achieving or even getting close to their designated targets. The statistics of success indicate that donors prefer to contribute to heroic interventions – dramatic, one-off, life-saving events – that can make them feel particularly virtuous about their philanthropy (Berliner and Kenworthy 2017). Crisis crowdfunding privileges compelling stories about those who can be perceived as innocent victims of a tragedy for which they couldn't possibly be blamed (Romm 2015).

This trend discriminates against the already moralized sufferer of diabetes: in a neoliberal regime in which individuals are considered responsible for their own welfare, those who are diagnosed with chronic metabolic disorders are often considered blameworthy for having made poor lifestyle "choices" (Phillips 2020). Going further, those who suffer from an amputation because of *uncontrolled* diabetes are assumed to have taken undue risks with their health and been medically noncompliant, undermining their perceived deservedness (Kenworthy 2024). In our story, as in most diabetes-related campaigns in Fiji, Avinesh and his friends are acutely aware of this moral economy, and thus deliberately reference Ashni's life-long work ethic and blamelessness to fend off such critique. Nevertheless, Ashni is also disadvantaged by the inherent race and gender biases on crowdfunding platforms. White men are disproportionately successful in medical crowdfunding campaigns, while people of color – especially women of color – are significantly underrepresented (Davis et al. 2023; Kenworthy et al. 2023). That Ashni will probably not reach the designated target accurately reflects a harsh reality.

Avinesh maintains optimism through an unbending faith in Hinduism, a spiritual strength that is common among carers and people living with diabetes across the Pacific (see also Hardin 2019; Phillips 2020). Both he and his mother are also surrounded by a strong, albeit gendered, social fabric that tightens in times of need: his oldest daughter, Preeti, still in high school, takes on the role of cooking and caring at home; his taxi-driver friends enlist in the quest to find a wheelchair, contributing their own social networks to help out; and neighbors and family visit Ashni during the day.

Despite repeated setbacks, Avinesh continues to tinker, eventually recycling other people's rubbish to craft a wheelchair for his mother. Although we present this as a form of entrepreneurialism, we reject neoliberal discourses that suggest informal settlers should – or can – simply bootstrap themselves out of hardship. Entangled with myths of "freedom" and "choice," such discourses romanticize and reinforce the current economic regime, from which the unequal toll of diabetes emerged in the first place. Instead, we tell Avinesh's story to highlight the brokenness of the system, the cracks that people with diabetes-related amputations often fall through, and the poignant ways in which communities work together to patch them up with whatever they can find.

REFERENCES

Berliner, L. S., and N. J. Kenworthy. 2017. "Producing a Worthy Illness: Personal Crowdfunding Amidst Financial Crisis." *Social Science & Medicine* 187: 233–42.

Clark, Candace. 1997. *Misery and Company: Sympathy in Everyday Life.* Chicago: University of Chicago Press.

Davis, A. R., S. K. Elbers, and N. Kenworthy. 2023. "Racial and Gender Disparities Among Highly Successful Medical Crowdfunding Campaigns." *Social Science & Medicine* 324: 115852.

Hardin, Jessica. 2019. *Faith and the Pursuit of Health: Cardiometabolic Disorders in Samoa.* New Brunswick, NJ: Rutgers University Press.

Hussain, Yasmin. 2019. "'I Was Professor in India and Here I Am a Taxi Driver': Middle Class Indian Migrants to New Zealand." *Migration Studies* 7 (4): 496–512.

Kenworthy, N. 2024. *Crowded Out: The True Costs of Crowdfunding Healthcare.* Boston: MIT Press.

Kenworthy, N., Z. Dong, A. Montgomery, E. Fuller, and L. Berliner. 2020. "A Cross-Sectional Study of Social Inequities in Medical Crowdfunding Campaigns in the United States." *PLoS One* 15 (3): e0229760.

Lal, Brij V. 1998. "Understanding the Indian Indenture Experience." Supplement, *South Asia: Journal of South Asian Studies* 21, no. S1: 215–37.

Liyanagunawardena, S. 2023. "Wrangling for Health: Moving Beyond 'Tinkering' to Struggling Against the Odds." *Social Science & Medicine* 320: 115725.

Mendenhall, Emily, Brandon A. Kohrt, Shane A. Norris, David Ndetei, and Dorairaj Prabhakaran. 2017. "Non-Communicable Disease Syndemics: Poverty, Depression, and Diabetes Among Low-Income Populations." *The Lancet* 389 (10072): 951–63.

Mol, Annemarie. 2008. *The Logic of Care: Health and the Problem of Patient Choice.* London: Routledge.

Mol, Annemarie, Ingunn Moser, and Jeannette Pols, eds. 2015. *Care in Practice: On Tinkering in Clinics, Homes and Farms.* Bielefeld: Transcript.

Narain, E., and T. Phillips. 2024. *Sugar: An Ethnographic Novel.* Toronto: University of Toronto Press.

Panepasa, G. 2022. "Fundraise or Die: How Fijians Are Crowdfunding Lifesaving Kidney Treatment." *The Guardian.* https://www.theguardian .com/world/2022/mar/23/fundraise-or-die-how-fijians-are-crowdfunding -lifesaving-kidney-treatment.

Phillips, T. 2020. "The Everyday Politics of Risk: Managing Diabetes in Fiji." *Medical Anthropology* 39 (8): 735–50.

Phillips, T., and A. Narayan. 2017. "The Healthcare Challenges Posed by Rapid Urbanisation in the Pacific: The View from Fiji." *Development Bulletin: Servicing the Cities* 78: 79. https://nauru-data.sprep.org/system/files/

Development%2520Bulletin%252078%2520Web%2520Version.
pdf#page=86.

Romm, C. 2015. "Is It Fair to Ask the Internet to Pay Your Hospital Bill?: The Ethical Issues That Come with Crowdfunded Healthcare." *The Atlantic,* March, 2015. https://www.theatlantic.com/health/archive/2015/03/is-it-fair-to-ask-the-internet-to-pay-your-hospital-bill/387577/.

Sarkar, M. 2019. "In a Taxi, Stuck or Going Places? A Bourdieusian Intersectional Analysis of the Employment Habitus of Pakistani Taxi Drivers in the UK." PhD diss., University of Leeds.

Trnka, Susanna. 2005. "Land, Life and Labour: Indo-Fijian Claims to Citizenship in a Changing Fiji." *Oceania* 75 (4): 354–67.

Wade, M. 2023. "The Giving Layer of the Internet: A Critical History of GoFundMe's Reputation Management, Platform Governance, and Communication Strategies in Capturing Peer-to-Peer and Charitable Giving Markets." *Journal of Philanthropy and Marketing* 28 (4): e1777.

Weaver, L. J. 2019. *Sugar and Tension: Diabetes and Gender in Modern India.* New Brunswick, NJ: Rutgers University Press.

Weaver, L. J. 2016. "Transactions in Suffering: Mothers, Daughters, and Chronic Disease Comorbidities in New Delhi, India." *Medical Anthropology Quarterly* 30 (4): 498–514.

CHAPTER FIVE

Ancestral Healing: Interconnected Legacies of Sugar in Brazil

D. Burnett

Mari is planning to visit her *mãe-de-santo*, spiritual godmother, Mãe Canela, for a divination in the morning. She was recently diagnosed with diabetes and has been noticing her energy wane, her work slow, and her unsteady blood sugar put her nerves on edge. In Candomblé, they seek the guidance of the *buzios*, or shells, used in divination when people face health conditions like Mari's. Candomblé is a complex and diverse group of Brazil's Black Indigenous religious and spiritual systems. Mãe Canela advises Mari of the energy that is surrounding her, what forces are speaking to and guiding her, and similarly, how Mari can recalibrate the forces and energies around her. Before she sleeps, Mari will pray and engage in rituals to prepare her mind and body.

In Mari's fatigue, however, she barely makes it through her nightly routine of dinner, cleaning, bathing, and preparation for the day ahead with her family. Each night, Mari feels so tired that it is almost as if she is floating through the night, moving above her body. Tonight, on the eve of meeting with Mãe Canela, Mari's body has already slipped into her subconscious. As soon as her head hits the pillow, she dips into a very lucid dream state. In her dream, Mari encounters an exceedingly maternal woman. She does not know this woman by name or face. When Mari hears her speak, however, she can tell she is not from this generation.

Mari has a profound connection with Isabella. In the dream, Isabella asks her if she can come closer so she can touch her and speak to her while looking in her eyes. Mari is hesitant, and Isabella sees it and says, "I am your grandmother's grandmother; it is my honor to connect with you. I am grateful to walk this journey with you. There are some things that I want you to know."

"Mari," Isabella begins, speaking in a lyrical dream voice that is both bold and gentle. "Healing is a life-long journey. One that requires daily effort." In her dream state, Mari smiles and calms. "There are no real shortcuts to healing work, and when you discover that you have healed one thing, something comes up in its place to assure you that there is more healing work to be done. The only safety in the healing process is confidence that true knowledge of a deeper sense of self lies on the other side."

Isabella continues to speak to her through the dream as she walks toward Mari and embraces her. "Healing is the most powerful work you can do for yourself, your family, your community, our world, and the planet. Healing work is life's gift to show you your own power, your own potential, your own giftedness. Healing work is sacred; it is your connection to divinity that is drawn from divinity. Healing work is sacred knowledge stored within you.

"You can turn the sweetness in your blood to sweetness in the world, if you learn to use your power right, Mari. Your sickness is bittersweet. Your sickness is sticky. Your sickness is courage. Your sickness is not your own; it reflects your experience. Mari, learn to master and wield your superpower with grace for all those who see you. I believe that if you do, you will be skilled in everything that you do."

Suddenly Mari wakes. She hears the voice of a vendor on the street selling gas ringing in her ear. Isabella's voice and image is powerful, although in her grogginess, it is hard to distinguish what is dream and what is physical. Nevertheless, the message is clear: this healing work is her duty, her gift, her power in the world. Mari is overwhelmed yet comforted by the energy of this maternal force reaching out to her. She is enveloped by the power of the spiritual forces that allow her to see herself, her life, her disease, and subsequently her healing in a new light.

Mari rises from the bed to wash, pausing briefly to record a quick WhatsApp voice note to herself. She describes what she can remember of the dream to document what she is hearing, seeing, experiencing from the other side. Also, she plans to describe it to Mãe Canela when she sees her later today and needs to remember details. Mari looks at her reflection in the mirror while she washes. When Mari thinks about Isabella, she is surprised to feel a comfort that she has not felt for some time: that she is not alone. Lost in the mirror's reflection of her face and her own wandering mind, she jumps when she sees her beloved eleven-year-old daughter, Julianna, staring at her.

Mari's face softens, and she embraces Julianna. "What are you doing up so early? Are you hungry, love?"

"Yes, I am, Mommy. I had a dream about you and wanted to see you"

"Oh, my darling, tell me all about your dream while I cook. Let's get you fed so I can get ready to see Mãe Canela."

"Yay, we're going to Tia Canela's house?"

"It's just me today, sweetie. You have plans with your cousins today, remember?"

Mari grabs Julianna's hand and walks into the kitchen to prepare breakfast for her family and spends time with her daughter before the rest of the family joins them. When her family members slowly file into the kitchen to eat, Mari fills their plates and cleans their dishes, never sitting down herself to eat. The family connects before going in different directions for the day. Mari dresses and then rushes out the door to Mãe Canela's house.

Mari leaves her home, heads down the stairs at a steep incline through the narrow pathway, and walks the few blocks down to the main road. She waits for the bus for twenty-nine minutes and knows she will arrive late to meet Mãe Canela. Her plan to make the eighteen-kilometer trip in two-and-a-half hours is ruined by the bus delay, and the tropical heat drenches her in sweat. Still, she smiles out the window of the bus station as she watches the multiple vendors selling street food to hungry commuters in the devastatingly beautiful, culturally rich, lush metropolis of Salvador da Bahia, Brazil. Mari is engulfed by the cacophony of scents in this gastronomical paradise while she navigates decisions around what food means to her insulin-resistant body. Her stomach growls on cue as the bus to her spiritual godmother's home finally arrives.

The massive bus is white and yellow with red, black, and green letters. The word *Axé* covers the outside of the vehicle, which brings residents from the peripheries of town into the city for work, business, shopping, and other affairs. The name of the bus company, Axé, is the Brazilian version of a Yoruba word, reflecting the long history of exchange of language, culture, and (often forced) migration. This history of forced migration, exchange of language and culture, has led to Candomblé traditions being culturally embedded in the foundation of the city. The word *axé* also links many in the city to a set of knowledge about a cosmological worldview that becomes familiar through the words, sayings, and experiences of practitioners across the city, nation, and world. *Axé*, while having many definitions, is generally defined as power, authority, command, a life force, a supernatural power, the ability to make something happen in the universe, an affirmation. Often, axé manifests as the ability to create certain outcomes with or through one's own milieu, the ability to express or affirm a commitment to "it will be what it will be" that lies in the power of the city.

It is Mari's axé that is at the center of her journey through life, through the city, and to spiritual community at her godmother's house. Mari is a Black Brazilian woman in her forties who works as a domestic worker and lives, like many Brazilian families, in a space added above her childhood home with her two children. On this day, she boards the Axé bus to make the long journey to her reading.

When Mari exits the bus, she is grateful to be free of the weight and heat of the people pressed so intimately against each other. She makes the relatively short walk from the bus stop to the gate of her godmother. When Mari arrives, she is greeted by the young children who reside at or near the *terreiro* (spiritual temple) and have a deep respect and love for her godmother. Mari spiritually and physically cleans herself off by wiping herself with the mixture of water, herbs, and perfume sitting at the gate, removing all the energy that was encountered on her journey, and then walks inside the temple.

Mari enters the terreiro and kisses her godmother on both cheeks. Mãe Canela, as a priest in Candomblé tradition, figures prominently in the anthropology of Salvador da Bahia, Brazil (Landes 1994), which has focused on the great power that women hold, especially spiritually in the terreiros that have been refuges for the care, protection, and strength needed to live in a city riddled with inequality (Harding 2000; Matory 2009). It is everyday Soteropolitanos, like Mari, who use the wealth of their traditions to promote their healing through herbs, cleansings, rituals, consults with the divine, and partnering spiritual knowledge with other medical knowledge. In this way, they address the ailments that manifest physically but have deeper and larger ramifications for each person and each community. In the traditional manner, Mari salutes Mãe Canela to honor her power in the tradition, the world, and specifically in her life. Afterward, they embrace, gaze into each other's eyes, and hug again. They have known each other for most of Mari's life, and they have found a special kinship with each other.

"How have you been?" Mãe Canela says.

Mari's eyes begin to water as she opens her mouth to speak and then breathes out heavily. Mãe Canela embraces Mari with one arm and with her other motions for her daughter to get water for her. Seamlessly, she guides Mari to a chair to sit down.

"Sit here, rest awhile, and when you're ready we'll go in the back."

"Okay," Mari releases.

"Did you eat anything today?"

Mari shakes her head no. A few minutes later, a bowl to wash her hands in appears in front of her. Then, a typical Brazilian lunch is served: a plate of black beans, rice, salad, farofa (golden ground cassava or yuca flour) with *pimenta* (a pepper sauce). Given that Mari is tired, she is provided with extra, and it is spiritually significant food. There was a festival yesterday, so that means there is a special meal. They serve her *acarajé*, a Candomblé classic sold around the city. They present a black-eyed pea fritter fried in palm oil that is served with *caruru*, which is a shrimp dish made with onion, okra, toasted nuts, and palm oil. On the side is *vatapá*, a delicious paste accompaniment made of coconut milk, palm oil, ground peanuts, dried seafood, cashews, chiles, onions, and tomatoes. To wash it down, Mari reaches for a glass of fresh *cajú*, or cashew fruit juice. After she has eaten, Mari stands and approaches the divining room, where Mãe Canela waits for her to do the divination.

As the shells fall, Mãe Canela silently makes a face. She looks up at Mari and asks a few questions about her health and recent visit to the doctor. They briefly exchange information for clarity, and Mari details her diabetes diagnosis.

"Your health is very vulnerable right now, and the spirits want you to know your health is draining from your body as a way to get your attention. Do you know that, my love?"

"No, but I do now. This is the second message about it I have received today."

"What was the first one?"

"I was visited in a dream by my great-great-grandmother Isabella. She spoke to me about healing and what I needed to do."

"That's exactly what they are saying you need. This is confirmation of what Isabella said. The *orixás* are also saying that to heal, you must connect with your ancestors. The *orixás* want you to treat yourself and occupy the world as if you were a wealthy white man," Mãe Canela tells her, referring to the knowledge from the divinities that guide, protect, and live with Candomblé practitioners.

"Use the privileges that these men have in society as a way to cater to yourself and to define how you allow others to treat you."

"How am I supposed to do that? A wealthy white man working as a domestic?" Mari replies.

"This is a part of major life changes needed for your own healing. The diabetes diagnosis is a function of a larger imbalance in your life. To achieve the healing you need, the spirits are encouraging you to connect with your direct ancestors. This is part of a more complete healing that is in addition to the healing needed to address the diabetes. They said this will settle the issues that the diabetes is causing in your life and rebalance what is going on with you spiritually. Your life and your path will smooth out greatly."

"It all feels overwhelming, like another responsibility, obligation to fulfill," Mari says.

"Along with me, they are here to assist and protect you on this journey of life. And they want the best for you, but also they want you to want the best for yourself as well, sweetness. Don't forget, let your ancestors help you heal, love; we are all here for you."

After Mari leaves Mãe Canela's house, tears stream down her face during the commute home. Although the message was hopeful and Mãe Canela worked to present it positively, Mari is emotional thinking about the imbalances in her life. Washing over her are all the feelings tied to a life of disease, the work of healing, and the depression Mari is experiencing from it all.

In the days that follow her time with Mãe Canela, Mari feels the highs and lows, with her blood sugar seemingly mirroring her mood. She reflects on the guidance Mãe Canela communicated to her and the mutual constitution and collaboration with spirit that their collective work introduced – such "communal production of healing in rituals relies on notions of self, body, and illness that seem radically different from the tenets of biomedicine" (Forde 2021). What does life look like from here? How can Mari find a way to overcome the experience of depression that accompanied her diabetes diagnosis? Mari is also wondering about the spiritual experience of imbalance that is showing up in her life. How will Mari's journey with spirituality place her closer to the healing that she needs to address the diabetes and other sources of disease in her life?

LIVING WITH "D(IABETE)S" AND SEEKING HEALING THROUGH ANCESTRAL KNOWLEDGE

Weeks later, Mari arrives home exhausted from cooking, cleaning, and caring for the people who provide the menial sustenance for her life. Amid her devotion to their lives, Mari neglects her own health. Mari knows this yet feels that her behavior is informed by deep patterns that go beyond the circumstances of her life, perhaps to an ancestral level. As Mari begins to connect ancestrally, she becomes more aware that the patterns and circumstances feel informed by a history of people who have had to make similar choices. She realizes that behaviors are learned and confirmed by society's animation of cycles that extend beyond herself, which Mari believes is the reason that spirit is requiring a life overhaul. On this night, Mari's best friend, Rita, calls her to see how she's doing.

"Hey, Mari, how are you doing?"

"Girl, I'm so tired, and I'm here dealing with the Ds."

"You're so funny, what are the Ds?"

"Diabetes, depression, devastation, disease, despair, and doubt."

"I'm so sorry to hear that, my dear friend. And I'm here for you through it all, and I hope you remember that you also have some other Ds that will be helpful to you as well."

"Which ones, Rita?"

"You know, divinity, devotion, determination, and don't forget your love of dance and getting dressed up."

"Thank you for saying that. How about we go dancing next weekend?"

"Sounds good. I'll let you go; I know you're tired from your long day, but love you."

"Love you too, goodnight."

Mari ends the call and reflects on the reminder from her best friend, which is the third confirmation that she must connect with others to heal, after the ones from Isabella and Mãe Canela. Mari is connected to family, community, networks, and the divine in this work that is uniquely Mari's, but also work that extends beyond Mari, as Isabella has reminded her. She realizes it is the maternal line and the women around her in her life who are leading her in the work of healing. This healing is a purposeful path in life that is critical not only to Mari's immediate survival through her – until recently, undiagnosed – diabetes, but also for a deeper, ancestral healing. Often the project of healing, drawn from Candomblé strategies, attends to a historical landscape of suffering and specific tools for healing that penetrate biomedical disease yet permeate the socio-cultural forces that structure disease. Therefore, the cultural tools of healing, the methodology of healing, and the impact of healing have certain targets that make an understanding of health in relationship to healing complex.

Mari's process of navigating through the diabetes diagnosis leads her to pursue a form of healing that engages her in a knowledge and wisdom far beyond diabetes. Mari devotes herself to learning Isabella's story by piecing together information from other family members, dreams, and consultations with spirit. Although healing is a part of the process of experiencing illness, Mari finds this level of healing to be far deeper than any treatment plan.

Mari discovers that Isabella was born in 1910 in the interior of Minas Gerais, a state just south of Bahia, to a family who worked in the sugar cane fields. Born to a poor family, only one generation after the official end of slavery in Brazil in 1888, she experienced great suffering through poverty, hunger, family violence, and violence toward families of a certain color (Telles 2014). Mari discovers that Isabella left Minas Gerais after marrying and came to Bahia, where her descendants settled.

Mari speaks with her grandmother about the few memories she has of Isabella. She learns of her premature death to illness, which left a fracture in the line of women who would follow her, searching for meaning and belonging in the loss, a deep need for healing in the mixture of grief and disease. Mari is discovering that ancestral healing means "reclaim[ing her] ancestor's resilience, and fortify[ing her] spirit so

[she] can do this work of healing. What we consider hereditary is, in fact, an inherited ancestral spiritual contract, and until we begin the work of ancestral healing, the agreement continues to exist inside our bodies. A spiritual inheritance or hereditary physical response offers us an opportunity to heal beyond ourselves, healing lineages" (Rose 2022).

This journey of ancestral healing is greater work than Mari ever imagined. Ancestral healing has been defined as "a type of spiritual healing that acknowledges that there are traces of trauma within the body that the person did not experience directly but were passed down or inherited (epigenetics). Acknowledging that you have traces of trauma that are not yours, your body can identify what is yours and what is not. The actual healing requires acknowledgment, intention to heal, and moving of the energy. It is a process in which you connect to an ancestor that experienced the trauma directly and you agree to be the living nexus to release this trauma for them and for yourself" (Martinez 2023). This form of healing also requires an openness and a presence to the pain, a witness to what happened, in order to imagine the possibility of what can be beyond the pain.

Brazil has been and remains a global force in the production of sugar. Sugar has often been a defining component of the economy of Brazil and was connected to the exploitation of the labor of the formerly enslaved and the stealing of land from those living in Brazil before colonial dominance. In Brazil's often devastating and prosperous history with sugar, we find that this global relationship to sugar has made its way inside the bodies and beings of those most vulnerable to the consequences of this history with sugar. Mari is not alone in navigating the consequences of diabetes in her forties: nearly one fourth of Brazilians will face diabetes as a chronic illness, and some, unfortunately, will suffer to the end from the fatal consequences of the illness (Bracco et al. 2021). Mari's connection, as a low-wage earner, deep-brown-skinned Black Brazilian woman in her forties, to diabetes reflects an entanglement with the cash crops of the nation. Anthropologists have long argued that flesh and bodies are related to Brazil's colonial history of sweet power, which was solidified through the bloody process of producing sugar (Johnson 2017; Mintz 1986; Spillers 1987; Weheylie and Wynter 2009). While Brazil produced sugar, its legacy seeped through as the sugar in the blood of those who turned sugar into gold for the nation.

For Mari, the transformative power of sugar ignites a deeper spiritual transformation that allows her to trace her family's history with sugar and suffering that marks her body and sears her flesh. The concept of ancestral healing shines a light on the urgency for Mari to recognize her intergenerational suffering and to move toward healing. However, ancestral healing is not unidirectional, meaning the healing is not just for Mari but also for Isabella and all those in between as well. The work of ancestral healing is, similarly, a method for engaging with epigenetic research in the spiritual dimension. Mari helps us to explore the spirituality of sickness relevant to diabetes in Salvador, Brazil. One can be healthy according to the measures of health as assigned by external sources; however, the ancestral healing that Mari undergoes can reach deeper than one's own trauma, imbalances, or disease. The kind of ancestral healing that Mari's guiding spiritual forces are leading her to is deeper than the treatment, management, or even the possibility of eliminating diabetes.

For many of those in Salvador like Mari, dealing with diabetes and co-occurring depression is a project of exorcising the history, legacies, and colliding forces of state formation alongside capitalism, among other forces, which involve people making through race and gender. These experiences are also closely tied to the construction of health through state-based health systems, necropolitics (Mbembe, 2020), and other forces. As the prevalence of diabetes spreads across Brazil, so too does the impact of the loss of years and quality of life and the forces that have made diabetes the projected third-leading cause of death in Brazil (Duncan et.al 2020).

Mari's experience with her *mãe-de-santo* is a demonstration of a spiritual, personal, political triad of health (Scheper-Hughes and Lock 1987). The connections of the spiritual world mirror the physical world in different aspects such as through the disruptions, discontinuities, and diseases in the world. By looking into the life of Mari, we find that the spirit is not exempt from the wounding that the flesh endures, being imprinted by the causalities and calamities of Brazilian society. The complexities of healing for people like Mari often involve deep spiritual transformation. Such transformation translates to one's mind, prompting reconfigurations at the level of self, spilling over onto the body, which incorporates the words of Mãe Canela to Mari to reconstitute the self for healing and repair.[1]

THE LIFE-LONG JOURNEY OF HEALING

Years later, when we visit Mari in her home in Salvador, we witness the process and practice of ancestral healing that has been critical to her journey of health and healing. Mari looks more vibrant than before, and when we sit down, we discover the reasons for the change. Mari has accepted and surrendered to the treatment of diabetes. Mari has a clarity about what it means to currently have diabetes and co-occurring depression and how to manage them. For her, the journey of healing looked like asking for what she needs. Mari was able to request, as a part of her wage, time to eat the healthier foods that she prepares for the family she works with. Moreover, Mari now walks with the eldest member of the family as exercise and has encouraged her family to have an exercise routine three times a week at home. However, Mari attributes the biggest change to her connection to Isabella.

Mari has devoted herself to ancestor reverence as a part of her healing, developing connections through dreams, feedings, learning family history, and visiting the lands where her family lived several generations ago. Mari has discovered that Isabella also had to navigate her own path to healing, although she did not have the same access to health care in the 1900s in the interior of the country. Changes through migration, changes in cultural patterns and practices, increased access to processed foods, and the absence of physical activities, along with the multiplicity of ways that suffering functions, affected not only Isabella but also Mari. Mari has determined that connection to Indigenous ways of knowing and pathways to a divine source, in addition to her direct ancestors, are important.

Mari's pathway to healing is as diverse and complex as the diabetes in one's body, which invades each system in a unique way that makes healing just as diverse. As Mari creates a daily practice of communing with the spirits of her ancestors, she develops a special connection with her great-great-grandmother, Isabella. Mari's notebook near the altar is a record of their connection. During the visit, Mari details the most recent encounter with Isabella.

> I was up late one night doing Julianna's hair. It was super hot.
> We were almost finished, and suddenly, the curtains blew and
> there was a cool breeze. I knew that she was here; I could feel her

energy. Immediately, I got up and began preparing myself with the rituals I normally do to receive Isabella and record what she is saying. I told Julianna to go get her grandmother, Ana, from downstairs and her older sister, Gabriela, from the other room. This was the first time I was able to show Julianna and Gabriela how to recognize, acknowledge, and receive the presence of the ancestors. Similarly, it was important for my daughters to understand what healing looks like for me and to understand the ancestors' role in this deep healing, for which I have been chosen.

As Mari seeks to heal and treat her diabetes, she uncovers a healing that is far greater than the doctor's orders of dietary and lifestyle changes, blood sugar monitoring, and medications through the interconnectedness of her life's story with that of her great-great-grandmother. By seeking out the life story of Isabella through others in her family and through spiritual methodologies, her devotion to the management and treatment of her diabetes becomes a spiritual practice that is connected to a larger project of healing for herself, her family, and her community. Mari discovers that her wellness, her health, and her relationship to sugar is far beyond the diagnosis she receives and is generative to a healing that is ancestral.

Mari's story of healing is distinct and prominent but, sadly, not uncommon for many people in Salvador who are navigating diabetes and other chronic noncommunicable diseases. Through interviews with Black women navigating a wealth of change in the city related to nutrition, lifestyle, and health, and through living among them, storytelling, photo elicitation, and other methods of data collection, it became apparent that the effort to address the illness, which is more prevalent each year, is a larger project than just disease treatment and management or health promotion. Through healing work, the deep excavation of the sources of sickness that might be sociocultural, historical, political, biological, or spiritual, they are seeking to address an illness in ways that exceed what biomedicine details. Therefore, the instruments, the rituals, and the outputs of healing often defy the principles of biomedicine as they seek to address the broader causes of suffering through work on the self, the body, and illness.

NOTE

1 Rebecca Seligman (2010) has detailed how Candomblé practitioners have utilized cultural tools and the dynamics of embodied forms of self-healing, which "in both cognitive and bodily processes of incoherence, ameliorate distress, and create positive looping effects that allow selves to recohere" and other healing transformations that "contribute to the construction, deconstruction, and repair of selves." Moreover, Maarit Forde's (2021) work highlights the complexity of traditions like Candomblé: "The commodification and racialization of bodies, various forced and voluntary migrations, and the development of plantation capitalism have produced culturally specific forms of suffering and healing."

REFERENCES

Bracco, P. A., E. W. Gregg, D. B. Rolka, M. I. Schmidt, S. M. Barreto, P. A. Lotufo, and B. B. Duncan. 2021. "Lifetime Risk of Developing Diabetes and Years of Life Lost Among Those with Diabetes in Brazil." *Journal of Global Health* 11.

Duncan, B. B., E. Cousin, M. Naghavi, et al. 2020. Supplement, "The Burden of Diabetes and Hyperglycemia in Brazil: A Global Burden of Disease Study 2017." *Population Health Metrics* 18, no. S1: 9.

Forde, Maarit. 2021. "Afro-Atlantic Healing Practices." In *The Routledge Handbook of Religion, Medicine, and Health,* 13–26. New York: Routledge.

Harding, Rachel E. 2003. *A Refuge in Thunder: Candomblé and Alternative Spaces of Blackness.* Bloomington: Indiana University Press.

Johnson, James. 2017. "Being and Becoming Human: Weheliye's Radical Emancipation Theory and the Flesh and Body of Black Studies." *The Earlham Historical Journal* 9 (2): 24–66.

Landes, Ruth. 1994. *The City of Women.* Albuquerque: University of New Mexico Press.

Martinez, Claudya. 2023. "Ancestral Healing Wasn't What I Thought It Would Be: #WeAllGrow Latina." WeAllGrow Latina. December 20, 2023. https:// www.weallgrowlatina.com/ancestral-healing/#:~:text=What%20is%20 Ancestral%20Healing%3F,down%20or%20inherited%20(epigenetics).

Matory, J. Lorand. 2009. *Black Atlantic Religion: Tradition, Transnationalism, and Matriarchy in the Afro-Brazilian Candomblé.* Princeton, NJ: Princeton University Press.

Mbembe, Achille. 2020. *Necropolitics.* Durham: Duke University Press.

Mintz, Sidney W. 1986. *Sweetness and Power: The Place of Sugar in Modern History.* New York: Penguin Books.

Rose, Karen M. 2022. *The Art & Practice of Spiritual Herbalism: Transform, Heal & Remember with the Power of Plants and Ancestral Medicine.* Beverly, MA: Fair Winds Press.

Smith-Morris, C. 2008. *Diabetes Among the Pima: Stories of Survival.* Tucson: University of Arizona Press.

Scheper-Hughes, Nancy, and Margaret M. Lock. 1987. "The Mindful Body: A Prolegomenon to Future Work in Medical Anthropology." *Medical Anthropology Quarterly* 1 (1): 6–41.

Seligman, Rebecca. 2010. "The Unmaking and Making of Self: Embodied Suffering and Mind–Body Healing in Brazilian Candomblé." *Ethos* 38 (3): 297–320.

Spillers, Hortense J. 1987. "Mama's Baby, Papa's Maybe: An American Grammar Book." *Diacritics* 17 (2): 64–81.

Weheliye, Alexander G. 2014. "Introduction: Black Studies and Black Life." *The Black Scholar* 44 (2): 5–10.

Telles, Edward E. 2014. *Race in Another America: The Significance of Skin Color in Brazil.* Princeton, NJ: Princeton University Press.

Wynter, Sylvia. 2003. "Unsettling the Coloniality of Being/Power/Truth/Freedom: Towards the Human, After Man, Its Overrepresentation – An Argument." *CR: The New Centennial Review* 3 (3): 257–337.

Diabetes *Always* Reflects Social Structures

Manuela, *a resilient immigrant mother from Mexico, forges a powerful friendship with researcher **Alyshia** as they navigate the intertwined challenges of motherhood, diabetes, and loss.*

Bà Son *transitions from a wealthy upbringing to navigating hardship and resilience, highlighting battles with diabetes and the evolving caregiver role of husband, Ông Năng, illuminating love's transformative power amid adversity.*

Pastor Rollins *emphasizes the necessity of community expertise in addressing health disparities, advocating for a supportive leadership approach within the church.*

Merlene *passionately champions culturally relevant diabetes education in the African American community, drawing from Caribbean heritage to bridge gaps in health awareness and traditional food practices.*

Tommey *underscores the Kinaaldá ceremony's significance in Diné culture as a vital connection between health, land, and ancestral teachings, advocating for the reclamation of identity and food sovereignty in the face of rising diabetes rates.*

Jesse *reflects on the Tohono O'odham community, revealing the transformative power of reclaiming ancestral food systems and cultural identity as essential steps in combating diabetes and fostering collective resilience.*

Social contexts create varying levels of risk for individuals based on cultural, embodied, and personal factors that reflect structural inequalities. A structural focus examines interlocking systems – economic, legal, educational, environmental, and health care – that marginalize communities. Inequalities compound when individuals experience multiple forms of difference, underscoring the need for an intersectional lens. Diabetes often emerges through disrupted relationality caused by migration, hunger, and economic marginalization. Racial capitalism provides a framework across these chapters for understanding diabetes risk, showing how historical and economic exploitation perpetuate health inequalities. For Indigenous communities like those of Tommey and Jesse, settler colonialism's lasting impact on land sovereignty, cultural knowledge, and health underscores the need for decolonization efforts.

Critical anthropology challenges individualized behavioral interventions, advocating for relational and structural health dimensions. As you read these chapters, keep these questions in mind: How do individuals and communities assess their circumstances to address structural inequalities? What steps can foster meaningful change in health practices? How might critical anthropology inform public health strategies to improve diabetes management and tackle broader structural issues?

CHAPTER SIX

Friends Can Heal Pain in the Midst of Trauma: Manuela's and Alyshia's Story

Manuela Fuentes and Alyshia Gálvez

Manuela was sitting on a piano bench in a second-floor meeting room at St. Jerome Church when Alyshia entered the room. She had just turned into the church from Alexander Avenue in the Mott Haven section of the South Bronx. It was 2002, and we were both attending a meeting of the Comité Guadalupano, a group of parishioners at the church who gathered to plan events around devotion to Our Lady of Guadalupe. It was both a religious group and a location for activism and information sharing for recently arrived immigrants. Most of the attendees were from Mexico, including Manuela. Father John Grange, the parish priest and child of Irish immigrants, had himself grown up in this parish and invited Alyshia to the meeting. Alyshia was visiting various Comités Guadalupanos in the Bronx, interested in them for her doctoral research as sites for immigrant rights activism and advocacy. Manuela carried her ten-month-old daughter, Lesslie, on her chest in a carrier. Alyshia smiled at this young woman and thought about her year-old son, Lázaro, who she had left at home but would be with her next time.

When Manuela migrated to the United States in 1997, she joined her partner in New York. Her partner, Saúl, had migrated two years earlier and sent funds so Manuela could pay for someone to transport her across the border and to New York City. In some ways, this was not unlike when Manuela's mother married her father and joined him in his community. These types of residential patterns are common in their community: typically, when a woman and a man partner, she leaves her natal family and moves in with her partner and his parents. A daughter-in-law does much of the domestic labor (cooking, cleaning, child and elder care) in her partner's natal family's home, while her ability to care for her natal family becomes contingent on whether her partner and his family are "kind" and "understanding." Some women never return to the community or family where they were born. Returning can even be seen as a "failure." Sometimes daughters-in-law are threatened with being "returned" to their parents if their marriage or their fulfillment of their duties as a wife fails. Yet, in Manuela's case, she had found a strong partner in Saúl.

"I remember that I came home and told Saúl," Manuela recalled as she reminisced about first meeting Alyshia. "I told him, 'Today we met a young woman who arrived [at church],' and [I referred to you as] 'a white girl.' I said, 'A white girl came and was listening to us there.' And I laughed because I told him, 'I don't know what she was doing sitting there; she must be thinking, "These people are really crazy … Talking about this." And I told him, 'I didn't really understand what she's studying, but hey, she was there observing us.' From there, I remember that you called to ask me for an interview, and suddenly, I don't know, I saw something in you. Your spirit radiates compassion and honesty. But the best part is you have a humble heart, and you gave me confidence to talk because sometimes, like, one also closes off in our world, and you don't say what you're going through. Sometimes I thought to myself, 'Why is she going to be interested in what you're going through?' It made me laugh because I think that in the first interviews we were talking and talking, and I said to Saúl I never even imagined that we were going to become friends."

For more than twenty years, we have kept talking. Our conversations are typically three times longer than we intend them to be. We talk about research, parenting, food, health, birth, diabetes, loss, and illness, and have become ever more connected as friends. Although we met through research, our friendship encompasses many themes. Manuela's first pregnancy was difficult; she experienced gestational diabetes and other complications that made even undertaking a second pregnancy, as she did several years later, a risk. Alyshia was still processing her first pregnancy and delivery, which were, according to her doctors, "normal," but felt like a confusing loss of autonomy and a damaging experience. We shared about our second pregnancies and births, breastfeeding, health scares, parenting debates, public school and college admissions, developmental and emotional crises, and our fears about our kids as they moved through the world before and during a pandemic.

"I said to him," Manuela continued relaying to Alyshia, "'She is from another world.' I didn't even know where you were from. But, I told him, 'Her world is different from mine.' I also felt like the English barrier separated us, in terms of the fact that I couldn't live alongside you. Then I saw that you were trying to get closer [to me], and I said to Saúl, 'I feel bad.' Yes, I did kind of reject you, right? I rejected you because I said, 'No, she can't. We can't be in the same world or in the same circle because they are different worlds.' But, in the end, I realized that I identified with you because of the human qualities you have. Even Saúl has identified this in you. He says, 'You are both kind-hearted. You both are always trying to help people. You have a heart.' He always says we have a chicken heart [*corazón de gallina*, or soft-hearted]. I feel like it brought us together, like we both have something in common."

Over the course of our friendship, we have supported one another in many losses, too. Our mutual friend Father Grange, who introduced us to each other, died, and we mourned together (Gálvez 2013). Manuela's mother became ill with diabetes and kidney failure and later died due to these conditions in 2016. Six years later, Alyshia's mother became ill and died from a different set of chronic health conditions framed by her doctors as "diet related." All three died, and the anniversaries of their deaths fall in a sequence of three consecutive days in the third week of October. Each year we console each other through these losses that had reverberating effects on our own mental health, physical well-being, and parenting. These experiences have sparked new conversations about where pain goes through time.

When we think about pain, we often think about pain relief. A pill or a hot compress for a headache. A disinfectant and a bandage for a surface wound. A hot tea with honey and lemon for a sore throat. Yet, what about pain that lingers in the mind and body and does not leave? What about pain that is not specific to a single part of the body but rather generalized to a condition or an experience of life? Or pain

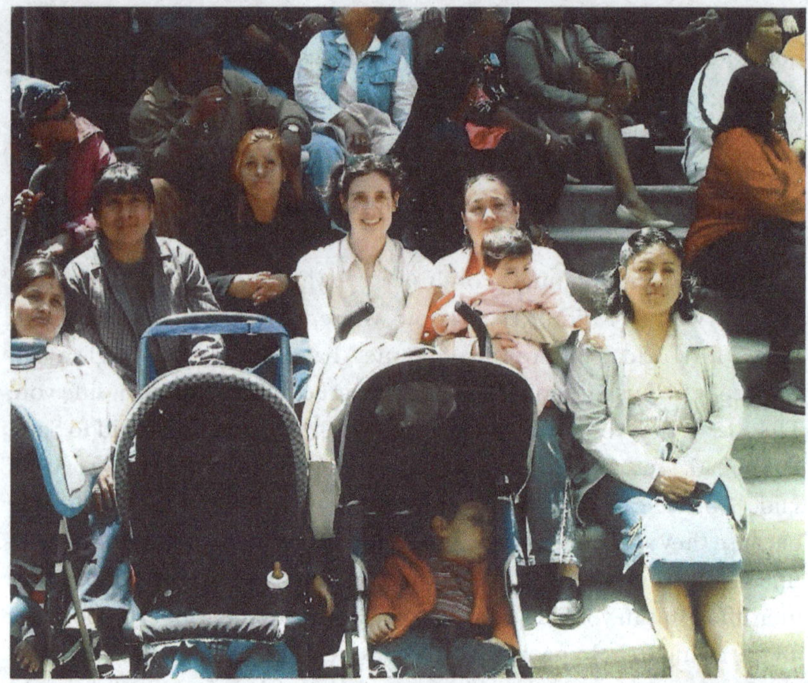

Figure 6.1: Manuela and Alyshia with our children, along with other women and children, at a protest at City Hall in Lower Manhattan, 2003

that comes from a single traumatic experience but winds up marking life into "before" and "after"? How does pain move in and take up residence in our bodies? How do our bodies and minds cope with time and distance, with the trauma of loss and migration?

Manuela helped frame Alyshia's second book, which focused on the experiences of immigrant women from Mexico navigating New York City's public health-care system. That book involved women's experiences in clinical settings as well as knowledge we were told by our mothers and mothers- and sisters-in-law, and how we navigated the differences between them. These conversations moved us toward discussions around diabetes and its complications. Manuela's difficult experience with gestational diabetes and her mother's worsening illness, and eventual passing due to complications from diabetes, have framed these conversations in deep and meaningful ways.

Alyshia said during one of our many conversations, "I remember that you said that one reason why you feel that you got diabetes during your pregnancies was the separation from your mother. Like with the trauma, and I remember that [Father Zarate, the priest in Mexico] –"

Manuela responded, "Oh yes, I saw him in an interview … right?"

"Yes." Alyshia nodded. "He said the same thing," she continued. "He said that diabetes is the disease of migrants because they live separated from their families. That was already nine years ago, when we recorded [those interviews] with you and the priest. I don't know why I'm forgetting the priest's name. He also passed away."

Surprised, Manuela responded, "Oh, he already passed away?"

"Mm-hmm," Alyshia confirmed. "But, at that moment, I heard it, and I sort of stood quiet; it was so new." Alyshia paused and thought about that moment. "That idea. I mean, I had never heard anyone say that other than you. And now the connection between diabetes [and trauma], specifically, is becoming more understood. Many diseases, but diabetes specifically as a disease that has a lot to do with stress, with depression, with trauma."

Understanding these complex relationships between migration and health became central to our conversations. We talked about how the food system Manuela grew up with in her hometown of San Antonio Texcala differed from what we could access in our supermarkets, corner stores, and farmers' markets in the Bronx and Manhattan. We shared ingredients, recipes, and ideas about where to get good tortillas or nopales locally. Manuela taught Alyshia to make memelas, also known as picaditas. But Alyshia's sons still think Manuela's memelas are best. Alyshia traveled with her family to visit Manuela's mother and siblings in Mexico, eating the food Manuela talked about missing and bringing back photos and information about how her mother was doing.

Manuela was a powerful voice not only in Alyshia's research but also her experience as a young mother. Returning to address the link between trauma and diabetes, Manuela said, "Yes, because I have verified it. Once, I had a problem. I was pregnant with [my son]. I wanted to have breakfast and because of that sadness from the problem, that anger, my sugar rose – so high and without eating anything. [Other times,] if I ate before, and sometimes that happened to me, like I indulged, and my sugar didn't go up to 200. I never raised it; my sugar was supposed to be below 120 when pregnant, with food. For a long time, it went up to 140 and with that anger, that sadness, and I couldn't tell anyone. I felt like I was exploding, and I checked my sugar, and I hadn't even had breakfast. So, I say … I feel that it is also our emotions that cause [diabetes]."

Although Alyshia was able to visit Mexico and sit at Manuela's mother's table, Manuela couldn't be there. Because of Manuela's immigration status, she remained far from her mother for the rest of her life. Alyshia flew with Manuela's son to visit his grandparents because Manuela could not cross the border. We still enjoy reminiscing about the trip. We laughed as Alyshia relayed how Manuela's three-year-old asked her for yogurt on the plane. We cried when we shared Manuela's heartbreak: the trip was the first and last time her son would meet his grandmother.

"And your mom?" Alyshia asked one afternoon in October 2023. We had sat down together to have, for the first time, a conversation about our conversations. "What do you think was the cause? In other words, if you had to put a date where … her life or her health changed."

Manuela replied, "It was when my dad died. She went into a depression. She didn't know what was happening; that's why. We didn't even know. She probably felt sad. But she was also from another town. Her town is big now, but she lived in the mountains, and there they didn't have what we had. She also didn't know the customs of our town. Our town, my dad's hometown, was closer to a city, so it had more urbanized customs. She said she grew up cooking with firewood, and she didn't know how to use a stove. So she was there, in my family, but her world was nothing more than our house. She didn't like to go out of the house. She didn't have friends. Just the family."[1]

Manuela understood that her parents' marriage had separated her mother from all she knew. Even though she was raised to understand her hometown as a more urbanized and even "better" place to live than her mother's hometown, she understood her mother dedicated years to her family as a stay-at-home mother and wife and was isolated from people and places she knew. When Manuela's father suddenly became severely ill due to leukemia and soon died, her mother became depressed. This, Manuela believed, was the triggering event for the onset of her mother's own health issues. Diabetes and kidney disease would, eventually, take her life.

Part of what made Manuela's mother suffer was the same thing that she herself had suffered from: her daughter had left her the same way she had left her own mother, the way daughters in their region are expected to leave their mothers. But the fact something is expected and normative does not mean it does not cause pain. After Manuela left for New York, her mother sought clues about how her daughter was doing. Many mothers worry about their daughters' well-being and safety when they leave home. She did not know Saúl well – he left when he was so young and when her daughter's relationship with him was young, too. Further, how would she keep an eye on her daughter all the way in New York? How would she know she was all right? The distance between mothers and daughters compounds anxieties about well-being. These are real traumas of separation and loss, not only due to death but also migration.

Moisés ("Moi"), Manuela's brother, has a visa and works as a *paquetero*, an informal courier, transporting goods back and forth between their hometown and the places where people from their hometown have migrated to: the South Bronx, as well as Illinois, New Jersey, and California. Moi's periodic trips to New York became fact-finding missions: their mother wanted to know if Manuela was okay. They talked on the phone all the time, but her mother feared that Manuela pretended to be okay on the phone when she was not. This is common practice for people who are trying to protect those they love: both those who have left and those who remain try to protect each other by pretending they are okay because they do not want to worry loved ones who are too far away to help.

Moi reported back: "Saúl is a kind and loving partner to Manuela. She's fine. She misses us, and life isn't easy there, but she's okay." Yet Manuela's mother knew this information was not enough, and it may not always be true.

When Manuela experienced gestational diabetes with both of her pregnancies, difficult births and post-partum recovery periods, Saúl received instructions for how to care for her and supplies from his mother-in-law and his own mother. No one thought this was a satisfactory substitution: both Manuela and her mother suffered. Manuela suffered not having her mother to take care of her and reassure her that she would get over feeling sad and broken by childbirth. Manuela's mother suffered not being able to be there in person for her daughter. Saúl suffered, trying to bridge the distance and fulfill both his mother-in-law's caretaking role and his own, caring for his babies, for Manuela, and trying to earn a living. Although Manuela and Saúl believe their own relationship was deepened by his willingness to care for her during their darkest days, it was still painful without her mother.

When Manuela's mother was ill, the situation was the same but inversed. Manuela wanted to be the one to take care of her mother. Blanca, Manuela's sister, who studied nursing, took their mother to her home in a nearby city, where she could more easily give her care and take her to her dialysis appointments. However, their mother was not happy leaving behind her home in their rural community, her plants, her birds, and her neighbors. She was depressed and beleaguered by the growing number of complications to her health. Manuela was frustrated because of the distance. She could send money for her mother's care (Saúl is indeed a kind and generous partner), but she could not hold her hand.

The cycle of pain, loss, and physical somatization of pain in the form of diabetes continued. Alyshia asked Manuela, "[When your dad died] ... your mom got depressed?"

Manuela nodded, "Mm-hmm."

"Alone, with three children?"

"My mom was always at home," Manuela responded. "So, I feel that that was the end for her. The depression was due to the fact she did not like going out. She liked being at home and was happy there. But with my father's loss, she entered a period of profound sadness. My father took care of everything. He was always such a doting husband. He took care of her, he loved her, and he wanted her to be happy and not worry about a thing. He was truly an excellent father and husband: loving, always taking care of his home and his family. I think that is truly beautiful.

"But he never realized that taking such good care of her left her not knowing how to take care of herself," Manuela continued. "She had to start from scratch, and it was very difficult for her to care for us alone. I think that was overwhelming for her: to play the roles of mother and father at the same time, to take care of us and guide us down a good path all alone. My brother, when he grew up, was a great support to her.

But that is why I have tried to be different, to be independent. I want to know how to do the things my husband does. He's a good husband and father. He loves us a lot. I want to learn and be prepared to be a support for my household because one never knows what the future holds."

Alyshia listened intently and mused, "Somehow, she survived. All that!"

Manuela smiled, remembering her mother's strength, "Yes."

"What an achievement!" Alyshia responded, remembering how difficult parenting can be, more so if your family is far away.

"Yes. So, I say that maybe if someone had been helping her, preparing her, giving her more information about her illness, like one receives here – someone prepared – she would have lasted more years," Manuela explained. "Giving her education about diabetes, [teaching] her to nourish herself, how to medicate herself. We all have the belief that if you give someone a medication, they will get dependent on it … But you also have to see that maintaining a healthy diet can help you, along with the medication. You can lower the doses. So, I don't know, I feel like that's what it was, the depression.

"And in reality," Manuela continued, "when an immigrant comes here – and I tell you [from experience], maybe I went through it and didn't feel it or didn't know. Now I know how to identify it. When you get here, you get depressed because you left your whole family, your customs. You arrive here and go out to the store, and they speak to you in English … It's curious. I don't know how it is in my town and other towns now. But do you know what custom we had? Our parents and grandparents taught us to have values, to be courteous. We would stop and see someone on the street and say, 'Hello, sister! Good morning. Sir or Ma'am, good morning. Good morning.' You come here and want to say hello, and no one pays attention to you. And you say 'How?' In other words, it's a radical change."

"And for your mom?" Alyshia questioned. "Do you think her life also changed when you came here?"

Manuela responded, "Yes, because it was a great sadness to not see me again. We never again could embrace. I can't imagine not being able to hug my children. I think I would go insane from the sadness. One falls into a profound depression. Our family members, I believe, if they love us, want to be with us. I think that this happens to all parents, spouses, children who stay behind in our communities, and it happens to those of us who have immigrated to the United States. We can suffer from terrible depression. It's like you know you're not going to see them for a long time.

"I don't know if it happened to you when you moved here," Manuela asked, looking at Alyshia. "But maybe some people will relate. But you battle to adapt, when you get here, with the sadness. You see the young people, you see their eyes. I tell Saúl, 'I look in their eyes, and you see the sadness they have because they are struggling.' That's the first year or two years that you spend battling with your sadness that you came here. I think that those that stay as well, the elders who stay behind, they suffer because you are not there, it is as if someone had died. You hope they're going to come back [eventually] … I mean, you say one year, two years, but you don't know …"

"And on the other hand, the person who is here may forget a little because they're making a life here," Alyshia interjected.

Manuela nodded. "They start working."

Alyshia affirmed, "Creating friendships, and you get used to it, and you get to know [the area] or have children. And the person there stays like that."

"They stay with pain and sadness," Manuela continued. "You know what I see, especially in single men and young people? That they come alone, without family, [and] fall into bad habits that are not healthy and can put their health at risk and harm their families. Someone in Mexico said to me once, 'There [in the United States] you all just go there and get sick and fall into bad habits,' and I answered that they don't know what one faces here: our sadness and how we fall into depression, our struggles with the language, with the food. The world you face here. And this makes me sad, they think that about those of us who are here because everyone who comes here passes through that painful situation.

"Sometimes I say we should make a group where we meet," Manuela added. "Because like the priest said, 'They just want someone to listen.' For example, we are here with family, and I say to Saúl, 'How was your day?' and he tells me [about it]. And sometimes I don't know, I have no idea [what he's talking about], but I'm listening. But people who come alone, are alone [here], what do they do? They don't have anyone to turn to. They don't eat well because they don't have time to cook. They have to work really hard to help the families they left behind.

[They say,] 'I'm going to eat fast food,' even though it's not healthy. We lose our foodways, that healthy diet we ate at home in our communities of origin. [They say,] 'Today, I'm just going to eat Maruchan [instant noodle soup] because I have to save money because the idea is to return home, right? So they eat the cheapest and quickest foods they can find."

Alyshia nodded reflectively. "And years [of their lives] pass like that."

Manuela agreed, "Mm-hmm." She continued her thought, "Then when we realize it, we are already sick. We didn't even know that we had a disease because we didn't eat well. Because we didn't take vitamins. Yes, that's what I've experienced in my own life, and I believe that it happens to many of us. I don't know, I call it a vicious system."

Alyshia confirmed, "Yes, it's all a cycle."

Manuela has been Alyshia's primary interlocutor in three books (Gálvez 2011; 2018; 2010) and many articles, but we have never before published together. Although our conversations reveal powerful interlocking dynamics of social and health conditions, we rarely use words like *syndemics, social determinants of health, disparities,* and *risk factors,* which are common in public health and anthropology. Yet the ideas behind these concepts have continuously been part of our conversations and in this way connect us to social science and medical understandings of diabetes research.

In her work on syndemics, Mendenhall, co-editor of this volume, has driven new understandings of the biosocial interaction between violence, immigration, diabetes, depression, and abuse – known as the *VIDDA* syndemic (Mendenhall 2012), building on prior literature on syndemics (Singer and Clair 2003; Singer 2009). She has also brought it into the mainstream of scholarly discussions, including a major special issue of the *Lancet* (Mendenhall et al. 2017; Weaver and Mendenhall 2014; Singer and Mendenhall 2022). Other authors in this volume and beyond use these concepts and further deepen our understanding of how diabetes cannot be understood only or even primarily as a disease of the endocrinological system (Hardin 2015; Kohrt and Carruth 2022; Carruth et al. 2019; Agudelo-Botero, Giraldo-Rodríguez, and Dávila-Cervantes 2022).

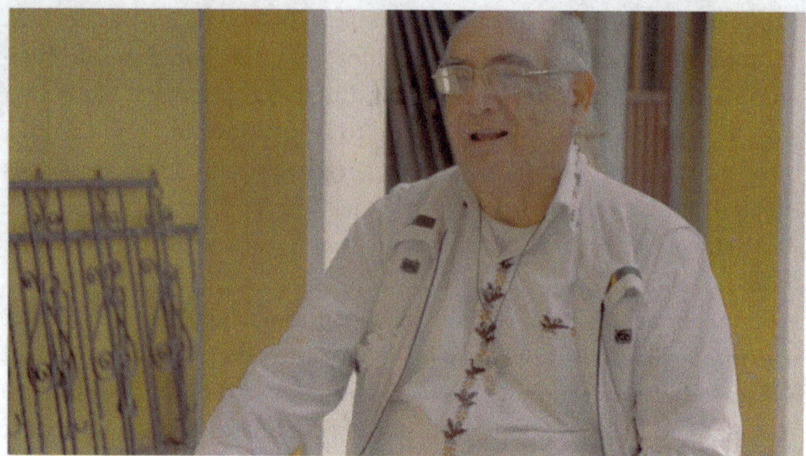

Figure 6.2: Father Gustavo Zarate, Malacatepec, Puebla, still from *¡Salud! Myths and Realities of Mexican Immigrant Health* (Schwittek 2017)

In 2023, we revisited conversations with Father Gustavo Zarate, known as the "pastor of the migrants." A Catholic priest from the state of Puebla, Mexico, Father Gus, at the behest of the Diocese of Puebla, initiated a pastoral project to serve migrants and their families. This involved a hotline that lonely migrants in the US could use to call and talk to someone if they were feeling homesick or depressed. He is someone who has come up in our conversations frequently over the years as an influential force of good in the migrant community in the Bronx.

Both Father Gus and Father Grange, the priest who introduced us, are part of a broader web of interlocutors with whom we have engaged in discussions on these topics. Father Gus said in an interview in a documentary that Manuela and Alyshia were involved in, directed by David Schwittek in 2015, that "Diabetes is the disease of the migrant." He paused for a moment. "Not just because migrants change the way they eat, but because it is the somatization of pain, trauma, and depression" (Schwittek and Gálvez 2017). It is possible that Father Gus read Mendenhall's work, but it is also possible that he arrived at this conclusion through his own interactions with migrant families, witnessing the way pain moves from heart and soul to body and back again, wreaking havoc in its wake. In similar ways, Manuela has witnessed this, too, in her own lived experiences with her own health and her mother's.

We have been in conversation now for two decades, but we do not have the answers to these extraordinary challenges. We do not have a cure or a solution or a remedy for grief or diabetes. We know that people say a hot compress or lemon-and-honey tea may help with a headache or a sore throat. Yet there is no simple solution for the lasting physical effects of the pain of trauma. There is no treatment for the pain one feels deeply within the heart and soul due to migration and family separation, particularly among those who cross borders and cannot return home. Unresolved pain and trauma have a way of moving across generations and borders, seeping into the bodies and hearts of those who have witnessed the trauma of their loved ones. This means that even those who have not directly suffered feel pain through their association.

One thing we know for sure because of our decades of collaboration is this: we can support and soothe each other. Friendship has healing powers. Talking through these ideas over the years and supporting each other in good times and bad has made our own lives better, and we hope our story can shape others.

Knowledge comes from all sides. In our case, it is constantly flowing within and between our work, movements, and intergenerational knowledge that we share, discuss, and write about, now in this chapter, together. Rural communities, Manuela has emphasized, have more knowledge than they are usually given credit for. People produce valuable goods, cultural productions, and wisdom. They maintain the well-being of communities, water, and land with little support or thanks. Through her writing and activism, Alyshia strives to make sure that her role as an academic writer and educator serves Manuela's community and beyond by urging that communities like hers be given greater respect, consideration, and resources. In the meantime, we are keeping each other company and working against the harmful effects of intergenerational trauma by building our love and respect for one another and our friendship.

NOTE

1 The authors met in Central Park in October 2023, and like so many of our conversations in the past, we started with a list of questions as a prompt for

getting started but did not follow them rigidly or in order. We recorded using a cell phone voice memo app and then uploaded the audio to Otter. ai transcription software for a Spanish-language transcription. The initial translation to English was done with Google Translate, but then both authors revised the English and Spanish versions on a shared document until we were confident they were accurate.

REFERENCES

Agudelo-Botero, Marcela, Liliana Giraldo-Rodríguez, and Claudio A. Dávila-Cervantes. 2022. "Type 2 Diabetes and Depressive Symptoms in the Adult Population in Mexico: A Syndemic Approach Based on National Health and Nutrition Survey." *BMC Public Health* 22 (1): 1–10.

Carruth, Lauren, Sarah Chard, Heather A. Howard, Lenore Manderson, Emily Mendenhall, Emily Vasquez, and Emily Yates-Doerr. 2019. "Disaggregating Diabetes: New Subtypes, Causes, and Care." *UMBC Faculty Collection.*

Gálvez, Alyshia. 2010. *Guadalupe in New York: Devotion and the Struggle for Citizenship Rights among Mexican Immigrants.* NYU Press.

———. 2011. *Patient Citizens, Immigrant Mothers: Mexican Women, Public Prenatal Care, and the Birth Weight Paradox.* Rutgers University Press.

———. 2013. "Padre John Grange: Un Ejemplo Ecuménico." *El Diario NY,* November 13, 2013. https://eldiariony.com/2013/11/13/padre-john-grange-un-ejemplo-ecumenico/.

———. 2018. *Eating NAFTA: Trade, Food Policies, and the Destruction of Mexico.* University of California Press.

Hardin, Jessica. 2015. "Everyday Translation: Health Practitioners' Perspectives on Obesity and Metabolic Disorders in Samoa." *Critical Public Health* 25 (2): 125–38.

Mendenhall, Emily. 2012. *Syndemic Suffering: Social Distress, Depression, and Diabetes Among Mexican Immigrant Women.* Left Coast Press.

Singer, Merrill. 2009. *Introduction to Syndemics: A Critical Systems Approach to Public and Community Health.* John Wiley & Sons.

Singer, Merrill, and Scott Clair. 2003. "Syndemics and Public Health: Reconceptualizing Disease in Bio-Social Context." *Medical Anthropology Quarterly* 17 (4): 423–41.

Singer, Merrill, and Emily Mendenhall. 2022. "Syndemics in Global Health." In *A Companion to Medical Anthropology,* 126–44.

Schwittek, David. 2017. *Necesitando al Otro.* Accessed October 4, 2024. https://schwittek.com/special-projects/necesitando-al-otro.

———. 2021. *21 Trucks of San Antonio Texcala.* Accessed October 4, 2024. https://schwittek.com/special-projects/21-trucks-of-san-antonio-texcala.

Schwittek, David, and Alyshia Gálvez, dirs. 2017. *¡Salud! Myths and Realities of Mexican Immigrant Health.* Accessed October 4, 2024. https://filmfreeway.com/1314729.

Weaver, Lesley Jo, and Emily Mendenhall. 2014. "Applying Syndemics and Chronicity: Interpretations from Studies of Poverty, Depression, and Diabetes." *Medical Anthropology* 33 (2): 92–108. https://doi.org/10.1080/01459740.2013.808637

Socio-Somatic Generativity: A Life Story from Vietnam

Tine M. Gammeltoft and Dung Vũ

BÀ SON'S LIFE STORY, CHAPTER 1: COMING OF AGE IN AN ERA OF SOCIAL UPHEAVAL (1950–1972)

I was born in 1950, here in Peaceful Hamlet, Thái Bình Province, Vietnam.[1] My family used to be one of the wealthiest in our village. When I was a little girl, my parents told me about the wealth of our ancestors. We owned large stretches of land with abundant rice fields, manioc, sugarcane, banana trees, and maize. But we were considered landlords, so when the state carried out land reforms in 1954, we had to share our land and assets with others in the community. But we were still better off than most families in our village. At the time, most houses had mud walls and thatched roofs, but our house was built with solid wooden planks. We never experienced hunger like other people at the time. But our lives were simple, and we worked hard. What I remember most from the first years of my life is work. I was the eldest child in our family, so I had to help my parents, take care of my brother and my sister, and do household tasks such as cooking, grinding rice, pounding rice, and raising pigs. I also helped to cultivate the garden. In our garden, we had lots of herbs – coriander, mint, lemon balm, basil, peppermint, and bountiful jasmine shrubs, too. Since I was a little girl, I have cherished jasmine; it reminds me of my childhood home. That's why you see we still have potted jasmines in our garden to this day.

My grandfather, the father of my father, belonged to a Confucian family; he was a man of learning. He was also a revolutionary veteran (*lão thành cách mạng*). In 1945, during the literacy campaign (*bình dân học vụ*), he went from house to house, teaching people how to read and write. My father, too, was a kind and respected man. He served as an accountant at our commune cooperative. But it was due to my mother's income that we did not starve. At the time, trading was illegal, but my mother traded nevertheless to ensure we had food. Many people wanted to do the same, but it was difficult as they had no assets. We owned a bicycle, so my mother could travel far and wide to buy and sell. She sold bamboo flutes and peanuts and supplied rice to noodle makers. She also farmed the land, working in our agricultural cooperative (*hợp tác xã*).

When I was fifteen, I was offered a chance to attend a teachers training college. I passed the entry exams. But since no one in our family had joined the army yet, our commune leaders did not allow me to go. I had to stay to work in the cooperative. These were difficult years for our country. We were at war with the US. We lived between life and death. Here in Thái Bình, they threw only a few bombs, but our men had to go to the front, and we women at home had to take care of everything, the land, the production, the children. We worked hard every day. We did not have machines to help with farming like we have today; we did everything by hand. Sowing, transplanting, harvesting. Back then, life was hard, but there were not as many diseases as today. People died either due to the war or due to old age; they did not die from disease. Today people die due to disease.

BÀ SON'S LIFE STORY, CHAPTER 2: BUILDING A FAMILY (1972–2000)

At the age of twenty-two, I was encouraged to join the youth pioneers (*thanh niên xung phong*) to support our army. But my family did not want me to go, so my parents asked a matchmaker to find me a husband. If I was married, I would not have to go. The matchmaker introduced Năng and his family to my parents. Our parents agreed that we should marry. We had grown up in the same commune, but we did not know each other, and we did not get the chance to get to know each other like young people do today. I did not know him at all, but he knew who I was. He said he had noticed me for my beauty, my height, and my dresses. I was known as the rich and beautiful girl in our village, he said. In 1972, Năng was in the army along with our other young men. He came home for a twenty-day leave, and we got married during his leave. It was a simple, war-time wedding with few guests. I was so young at the time, and I did not think much about anything, I was clueless and naive (*ngẩn ngờ, dại khờ*). I had no idea about love; I just did not want to join the army. Our parents agreed, so we got married, and that was all.

I moved into the house where Năng and his parents lived. His parents welcomed me, treating me like a daughter. I was lucky. Many of my girlfriends were treated harshly by their parents-in-law, being ordered around like a servant, but Năng's parents were gentle and kind to me. Shortly after our wedding, I got pregnant, and in 1973 I gave birth to our first child, a girl. People say, "Even deep rice fields and female buffalos cannot compare to the value of the firstborn daughter" (*ruộng sâu trâu nái không bằng con gái đầu lòng*). That's how I felt. My parents-in-law were disappointed that she was not a boy, but to me, she was so precious. Holding her in my arms, I felt so happy. We named her Tươi [Fresh]. She was always smiling and trustful, even with strangers. I only wish Năng had been here, to welcome her into life. He did not meet his daughter until she was three years old. Until then, I took care of her alone.

In 1975, the war ended, but it was not until 1982 that Năng came back to live with us. Until then he pursued his career as an army official in Hanoi. In 1977, our son was born. We named him Tỉnh [Alert]. At that time, it was very hard to bring up two small children. After the war, we starved. We lived from rice, peanuts, and water spinach (*rau muống*), which was easy to grow. If we could find some shrimp in the rice fields to add to our children's meal, we felt grateful. Every morning, I got up while it was still dark, lit the fire in the kitchen, and prepared rice gruel for the children. During the day, I worked hard in the rice fields, carrying manure, rice seedlings, harvested crops, and tools to and fro on my shoulder poles. In the summer, the sun was scorching; in the winter, the rain was drizzling and cold. I also sold vermicelli to generate extra income for us. I was young and strong, but it was hard. In 1982, I gave birth to our third child, a beautiful little girl we named Bích [Jade]. Without Năng at home, I felt so alone. He then decided to give up his military career and returned home to us. Being two in the house made everything easier. We helped each other produce vermicelli, and I would go to sell it in the market every morning. As our finances were strained and we could not afford to have more children, I had an intra-uterine device. But still, I got pregnant again, and in 1985 I gave birth to our third daughter, Trang [White]. Her skin was so fair, so we named her Trang.

Of course, Năng had hoped to have another son. I gave birth in the hospital, and when Trang was born, he went to visit us. On his way, crossing the Nề bridge, he met my sister, who told him our baby was a girl. He handed the food he had brought over to my sister, turned around on the spot, and returned home. It took three days before he came to see the baby and me. He was so disappointed. Three daughters. Our children grew up day by day, went to school, and found their ways in life. Now, they are all married and have children. Our three daughters live here in our village with their families. They are busy. Trang has struggled with breast cancer, and Bích is taking care of her mother-in-law, who is paralyzed after a stroke. Our girls belong to their husbands' families now (*xuất giá theo chồng*). So we cannot expect much of them. Our son lives in the south of Vietnam with his family. We had hoped he would stay in our village so that we would have our grandchildren here, together with us in this house, like other people have. A house with small children is so lively and joyful. But he moved to the south, and since then we have managed on our own, day by day. Our son is not always reliable. He and his family come to visit us once a year. Some years they do not come. But it's not a problem for us. We have Năng's pension and our savings, so we can live independently. We do not need to ask our children for help. We can manage. We have each other.

BÀ SON'S LIFE STORY, CHAPTER 3: GROWING OLD WITH DIABETES (2000–2022)

When our son had his second child, in the year 2000, I went to the south to help take care of the children. I stayed there for eight months. It was at this time that my diabetes started. The first sign was the ants. I found it strange that there were so many ants in the bathroom. At first, I thought the children might have dropped some biscuits on the floor. But later I realized it was because of the sugar in my urine. One day, my daughter-in-law checked my weight. When I stepped down from the scale, she told me I was 48 kilos. "No," I said, "my weight has always been 58 kilos. I'm 58 kilos, you must be wrong." But she was right, I weighed 48 kilos only. I had lost ten kilos in a few months. When I returned home, my diabetes was diagnosed. They said my blood sugar count was 29. There was so much sugar in my blood. At the time, no one had heard about diabetes. It was a new disease; it was known as the disease of the rich. People did not know what it was, and they were scared. No one wanted to come near me. They also shunned my husband and children, thinking it was contagious, like leprosy. They forbade me to sell vermicelli in the market. A few years later, the official who did not allow me to enter the market was diagnosed with diabetes himself. And now, many people have diabetes. There is not a single family without someone with diabetes. But to begin with, I was the only one.

When I got the diagnosis, the doctors at the hospital prescribed some pills. But Western medicine is very harsh. So instead of taking the pills, I went to a traditional healer in Hanoi and took the herbs he gave me. Traditional medicine is gentler, and I felt fine for many years. I lived normally, like everyone else. We did not have much money, so I did not go for diabetes checkups or examinations. But then the complications started. One day I woke up with acute pains in my side and my stomach; it felt as if I was being stabbed. Năng took me to the hospital immediately. They said it was kidney stones, and I had to undergo an operation. The operation was costly, and our insurance did not cover it, but we managed. This was in 2008. After the operation, doctors at the hospital told me to measure my blood sugar regularly, but how could I do that? Only the hospital had the equipment to measure blood sugar; we had nothing at home or at our commune health station. The hospital is far away, and I do not want to burden my children or Năng by asking them to drive me. I could not measure my blood sugar every day, but I took the medicine. After a while, the doctors gave me insulin to inject every day. Since then, Năng has been taking me to the hospital regularly, one day each month, for checkups. I sit on the back of his motorbike, and then we go.

One summer, my feet started to grow numb. Some days, I could not feel my feet at all, and they felt so cold. They were not warm like normal feet at all. I felt unsure when I walked, and I did not dare ride my motorbike anymore, so I started riding my old bike instead. I tried to care for my feet by bathing them in water with ginger and always wearing socks, but it did not help. They were numb. During those years, my eyesight also weakened. Suddenly I could not read the sign above the shop across the alley. It was as if there was a curtain in front of my eyes. It was frightening. Day by day, my feet got worse. My right foot felt as if ants bit it. At the hospital, they told us it was necrosis. My diabetes had caused the tissue to die, and they said there was nothing they could do about it. Then strange sores started appearing on my arms. The doctors did not know what it was. At night, I could not sleep. I had to go to the bathroom every hour. I often heard about new kinds of diabetes medicine, sometimes Western medicine (*thuốc Tây*), sometimes traditional Vietnamese medicine (*thuốc Nam*) or Chinese traditional medicine (*thuốc Bắc*). When I told Năng about a new kind of medicine, he would go to get it for me. Sometimes he traveled very far, even to mountainous areas, to buy a new medicine I could try. But nothing worked. Last summer the doctors told us that they had to amputate my right leg. There was nothing else they could do. So that's how I lost my leg. Now, I spend my days in front of the television, sitting in my wheelchair. Năng helps me every day, and our neighbors often pass by to chat, and our grandchildren come, too. I'm okay. I only hope I can keep my left leg. It helps me to keep my balance when getting in and out of bed.

I feel I'm a burden on Năng. He does not complain, but I can see how hard he works and how worried he feels. My disease takes a toll on him. There is so much he must do. He is the one who goes to the market to buy groceries for us. I tell him what to buy, and then he goes. He also cooks, cleans the house, takes care of the garden, and helps me bathe and get into my wheelchair every day. While he was away serving in the army in Hanoi, I struggled alone to take care of our children and our parents. Those years were the hardest in my life. There was so much work. The children were small; they were often sick. And we lacked food, clothes, medicine, and even the most basic things. Today we have machines to help us with laundry, cooking, and farming – but back then we had nothing. Those were the years of war and the years of the subsidy system (*thời bao cấp*).[2] Being away, living in Hanoi, was hard for him, too, but we both know that I was the one who suffered the most. He had only himself to take care of, going to work in the morning and coming home in the evening. I was looking after everyone, our children, our parents, our chickens, pigs, and paddy fields. I was strong and hardworking, and I brought up our children and took care of our parents without complaint. He is grateful to me for that. Together, we lived a life of love and meaning (*một cuộc đời trọn nghĩa vẹn tình*).

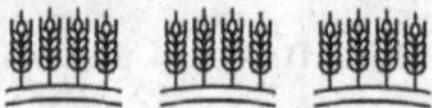

"In our entire country, there was no one like her."

This is Bà Son's life story, which we told in a first-person voice.[3] The story illustrates the dramatic social and economic changes that Vietnam has gone through since Bà Son was born in the mid-twentieth century: within less than one generation, the country has transitioned from a situation of hunger, war, and deprivation to peace and relative affluence. Our work with Bà Son's life story began in the house where she and her husband, Ông Năng, lived for nearly fifty years and raised their four children. They bought this plot of land and built their house in 1976, a few years after their wedding. Located at the heart of the village, it is a classical Red River Delta house with a porch in front of it, built on a spacious plot of land that allows for a luscious garden with banana trees and potted plants, a large fishpond, an outhouse for chicken and other livestock, and an extra outdoor kitchen where Ông Năng used to brew alcohol. The couple lived together in this house from 1976 until Bà Son's death in 2023. Less than a year before her death, she lost her left leg, too – it was amputated in April 2022, one month after our life-story conversations. Shortly after, she suffered a stroke. Năng was with her as she took her last breath on April 3, 2023, sitting by her side in this house where they spent a lifetime together. "She still wanted to live," he told us. "Until the very end, she knew how to endure" (*chịu đựng rất là giỏi*).

We first met Bà Son and Ông Năng during ethnographic fieldwork in their village, Thôn Bình An (Peaceful Hamlet), in Vietnam's Thái Bình Province in 2018. On February 28, 2024, we visited to burn incense for Bà Son. It was early in the Lunar New Year, and, following local tradition, the yard in front of the house was decorated with fresh green ornamental plants, welcoming the new year. As we entered the house, we sensed that Bà Son was still here, watching over us from the ancestral altar. Ông Năng had placed the altar where Bà Son's bed used to

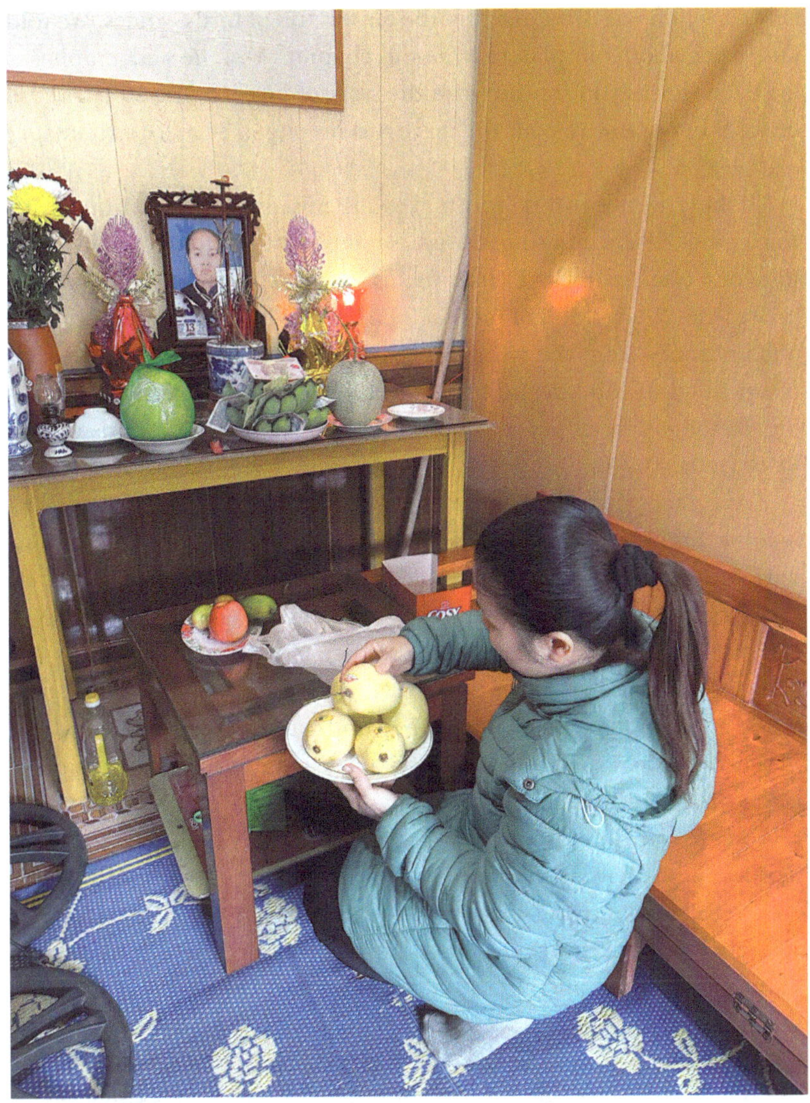

Figure 7.1: Remembering Bà Son (Photo by Tine M. Gammeltoft, 2024)

be, on the left side of the main room. We lit incense sticks and placed them on the altar, along with five round and ripe mango fruits. After a silent moment of watching as the incense spiraled upward carrying our words of respect and good wishes to Bà Son, we accepted Ông Năng's invitation to tea. We sat together on the porch, at the exact spot where Bà Son used to sit in her wheelchair, looking out over the garden. Fine

February rain was drizzling, and the air was full of birds' voices. We told Ông Năng about our plan to write this chapter. "Yes," he said, emphasizing each word, "you should write the story of her life. Her story should be told. In our entire country, there was no one like her (*cả nước không có ai như bà*)."

"Talking to the two of you makes me miss her," he continued, his voice quiet. "We spent so many years together. I will not go looking for someone else. All my love (*tình cảm*) is for her." He fell silent. From the house, the woody smell of incense reached us. In the garden, the high-pitched tones from the white-throated fantail bird (*chim rẻ quạt họng trắng*) filled the air, ascending, then descending. Ascending, descending. In the neighbor's yard, a rooster was crowing. The sounds of Red River Delta villages.

Until recently, rice farming was the only substantial source of income for people in Thôn Bình An. Today, occupational options have multiplied, with many people making their living from trade or industrial work and many seeking employment in other provinces or countries. An avalanche of consumer goods and new foods has expanded consumption options, turning sugary items such as "milk tea" (*trà sữa*), juices, and sweetened milk and cereal products, and highly processed foods such as fruit snacks, biscuits, and cup noodles into attractive diet options for many people. While these expanding options for work and consumption are generally appreciated, these developments have also led to new problems, including a rapidly rising prevalence of type 2 diabetes and other chronic health conditions (Biswas et al. 2022). From being a rare condition a few decades ago, diabetes is now, as one elderly villager put it, a disease that "everyone suffers from" (*ai cũng bị*).

Sitting on the porch, we talked about Bà Son's life with diabetes. How she fell ill with a disease nobody knew of at the time; how she lived an ordinary life with it for many years; and how her complications eventually intensified, resulting in the loss of first one and then the other leg. While talking, we studied the identity cards that Ông Năng had placed on the table in front of us – each depicting Bà Son's face at different times of her life. A young, a middle-aged, and an old woman moving through life. She lived through this life in a society where the social and moral expectations placed on her as a daughter, a daughter-in-law, a wife, a mother, and a grandmother were clear and explicit, articulated

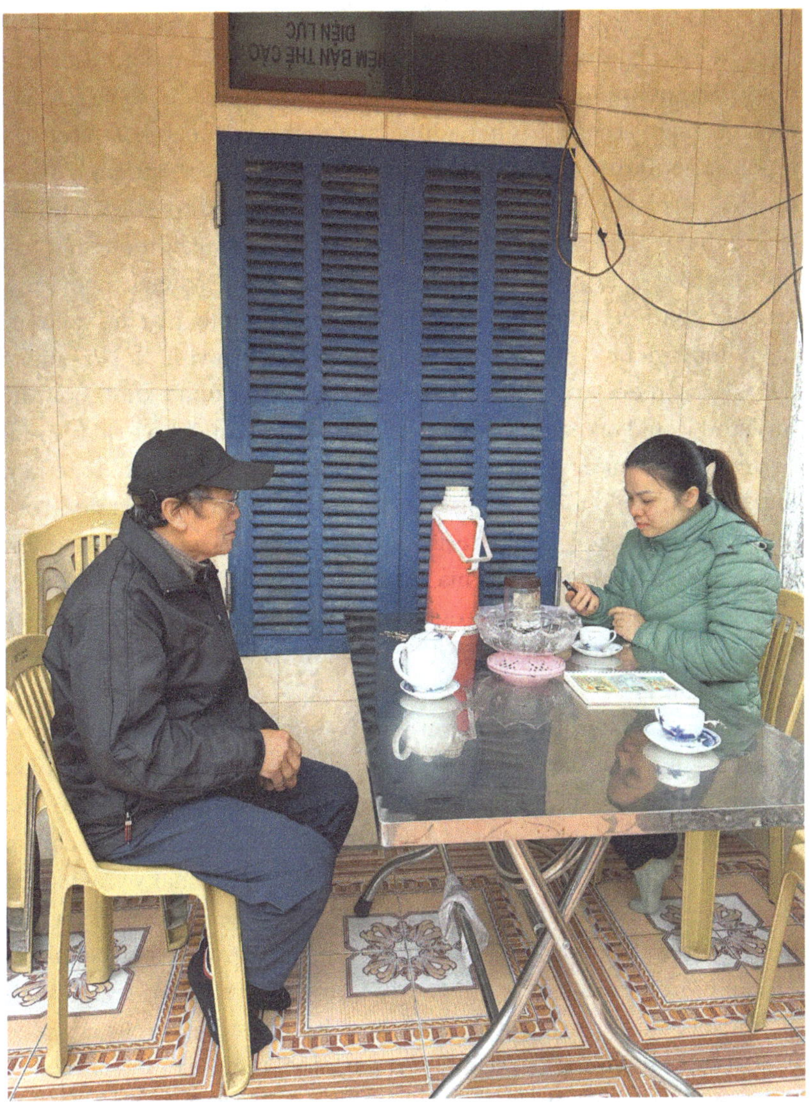

Figure 7.2: Ông Năng and Dung in conversation (Photo by Tine M. Gammeltoft, 2024)

in sayings, proverbs, political slogans, and social interactions, and where everyday lives in her village were organized along lines of kinship (Hy Van Luong 1989; Shohet 2021). As a mode of everyday social organization, northern Vietnam's patrilineal and patrilocal kinship system has far-reaching implications for women's lives (Gammeltoft 2021,

2022). Bà Son felt this poignantly, spending the first years of her married life in the house of her parents-in-law; confronting her husband's deep disappointment when their fourth child turned out to be female; and having to accept that her adult daughters were unable to offer her much support during the years she lived with diabetes. Although living physically close to her, her daughters now belonged to other families where their roles as wives, mothers, and daughters-in-law took their toll on time and energy. In this male-oriented kinship system, their son's absence rendered Bà Son and Ông Năng vulnerable, placing them in deep dependence on one another. During our first visit, in November 2018, Bà Son declared in a firm voice, "Honestly, I don't know how my husband would manage without me." She was the one who held responsibility for the many practices of care that sustained their life together. She kept an eye on Ông Năng's health, brought home groceries from the market, cooked their meals, and cared for their grandchildren. Their daily life together was maintained through the labor of Bà Son, as millions of human lives across the globe are sustained by women's – often invisible and unrecognized – care work (Daniels 1987; Seedat and Rondon 2021).

A few years later, the situation had changed. Now, a year after the death of his wife, Ông Năng said, "I did all I could to help her. I served her completely. Without me, she would have died much earlier." Bà Son's diabetes and Ông Năng's responses to it entailed a transformation of long-standing gendered caregiving roles. Over the many years when Bà Son struggled with the complications of her disease, losing first one leg and then the other, Ông Năng became her main caregiver – taking on not merely tasks that are defined as lying within a male realm, such as transportation and heavy lifting, but also tasks that are usually delegated to women, such as daily shopping, cooking, cleaning, and emotional support. As *her* body waned, *his* took over, in an embodied process of generativity or *poiesis*, as described by Robert Desjarlais (2015, 653): "There is a creative tendency in life itself. Poiesis is found in moments of joy and suffering, and of life and death … Something is made present when something else is no longer present."

Processes of poiesis often take place, as Desjarlais notes, in the company of others; they are communal endeavors: "Most often what is involved is a kind of *co-poiesis*, of a collaborative fashioning and unfashioning of self and other, as well as of a *poiesis-on-behalf-of-another*. What

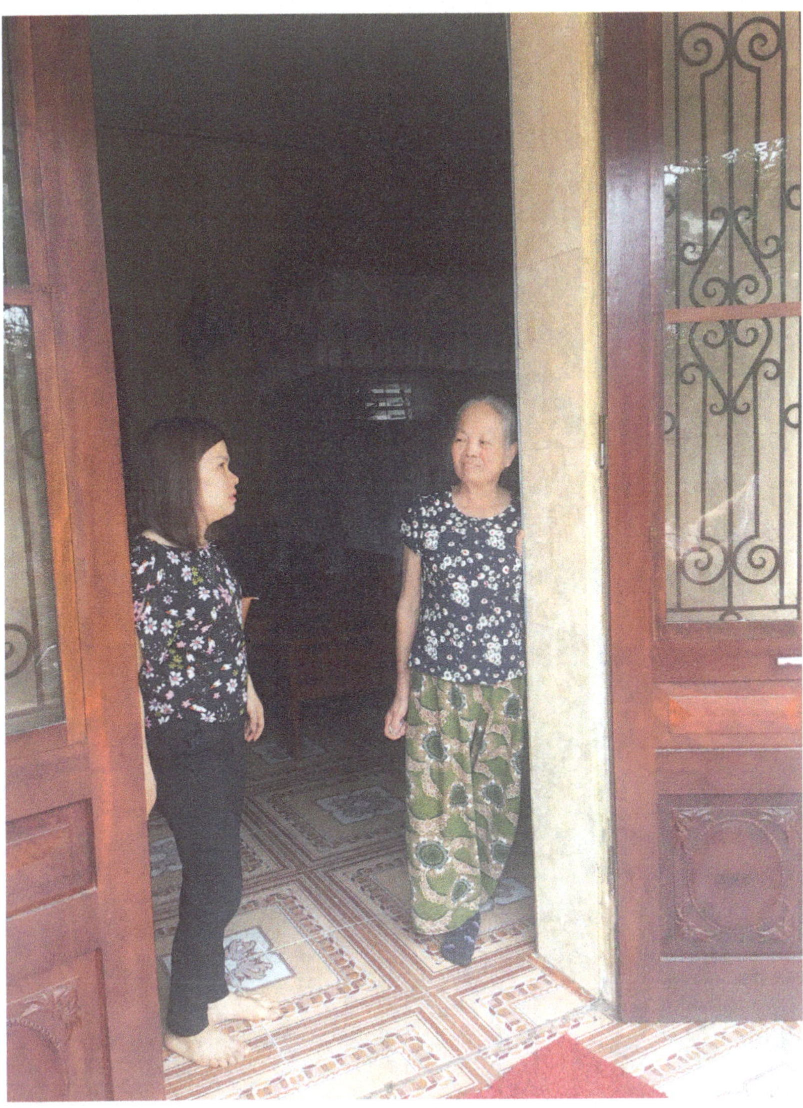

Figure 7.3: Dung and Bà Son at home (Photo by Tine M. Gammeltoft, 2019)

people often bring forth, or dissolve, is on behalf of others" (Desjarlais 2015, 655). Striving not to burden their children, Ông Năng transformed conventional gendered patterns of domestic caregiving. This was a quiet gender transformation – not one that attracted public attention as when young women in Vietnam resist marriage (Thanh Huyền

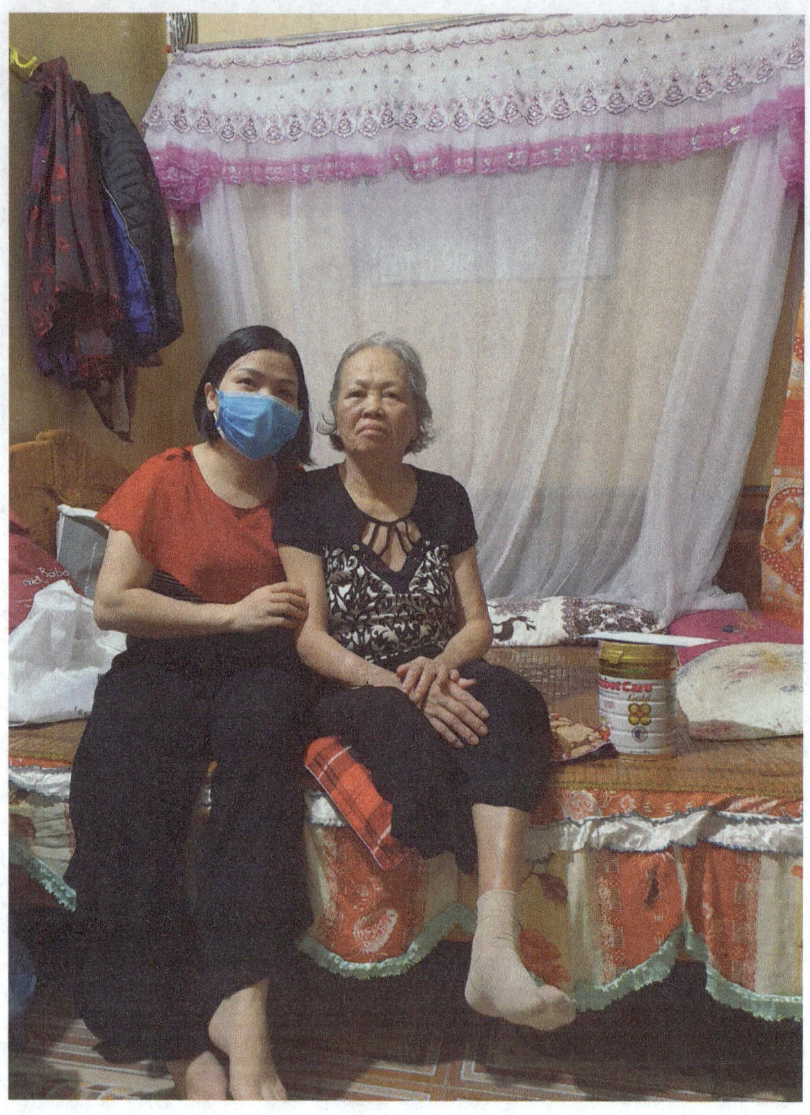

Figure 7.4: Dung visiting Bà Son at home, shortly after her first amputation (Photo by Vũ Phong Túc, 2021)

2024) or LGBT community members advocate for sexual and marital rights (Nguyen and Doan 2022). Yet despite its quiet nature, this was a significant transformation, shifting habituated modes of distributing domestic care tasks within village households in this Red River Delta area (Guilmoto 2012; Phan Anh 2021).

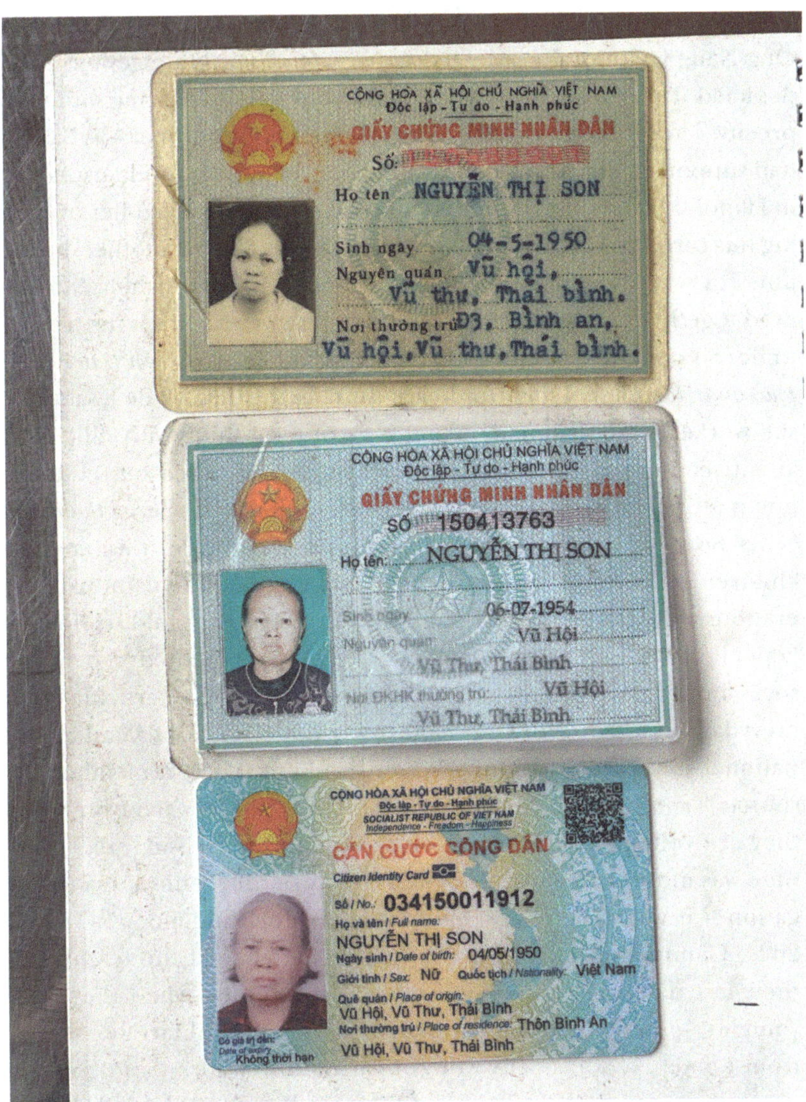

Figure 7.5: Three ID cards, one life (Photo by Tine M. Gammeltoft, 2024)

The transformation that took place in the household of these two elderly people testifies to what Oliver Sacks terms "the paradox of disease." Disease, Sacks observes, is not merely destructive, but can bring out "latent powers, developments, evolutions, forms of life" (Sacks 2012, xiv). Disease holds generative and creative capacities. In the case of Bà Son and Ông Năng, these capacities unfolded in a domestic atmosphere suffused with past experiences – experiences that made Ông Năng feel morally indebted to his wife. Their life together, as he depicted it on this February day, had been a life of sharing and reciprocity. They had supported and sacrificed for one another – as Bà Son had supported her husband, enabling him to pursue a military career in Hanoi through her labor at home, so he had supported her by ending this career and returning home when life as a single mother during times of scarcity became too hard for her. As he put it himself: "We lived together for a long time, for fifty or sixty years. This is not a short while. So one must attend to matters of the heart (*chuyện tình cảm là phải quan tâm*). I feel sorry for her because in the past, while I was away, she worked hard at home, taking care of everything with diligence, attentiveness, and responsibility (*chắt chiu*). She raised our children into mature and responsible adults (*nuôi con khôn lớn trưởng thành*)."

Bà Son carried their shared lives into the future, raising their children to become independent adults, ensuring that future generations would take over where they left. Ông Năng told us how he kept all of this in his heart, feeling grateful and indebted to her. The social importance of such moral debt is often explicitly articulated in everyday worlds in Vietnam, held up as the essence of familial and national ethical obligations. "When drinking water, remember the source" (*uống nước nhớ nguồn*), children are admonished from when they are young. Yet in the life of Bà Son and Ông Năng, this gratitude was more than a matter of moral duty or mechanical social obligation – it was visceral and emotional, a "domestic mood" (Danely 2024; Gammeltoft 2018; Throop 2014) that shaped the textures of their last days together. The events that unfolded when they were younger – their wedding, the war, Ông Năng's military service far from home, Bà Son's daily work of caring for children and crops in times of extreme scarcity – were still spectrally present in their home, suffusing each day, shaping emotions and moral orientations, and forming the groundwork for Ông Năng's daily caregiving (Gammeltoft 2024; Kavedzija 2020).

This everyday moral fabric of life – characterized by a finely tuned attentiveness to and acknowledgment of others' gestures of kindness and support – became the cultural ground from which Bà Son's diabetes emerged socially as so much more than merely a devastating chronic disease. Rather than simply a force of disability and death, as it is often represented in national health statistics and epidemiological accounts, Bà Son's diabetes was also a force of life. We have recounted her life story here to honor her and to draw attention to the significance of socio-somatic generativity, to the transformative and generative capacities of a biologically degenerative disease.

NOTES

1 Our recounting of Bà Son's life story is based on ethnographic fieldwork conducted in Vietnam's Thái Bình Province from 2018 to 2024 by a team of Vietnamese and Danish researchers. The fieldwork formed part of the interdisciplinary research project VALID (Living Together with Chronic Disease: Informal Support for Diabetes Management in Vietnam) (17-M09-KU), funded by the Ministry of Foreign Affairs of Denmark (DANIDA). For details, see https://anthropology.ku.dk/research/research-projects/current- projects/living-together-with-chronic-disease/. The moment in time from which Bà Son tells her story is early March 2022, when we conducted a series of intensive life-history conversations with her. Over eight days, Dung visited her every day, bringing a voice recorder and her notebook. Tine was in COVID-19 quarantine in Hanoi at the time and took part in the conversations via the Vietnamese online messaging app Zalo. We have divided Bà Son's story into three chapters, each covering a life stage as she conveyed it to us.
2 "The subsidy period" refers to the years when Vietnam's economy was centrally planned, from the end of the war in 1975 to 1986, when economic reforms were launched. This period is generally known as a time of poverty and hardship (see for instance MacLean 2008).
3 In terms of writing genre, the life-story part of this chapter can be characterized as "ethnographic creative nonfiction" (Narayan 2007; Wulff 2023; see also Butler 1994). The account describes life events that Bà Son told us about or that we observed during fieldwork, such as childbirths, shifting forms of work, family relations, and experiences of disease. In recounting these events, we tried to stay close to the tone of Bà Son's voice as we have come to know it. Her life story as we tell it here is thus firmly grounded in ethnographic fieldwork, yet it is also *creative* in that we have added sensuous details such as sounds, smells, sentiments, and the names of fruits, birds, crops, and flowers.

REFERENCES

Biswas, T., N. Tran, H. Thi My Hanh, P. Van Hien, N. Thi Thu Cuc, P. Hong Van, K. Anh Tuan, T. Thi Mai Oanh, and A. Mamun. 2022. "Type 2 Diabetes and Hypertension in Vietnam: A Systematic Review and Meta-analysis of Studies Between 2000 and 2020." *BMJ Open* 12 (8): e052725.

Butler, Robert Olen. 1994 [1992]. *A Good Scent from a Strange Mountain.* London: Minerva.

Danely, Jason. 2024. "In the Shadows of Gratitude: On Mooded Spaces of Vulnerability and Care." *Ethos* 52: 20–36.

Daniels, Arlene Kaplan. 1987. "Invisible Work." *Social Problems* 34 (5): 403–15.

Desjarlais, Robert. 2015. "A Good Death, Recorded." In *Living and Dying in the Contemporary World,* edited by Veena Das and Clara Han, 648–661.

Gammeltoft, Tine M. 2018. "Domestic Moods: Maternal Mental Health in Northern Vietnam." *Medical Anthropology* 37 (7): 582–96.

———. 2021. "Spectral Kinship: Understanding How Vietnamese Women Endure Domestic Distress." *American Ethnologist* 48 (1): 22–36.

———. 2022. "Marriage, Family, and Kinship in Vietnam: Shadows and Silences." In *The Routledge Handbook of Contemporary Vietnam,* edited by Jonathan London, 437–47. London: Routledge.

———. 2024. "Calibrating Care: Family Caregiving and the Social Weight of Sympathy (*Tình Cảm*)." *American Anthropologist,* 126 (4): 596–607.

Guilmoto, Christophe. 2012. "Son Preference, Sex Selection, and Kinship in Vietnam." *Population and Development Review* 38 (1): 31–54.

Luong, Hy Van. 1989. "Vietnamese Kinship: Structural Principles and the Socialist Transformation in Northern Vietnam." *Journal of Asian Studies* 48 (4): 741–56.

Kavedžija, Iza. 2020. "An Attitude of Gratitude: Older Japanese in the Hopeful Present." *Anthropology & Aging* 41 (2): 59–71.

MacLean, Ken. 2008. "The Rehabilitation of an Uncomfortable Past: Everyday Life in Vietnam During the Subsidy Period (1975–1986)." *History and Anthropology* 19 (3): 281–303.

Narayan, Kirin. 2007. "Tools to Shape Texts: What Creative Nonfiction Can Offer Ethnography." *Anthropology and Humanism* 32 (2): 130–44.

Nguyen, Thi Thu Huyen, and Long Doan. 2022. "The Prospects for the Legalization of Same-Sex Marriages in Vietnam." *International Journal of Discrimination and the Law* 22 (4): 347–70.

Phan, Anh. 2021. "Red River Delta Gender Imbalance Highest in the Country: Report." *VnExpress International,* October 27. https://e.vnexpress.net /news/news/red-river-delta-gender-imbalance-highest-in-the-country -report-4377886.html.

Sacks, Oliver. 2012 [1995]. *An Anthropologist on Mars.* London: Picador.

Seedat, Soraya, and Marta Rondon. 2021. "Women's Wellbeing and the Burden of Unpaid Work." *BMJ* 374: n1972.

Shohet, Merav. 2021. *Silence and Sacrifice: Family Stories of Care and the Limits of Love in Vietnam.* Oakland: University of California Press.

Thanh Huyền. 2024. "Nhiều Hệ Lụy khi Người Trẻ Ngại Kết Hôn" [There Are Many Consequences When Young People Are Afraid of Getting Married]. *VOV2,* March 6. https://vov2.vov.vn/doi-song-xa-hoi/nhieu-he-luy-khi -nguoi-tre-ngai-ket-hon-47434.vov2.

Throop, C. Jason. 2014. "Moral Moods." *Ethos* 42 (1): 65–83.
Wulff, Helena. 2023 [2021]. "Writing Anthropology." In *The Open Encyclopedia of Anthropology*, edited by F. Stein. Facsimile of the first edition in *The Cambridge Encyclopedia of Anthropology*. http://doi.org/10.29164/21writing.

CHAPTER EIGHT

Footsteps: How Did We Get Here?

James Doucet-Battle

One sunny Sunday morning, my partner and I attended a church service in Oakland, California. Invited by a close friend and her husband, we gathered there to celebrate their daughter's public declaration of faith. The church's congregation, diverse but primarily African American, conveyed a progressive, middle- to upper-middle class ethos of liberal individualism and robust community engagement. After the service, I asked the African American pastor if their church had an organized health ministry (they did not), and in particular, if she played a leading role in efforts to address health disparities (she did not). "I don't *lead*," Pastor Rollins[1] said. "I *follow* wherever the congregation's *footsteps* take me. From behind, I push forward in support of them."

So when I met Pastor Rollins in 2018, I thought I had perhaps found a church untouched by either biomedical or social-scientific gazes. Instead, I encountered their preemptive refusals, not due to the nature of any singular concerns or questionable bioethical histories, but from the lack of any organic emanations of interest emerging from within the congregation itself. This despite type 2 diabetes and, by inclusion, obesity being well-known and arguably accepted biosocial facts plaguing the African American community. While I recognized and understood Pastor Rollins's response to my question, the social scientist in me found it insufficient, leaving me wanting to know more about this strategic but contingent refusal to engage in a discussion about health in the congregation. She punctuated her response with a hushed tone conveying a counseled silence that foreclosed a widened conversation with church members. I was reminded that health disparities, particularly within the African American community, emerge from entangled histories of injustice, inequality, and exploitative and extractive labor, leaving churches as the institutional bulwark against these recurring traumas and silencing insults to human dignity.

Diabetes education efforts aimed toward African Americans often center on churches as dissemination points of biomedical information. Yet what often goes unnoticed, in both public health and social-scientific scholarship, are the historical continuities between *diabetes* as a medical condition and its metaphor, *sugar*, as a racial project. More provocatively, in what follows, I will argue that both the condition and the project share linked continuities within transmutable forms of racial capitalism.

FOOTSTEPS ONSHORE AND OFFSHORE

A journey of a thousand miles, as the saying goes, begins with a single step. The blackened footsteps leading to church and clinic began their march from distant shores far away and long ago. These episodic journeys, for example, from Elmina Castle in present-day Ghana to Charleston, South Carolina, traversing over five thousand miles of open sea … Stepping through doors of no return and around trees of forgetting, the conscripts treaded onto ships destined for foreign ports, where they disembarked, headed toward slave markets ranging from New Amsterdam to Buenos Aries and Montevideo, New Orleans to Cartagena, Acapulco, and Santiago. With feet standing still, they were auctioned to the highest bidder. Thus began the exchange of one's "country marks" in new regimes of labor, (mal)nourishment, and a plethora of associated relations to both the body and the mind, absorbed and diffracted into and across dozens of biopolitical systems from Canada to Cape Horn.

The Slave Voyages website, slavevoyages.org, provides a graphic example of the millions of footsteps taken on these arduous journeys into metabolic modernity. The site's time-lapse feature gives visual evidence, based on documented voyages, of the extent of a slave-trading industry of voracious and addictive import, which existed for nearly four hundred years. Footsteps from savannahs to the coast, and from forests to the coast, walked to the docks of flotillas of ships awaiting their human cargo. On the other side of the Atlantic Ocean, the enslaved African would traverse new terrains toward the plantations, haciendas, mines, encomiendas, and *colonias* in the, *a*, New World.

Most notably, for our purposes, the incessant demands of the sugar-industrial complex generated obscene profits while changing nutritional destinies around the world. The long durée of slavery and eventual emancipation also initiated a movement toward rapid urbanization, a process that would accelerate during the twentieth century. In the United States, the Great Migration of African Americans exemplified this drive to urban spaces of greater but contingently available opportunities, places to imagine anew and to hope again. W. E. B. Du Bois chronicled these early movements of the footsteps that trekked to Philadelphia, who along with the pre-existing Black population, revitalized both the racialized community and its racialized category.[2] Using data based on health statistics comparing urban blacks in the North with whites in the South, Du Bois later argued against prevailing claims linking race with disease risk (1906).

Thus, Black footsteps to the city signified an increasing visibility for black Americans under both racial and medical gazes. These dual lenses onto reading black bodies in the Fordist context of the city would continue apace during the remainder of the twentieth century. The footsteps of the plantation Negro, pathologized by Samuel Cartwright, who, unperturbed by the absence of biostatistical evidence, coined the term *drapetomania* to describe and ostensibly diagnose the afflicted slave compelled irrationally to run away from her master. In other words, footsteps toward freedom were seen and accepted by many medical *men* as a pathological condition requiring active surveillance and bioregulation. Ironically, within a few years of Cartwright's ideological assertion, the footsteps of the Union Army would upend the plantocracy Cartwright sought to legitimize through science, as General Sherman's soldiers marched toward the sea, fulfilling his promise "to make the South howl." Some of the formerly enslaved followed the Union troops across the Southern US, while others remained where they lived previously and would continue to toil. Both groups, the wanderers and the settled, would later converge over the next century in a massive demographic shift from the South to the North and West of the country.

Sugar, a precious commodity during the Civil War that served as the problematic catalyst for the slavery industry and global capitalism, became known and referred to as a metaphor for diabetes, particularly within and articulated by the African American community. For those ensconced in cities, the black population was now a visible community whose biobehavioral reputation had already preceded them. However, during the early twentieth century, Jewish immigrants, not African Americans, were seen as most susceptible to developing what we know today as type 2 (formerly *adult-onset*) diabetes.[3] Actually, African Americans were not considered a high-risk type 2 group, with the US Army going so far as to assert this finding based on its comparative analysis of physical examinations of black and white troops that served in World War I. Therefore, in terms of "racial risk," those with Jewish ancestry served as the *prima facie* example of the subpopulation most prone to becoming diabetic.

Yet, Du Bois presciently pointed out that the nutritional insufficiencies of the urban Negro diet remained embedded in an encultured relationship to food formed during slavery. The realities of the subsistence-level deprivations of the slave diet, meant to barely ensure survival and definitely not intended to promote health, were transported by the footsteps of these internal refugees in the United States along those roads and railways leading out of the South. Now living within demographically and residentially dense areas of mostly segregated cities, black Americans came increasingly under the purview of public and community health professionals, where medicine and health literacy efforts went about the work of further interrogating the Negro body.[4]

Over the course of the twentieth century, the growing attention toward the ever-more visible US black body in urban spaces, most notably in the case of sickle cell disease, would redound to type 2 diabetes. African Americans, seen by the US Army after World War I as less prone to metabolic disorders than whites, came to symbolize (along with Indigenous and Latinx groups) a high-risk diabetes population. The topics of hypertension, obesity, and later food access came to subsume any significant analytical consideration of the inescapable racism some black people thought the North and West would ameliorate. These domains, while generating reams of statistical data, reinforced racial categories and buttressed racial categorization as a plausible method for improving health outcomes and achieving health equity. In the relative absence of a foregrounding discussion and examination of racism, race and risk found new forms of articulation in science, medicine, and society at large.

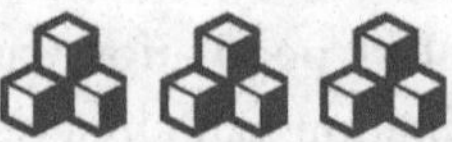

How did we get here? I posed questions to Pastor Rollins that were admittedly tinged with a mélange of self-interest and ethnographic curiosity. Although my larger project on type 2 diabetes had been completed and the manuscript written, I stumbled, curiosity still alive, into meeting Pastor Rollins. Up until that Sunday, my search for a church health ministry in Oakland with which to examine African American community trust toward biomedicine had seemed futile and was subsequently abandoned. Ten years earlier in 2008, I wanted to hold a conversation about type 2 diabetes and allied efforts to recruit African-descent populations for genomic clinical research into cardiometabolic disparities. Rebecca Skloot's *The Immortal Life of Henrietta Lacks* had just been published the year before, causing a buzz in both scientific and popular media circles. In the book, Skloot retraces the history of a black mother from Maryland, and the circulation of her cervical cancer cells from the early 1950s to the 2000s. These cells, taken without consent, became the foundation of biomedical research, populating petri dishes and invading laboratories around the world, revitalizing the discipline of cell biology, providing extraordinary profits to those who sold these cells, and opening new areas of career expansion among those who came to work with them. Henrietta passed away shortly after her diagnosis, but over the next five decades, the family remained unaware of the use of their mother's cells and never saw a dime. The book resurrected conversations about past and current bioethical injustices toward African Americans, of which the Tuskegee Syphilis Study looms prominently in community memory.

As I discovered, the apparent futility of my search for a health ministry to work with stemmed from the fact that, as one clinical researcher later told me in 2009, "Clinical researchers have descended upon African American churches in droves in Oakland to hold discussions and conduct focus groups about *The Immortal Life of Henrietta Lacks*, what that means to the community in terms of trust in scientific research, and how best to leverage that knowledge toward shaping future clinical recruitment strategies geared toward African Americans." According to her, "Most of the black health ministries in Oakland have been contacted [concerning the *Immortal Life of Henrietta Lacks*]; of these, nearly all of them have become involved." To be clear, a "health ministry" is composed of members of a particular congregation. They reflect the professional and socioeconomic diversity (or range) within that congregation. In this respect, health ministries reflect a broad spectrum of African American religious and community life. So when I began my research into type 2 diabetes in the African-descent community in 2008, most of these church entities were tied up in the busy work of facilitating extant institutional researcher clamorings to establish discussion, focus, and even reading groups on *The Immortal Life of Henrietta Lacks.*

I must admit to having had a serious rethinking of my research at the time, debating whether I should temporarily shelve my type 2 diabetes project and intellectually surf the social wave *The Immortal Life of Henrietta Lacks* had brought forth. My rethinking arose not out of any opportunistic sense or careerist strategy, but out of the sheer gravitas of the story and the profound ongoing and future bioethical implications for African-descent participation in genomic research trials, both as researchers and the researched, that it raised. I decided to reprioritize my research focus onto type 2 diabetes in African-descent communities. I saw the illness as a growing phenomenon that loomed as a clearer and more present threat to all communities. Despite the metabolic democracy that obesity and type 2 diabetes offer equally across populations, new algorithms and technological advances had served to buttress older claims linking race, biology, and risk. As part of anthropology's disciplinary refusal of arguments equating race with biology, I recommitted to the project of unmooring type 2 diabetes risk from racial biology. Moreover, I remained committed to this examination through fieldwork in a black church.[5]

So the 2018 church in Oakland wasn't my first venture into understanding the role of health in the church. Given the situation in Oakland mentioned earlier, I relocated my project to Rochester, New York, where I serendipitously found myself invited to a health ministry workshop on type 2 diabetes and Alzheimer's (now referred to as type 3 diabetes by a growing number of clinicians). Since it was conducted by a local church that I knew well, having grown up in the area, Mt. Zion Baptist Church, I thought attending would provide an excellent opportunity to meet and re-meet a significant cross-section of the African American community. The demographic and geographic density and diasporic diversity of the African-descent population in the area provided a somewhat socially known but anthropologically unfamiliar community in which to dive headlong into an intensive period of fieldwork. The two main workshop leaders were both church members: Merlene Bailey of the American Diabetes Association and Robert Mann of the Alzheimer's Association of Monroe County. Mt. Zion's pastor, Reverend Hargreaves, expressed keen interest in my work, going so far as taking time to give me a tour of the newly remodeled church and facilitating introductions to workshop leaders and other members of the congregation attending the event.

Reverend Hargreaves also introduced me to a third workshop leader, a diabetes educator from the University of Rochester Medical Center. Margaret Richards gave a well-received presentation on the diabetes education classes and clinical resources provided by the University of Rochester. In addition, she discussed glucometer technologies, hemoglobin A1C diagnostic tests, and pharmaceutical guidelines. Yet, despite a quite capable and impressively portable presentation, no footsteps from any of the more than fifty congregation members in attendance led to Margaret Richards's information table post-workshop. I did, and found Margaret, a white woman, quite affable and open to discussing the Medical Center's diabetes research, therapeutics, and diagnostic technologies. Merlene Bailey later pointed to an ambiguously ambivalent relationship between the university and the community, accusing it of engaging in a top-down conversation that failed to meet the community on its own cultural terms. A child of parents from Guyana and Barbados, Merlene, who grew up in Rochester, had an adaptive competency in both African American and Afro-Caribbean cultural understandings about type 2 diabetes, foodways, and religious values.

I left Margaret Richards's table convinced she had information of value to the workshop participants. Returning to a table of five middle-aged to elderly women, I asked if any of them were interested in speaking with Margaret Richards. All shook their heads no, punctuated by the same demonstrably palpable hushed silence Pastor Rollins would communicate ten years later. A silence that speaks, but which can never tell, in a language it was assumed, and quite correctly, that I understood.

At that time, I had envisioned executing a comparative ethnographic project that would examine issues of trust, health literacy, and diabetes technological uptake among African Americans in the community, in tandem with the efforts of a local research recruitment organization to attract African Americans for enrollment in type 2 diabetes clinical drug trials. I thought, perhaps naively, that the incidence of type 2 diabetes in the African-descent and Latinx communities in Rochester would generate interest in and attendance to diabetes education classes. This proved not to be the case. Dr. Asela, then medical director of the Clinical Research Center, lamented the relative absence of African Americans attending their type 2 diabetes education classes. These classes, offered at no cost, were held on-site, less than a ten-minute drive from a large African American and Latinx community on the city's northside. Frustrated by the apparent lack of African American attraction in the center's work, Dr. Asela saw a plaintive appeal through black churches as the only way, the only fora, the only viable means to perform outreach toward a seemingly intractable community. Though he was a fairly recent immigrant from Sri Lanka, he was aware of the history of African American distrust in biomedical research, most notably the Tuskegee Syphilis Study. "I just want them to come to the classes," he maintained. "We have so much to offer here." But the classes were meant and designed, under the banner of care and concern, to serve an introductory and ultimate purpose – to generate African American interest in participating in type 2 as well as other cardiometabolic illness clinical drug trials.

One wonders whether the interest and entreaties to care Dr. Asela professed had sustainable legs upon which to evidence footsteps taken toward establishing a long-term commitment to minoritized communities: Dr. Asela no longer works at the Clinical Research Center; today, the CRC's medical team and administration is one-hundred-percent white. Sixteen years later, the center seems to have made little progress in achieving greater professional diversity and ethnoracial concordance between its staff and the wider community. The working assumption, mirroring Merlene Bailey's critique, is that institutions will attract curious, and hopefully willing, feet, stepping *to* them, in numbers, by the sheer magnetism of their biotechnological pull, racialization of risk, and authoritative expertise.

Merlene Bailey and I met for breakfast nearly every year between 2009 and 2017. Her keen interest in my project did not equate to a steadfast commitment to her continuing teaching diabetes education classes and performing outreach to the African American community. Although she remained a member of the Mt. Zion Health Ministry, she left the American Diabetes Association and took up a directorship at a local university, building her own community consulting business.

STEPPING INTO DARKNESS

Conscripted into internally displaced modernity, footsteps tracking north, west, and places in between settled into redlined, gerrymandered, and residentially segregated spaces. Demarcated by political and racial capital and sacrificiable as racial labor, African Americans' geosocial proximity to quality food, medical care, and the attendant observational gaze of the clinic took on novel dimensional contexts. These domains continue to occupy the attention of scholars, activists, physicians, scientists, pharmaceutical companies, and venture capitalists alike.

It is into this moment in black modernity my multi-sited research into type 2 diabetes began. In Oakland and Rochester, I situated my work within two disparate nodes of migration from the South, each containing newer arrivals from the African diaspora that energized, reconfigured, and dynamized a contested racial category. The category, "African American," as a living social body, gained new relevance as a desirable but, for those in public health and clinical research, strategically and analytically unknown community toward which to formulate a coherent language of outreach. The more recent diasporics did not arrive in the US through the slave trade, an enterprise driven and made most profitable by the sugar plantation industrial complex.[6] Unlike their earlier black immigrant predecessors from the Caribbean, sugar was not their capitalist raison d' être historically.

Therefore, Rochester served as an ideal field site precisely due to the diversity of African-descent groups resident in the city and surrounding areas. It is a city where one could meet a Jamaican, Trinidadian, Haitian, or Nigerian just as easily as one could meet an African American with parents or relatives from any of those countries (and others), something you would not know otherwise unless they told you or you knew their families. My family moved to the city from Louisiana during the 1950s, speaking both Black American English and Afro-French Creole, part of a migration from throughout the Black Atlantic that increased the city's *Negro* population nearly eightfold over that decade. So ongoing periods of intensive migration from the US South and dynamic pulses of subsequent immigrant entry make it difficult to impossible to speak or to write univocally about either the category or the community in singular terms. What can be said is that no matter the category or the community, all are embedded within capitalist modes of consumption in the midst of an availability of excess calories, technologically enabled physical inertia, and the nearly inescapable media saturation influencing obesogenic and diabetogenic behaviors. This redefinition by recomposition of the category was enabled by footsteps taken from shore to shore, largely by airplane, not by ocean-going ships. Now comprising over ten per cent of the African American category, they represent groups of diverse "blackness" embedded firmly within the shared metabolic destiny of the global West. They have been lumped together in a racial category, and the historical burden of racial science – its persistence and ongoing claims and queries about the black diabetic body – now rests on their collective diasporic shoulders.

In the preceding, I digressed intentionally to point toward a focal shift in historical inquiry: from the "Heart of Darkness" to the "Body of Darkness." Conrad's classic (and infamous) *Heart of Darkness* chronicled his nineteenth-century journey into Africa, searching for riches but only finding horror in Europe's obsessive project of extracting wealth from Africa, in the absence of interest in knowing the African as a human being.[7] Mirroring this story, I came to better understand Dr. Asela and other clinical research, private sector, and public health stakeholders' incessant search to find language or, more accurately, a linguistic entrée that would convey interest, care, and concordance with African Americans (broadly defined). As implied above, finding a coherent narrative confronts the struggle of achieving legibility across communities. These efforts evoke a reverse analytic of Hortense Spillers's notion of the "decipherability of black flesh" as first requiring a code, an alphabet, a formulaic, that would make the black body intelligible through its presumed darkness.[8]

The footsteps taken by recent immigrants did not automatically relegate them to blackened or racialized spaces, and they benefitted, according to the data, from the "healthy immigrant effect," a measure of better health in comparison with domestic-born African Americans.

However, the healthy immigrant effect offers a time-sensitive shield of protection, and only compared to African Americans. Language and culture, often seen as prophylactic, cannot, over time, withstand the pernicious effects of racism and consumption adversely affecting both the category and its longer interred occupants. In the US, a correlation has been made between degrees of acculturation and diabetes risk in African immigrants (Mukaz 2022).[9] While these new immigrants may not have initially identified with either the African American or Black category, their children and grandchildren increasingly have through shared racializing experiences, language acquisition, and cultural assimilation. In other words, people become the category based on what they see, say, and do. For these young people, Black Lives Matter.

I continue to meet students from families originating in the Horn of Africa, West Africa, Egypt, and the Maghreb, who along with legacy Caribbeans, see themselves as African American or Black. From campus student groups to the lab, these students articulate an identity shaped by their own racialized experiences and the social contexts in which they occur, cultural spaces their parents most likely cannot imagine, much less conceive. This is the process of acculturation alluded to earlier, as well as its costs. Over pizza, burgers, fries, tacos, and bubble tea, bodies arrayed in racial formation march in step along a shared cultural highway of market-driven consumption, care, and a seemingly incontrovertible pharmaceutical destiny amid the obesogenic spoils of capital and empire. Body mass index charts for children have been doubled from 30 to 60 BMI. Again, "How did we get here?"

Taking a cue from the film of the same name: How do we "get out"?

STEPPING INTO EXPERTISE

A map that might lead to a way of getting out starts with a narrative retracing of the footsteps taken in this chapter. I began this excursion in the church, a nominal site of these conversations about diabetes and health, of conversations taken up in Rochester, and of footsteps not advanced in Oakland. The church serves as a convergent site of diverse strands of the African diaspora, a translational space for acculturating slowly but surely into mainstream US life. Pastor Rollins advisedly cautioned that footsteps taken toward medical justice first require strategic thinking by those who would lead such an effort. She made it clear that true leadership begins from within the congregation and wider community – that the role of the *pastor* is to *shepherd* the flow of that social energy, not direct it, a difficult exercise in balancing the levers of power in fields of socioeconomic combat. Using the symbolic and political capital of the church, the pastor can then lead from the back, making legible the voices of the unheard in articulating the rights of citizenship for all. In Rochester, Merlene Bailey's Caribbean background added cultural legibility to her message about type 2 diabetes. On the other hand, the Clinical Research Center has done little to diversify its professional cadre of experts, in a city that is majority African American and Latinx, two of the largest at-risk groups for type 2 diabetes. Footsteps taken, conversations had, and knowledge shared with skill and care epitomize the true definition of an expertise that strives to achieve greater legibility and deepens trust in underserved communities. Arguably, this is the bare minimum starting point for addressing and eliminating health disparities.

Expertise, and who is considered expert, particularly for underrepresented minorities, requires a heightened public visibility that reinforces both their status and their authority. In Rochester, local media rarely (if ever) feature black physicians, clinicians, and social scientists to explain the nature and the culture of health disparities, much less the social dynamics within and needs of the communities at risk. Meanwhile, black physicians in the San Francisco Bay Area complain of hypervisibility in the workplace in terms of micromanaging, bullying, and presumed incompetence.[10]

Diversifying the necessary steps to expertise is no easy task. Black and brown students continue to face challenges in STEMM disciplines. K–12 education in the US is not resourced equitably; that said, Historically Black Colleges and Universities (HBCUs) punch far above their weight in training excellent physicians, engineers, and biologists.[11] They serve as central avenues and intellectual nodes for diverse black, brown, and white footsteps to traverse across constructed boundaries, where they engage in the perennial grappling with the inherent paradoxes of science as truth and race as social fact. Hopefully they will gain true expertise, relevant to the communities they work with in the future, which affirms their identities, expands spaces of care and trust beyond churches, and fulfills the ancestors' footsteps toward a healthier, more dignified life.

NOTES

1 Pseudonyms used for all individuals and institutions named.
2 I continue to struggle mightily with usage of uppercase *Black* and lower-case *black*. In this chapter, I use the term *Black* in reference to its deployment as a categorical label, and the lowercase *black* as a descriptive label. I proceed mindful of the questionable relevance of these two terms as political and identarian referents, both of which offer little explanatory power once emptied of their respective categorical and descriptive labeling.
3 For an in-depth medical history of this era, see Tuchman (2020).
4 Wailoo (2014) offers a cogent illustration of the ways twentieth century African American urban settlement gave visibility both to sickle cell disease as well as its racialization.
5 The story of Henrietta Lacks and HeLa eventually found resonance in my project: The precipitous decrease in genomic sequencing costs that began in 2011 was following the mapping of the genome and epigenome of HeLa in 2013. As I relate in my book, these developments have contributed significantly to research examining human metabolic adaptation to environmental change.
6 For a comprehensive treatment of the sugar, slavery, and modernity triangulation, see Mintz (1985).
7 In fact, the only words uttered by an African, a servant, "Mistah Kurtz – he dead," occur toward the end of the book.
8 I address Spillers's ideation more fully in *Sweetness in the Blood: Race, Risk, and Type 2 Diabetes* (2021).
9 Lest one misinterpret this finding as an argument for racial risk, the authors clarify that this risk is mitigated by reduction in BMI.
10 Off-topic but worthy of mention – a colleague who wears a hijab experienced post-natal problems shortly after giving birth. Her pleas and complaints went unheeded by white doctors and nurses. She said that, only and finally, it was black women doctors that listened to her and provided the necessary care. See also NBC Bay Area News (2023).
11 At the time of this writing, I am in the Netherlands, mindful that neither HBCUs nor comprehensive STEMM diversification efforts exist in the European Union. "Diversity" in the EU is limited to gender, not race or ethnicity (which are unrecognized categories in EU countries). See Science Europe (2024).

REFERENCES

Conrad, Joseph. *Heart of Darkness*. (1899) 1996. New York: Palgrave Macmillan.
Doucet-Battle, James. 2021. *Sweetness in the Blood: Race, Risk, and Type 2 Diabetes*. Minneapolis: University of Minnesota Press.

Du Bois, W. E. B. 1906. *The Health and Physique of the Negro American*. Atlanta: Atlanta University Press.

Gomez, Michael Angelo. 1998. *Exchanging Our Country Marks: The Transformation of African Identities in the Colonial and Antebellum South*. Chapel Hill, NC: University of North Carolina Press.

Mintz, Sidney W. 1986. *Sweetness and Power: The Place of Sugar in Modern History*. New York: Penguin.

Mukaz, Debora Kamin, Melissa K. Melby, Mia A. Papas, Kelebogile Setiloane, Nwakaego Ada Nmezi, and Yvonne Commodore-Mensah. 2022. "Diabetes and Acculturation in African Immigrants to the United States: Analysis of the 2010–2017 National Health Interview Survey (NHIS)." *Ethnicity & Health* 27 (4): 770–80.

NBC Bay Area News. 2023. "How Does This Happen to All of Us?": Black Doctors Allege Discrimination at Sutter Health. May 13, 2023. https://www.nbcbayarea.com/investigations/how-does-this-happen-to-all-of-us-black-doctors-allege-history-of-discrimination-at-sutter-health/3228823/.

Science Europe. 2023. "Science Europe's Work on Equality, Diversity, and Inclusion." https://scienceeurope.org/news/se-work-on-edi/.

Spillers, Hortense. 2009. "Mama's Baby, Papa's Maybe." In *An American Grammar Book*.

Tuchman, Arleen Marcia. 2020. *Diabetes: A History of Race and Disease*. New Haven, CT: Yale University Press.

CHAPTER NINE

Disruption: Centering Native Youth Voices for Health and Healing in Arizona

Tommey Jodie, Jesse Pablo, Laurel Bellante, and Megan A. Carney

Our story begins with Tommey and Jesse. Tommey, twenty-one years old, grew up with the Diné tribe in northern Arizona. Her father was diagnosed with type 2 diabetes when she was very young. Her mother was diagnosed more recently, only a few years ago when Tommey was in high school. Jesse, thirty-one, has lived most his life on the Tohono O'odham reservation in the Sonoran Desert of southern Arizona, where more than 50 per cent of the population lives with adult-onset diabetes. Jesse spent much of his childhood with his grandparents, both of whom were diabetic, and very recently his dad was diagnosed with the disease.

In 2022, the four of us – Tommey, Jesse, Laurel, and Megan – met in the context of a year-long youth storytelling project centered on the themes of food and social justice at the University of Arizona. Laurel and Megan, as faculty members and mentors, coordinated various aspects of the project while providing support to the inaugural cohort of fourteen undergraduate student interns, which included Tommey and Jesse. As with other land-grant institutions, the University of Arizona resides on unceded land that was acquired through settler colonial violence, specifically toward the Tohono O'odham and Pascua Yaqui tribes.

In our chapter, we approach storytelling as a creative and collaborative method that can illuminate the complex dynamics behind the emergence of diabetes, the many ways of living with diabetes (and living well), and the power of youth in disrupting hegemonic epistemologies around health and food systems. We use storytelling to reflect upon the devastating disruptions of living with diabetes for Native peoples today and elucidate how they are directly linked to disruptions initiated by settler colonialism. However, we develop a practice of *disruption* as a necessary step in seeding counterstories that articulate different ways of understanding the roots of the problem and new visions for how to move forward. In other words, this chapter, and our stories, represent an effort to *disrupt* hegemonic narratives about this disease. Here, *disruption* through the creation of counterstories becomes a tool to steer us away from harmful narratives that position Native peoples as victims or frame metabolic diseases as solely a problem of individual choices and behaviors.

We center the voices of Native youth (Diné and Tohono O'odham) in narrating lived experiences with diabetes as they have witnessed the disease disrupt their communities while also finding ways to flourish otherwise. In Tommey's and Jesse's stories, we focus on three distinct aspects of this disruption: the disruptive harm presented by settler colonialism to Native ways of living with the land, the necessity of foregrounding counternarratives to disrupt hegemonic epistemologies around food and health systems, and disruption as a form of resistance, or a means of living well and flourishing otherwise. In what follows, first Tommey and then Jesse share poems and artwork followed by reflective prose to describe their struggles and to reassert their Indigenous identities, wisdom, and food practices to disrupt patterns of harm and sow possibilities for healing. Both storytellers offer observations of the legacy of colonialism in their communities, particularly as it relates to the disruptions of their food traditions and food access. They draw attention to how diabetes has emerged alongside an increased reliance on government allocations of commodity foods and the ongoing displacement of Indigenous communities from their original homelands, foods, and food practices. Readers are encouraged to follow the threads of current harms back to their historical origins. Both Tommey and Jesse emphasize storytelling as a vital tool for not only preserving ancestral knowledge, but also for devising more comprehensive understandings of, and solutions to, diabetes within Indigenous communities. Despite the overwhelming and ongoing challenges of managing diabetes within their families and communities, both authors also find hope in returning to, expanding, and sharing Indigenous foodways through both practice and story.

HELD BY THE LAND: TOMMEY'S STORY

When Diné (Navajo) girls have their first menstruation, we hold a ceremony called a Kinaaldá to mark the transition from girlhood to womanhood. This ceremony, first performed by Changing Woman, a central deity in Diné culture, symbolizes the four stages of life: infancy, childhood, adulthood, and old age. The poem below reflects this life journey and speaks to the critical role traditional practices play in maintaining health and well-being in the face of disruptions like diabetes. The Kinaaldá, a part of other life cycle ceremonies in Diné culture, fosters a deep connection to the land, our bodies, and our ancestral teachings, grounding us in the principles of balance and holistic health. These teachings emphasize the importance of nurturing ourselves and our communities, eating with reverence for the land, and practicing physical movement – core aspects of diabetes prevention.

The disruption of these life cycles and our associated practices of care and sustenance, whether through colonial violence, loss of food sovereignty, or disconnection from traditional knowledge, has contributed to the rise of diseases like diabetes in our communities. As a Navajo woman with a marginalized identity, the below poem reflects how I see myself moving through this world – carrying the responsibility of preserving my community's foodways, traditions, and health, while navigating the challenges of erasure and disruption. The character Morning Dawn represents all of us in this shared responsibility, reminding us that by honoring these life cycles, we fortify our communities and reclaim the balance necessary to protect ourselves from the rise of diseases like diabetes. As you read the poem, consider how ancestral knowledge is woven into our health, and how maintaining these connections offers a path toward healing for my people.

I. Birth

Gleams of glitter across the land signal the gift of Morning Dawn.
   Sleeping in the clouds, she was born in the closing hour of spring.
Molded by Talking God, she was a thought, a dream, a prayer, a remnant
   of the future.
   Some sudden wind at the vesper awakened her beauty.

Her first breath was always hers, half they took as joy.

    Medicine trickled onto holy grounds from above.

They river all around the lovesick dwelling, wrapping her in a blanket of

    home.

    Still lost in the holy world she cried, symphonies with no words.

Her hands shimmered through the air, catching coyote's many stars.

    Easily transcending a swell of blues to a mischievously sweet smile

that mimicked her ancestors' timeless quips.

    Clouding our anxious world for just a few minutes.

She is rematriation to this extracted desert.

    We praise the cord that would tether her heart to the land.

She will bring the rain to her people,

    as I linger within the mist.

II. Girlhood

Every day there is a praise song.

    The land sings a monument of songs for its children.

For its messengers of this colored earth

    The children whistle the tune of an ancient war.

Reminding our bodies of the turquoise drop, the arrowhead pointing

    Towards each field, an extension of our body

They welcome us home as a mother.

    As they welcome the naayízí, the naadą́ą́', the ch'ééhjiyáán in the

        spring.

Our palms smooth the sand, the pounding of vein, thunderstorms lather

    our field.

    And now everything is taboo/gluttonous bellies that consume every

        gathering.

Uncovering a violence within ourselves, while humming the words of

    forgotten hané.

    Because I cannot speak my own language, only the sound of a seed

        growing.

But I will still yell that the commodification of my tongue yields nothing.

    And whisper to ancestral stars for solace on unfamiliar lands

        This is somebody's home, yet I ache for mine.

At this age, we only know our homes, our siblings, and how far away they are.

III. Womanhood

In the quiet moments between dusk and dawn,
    When the world holds its breath/I feel the pulse of the land
A soft whispering wind that carries generations of voices across the
    canyons.
    Even as I stand on unfamiliar ground, my roots dig deep into the soil
Entwining prehistoric language to the persistence of our communities
    With winds that hold us in the gaps of our heartbreaks.
Even on horseback, our eyes will watch the stars.
    We see Morning Dawn aligning constellations.
Reconfiguring our world and plentiful fields to learn how the water flows
    together,
    How to carry the rushing inside of me.
I ask her not to forget how the wind whispers our NDN names. How
    America is a myth.
    Telling us sugar-coated lies about how I entered the Earth, how I'm sup-
        posed to die.
We laugh at the possibility of it. Land back. Swimming backwards in time.
    To light as light, food as food, and story as a reflection of time.
There has always been a resistance within us.
    An Indigenous regime of rematriation.
When we speak of sacredness, we speak of our own power from the land.
    Sacred mountains, sacred rivers, sacred medicines, sacred foods, sacred
        bodies.
It's in our cosmology.

IV. Old Age

We are now our stories foretold.
    We still stand on the shoulders of those who came before us.
Morning Dawn etched into our hearts, as a light that flows like rivers
    through our spinal cord.
    Yesterday, we were a mirage, but today we are moist with female rain.
Our fields seeping out the Earth's most radical bloom, remembering.
    This spring's thaw untangles my thoughts.
The Earth begins to soften beneath my feet as I speak of her beauty and
    persistence.
    The land likes hearing fond stories of herself too.

I tell her what I've learned:

Body and land are the same, maimed by one another.

Also known as tough love.

I am you, homeland to my heart; we cannot forget our own bodies.

Because you have also greatly suffered to return to me

Our bodies are innocent.

They will only show you what they know.

Let me show you what I know.

Reverting to the teachings of our ancestors and adapting these practices to meet contemporary threats has been a central solution for Indigenous food sovereignty scholars and a cornerstone of our resistance and survival. This ancestral knowledge, passed down through generations, has sustained us because our ancestors always knew the way. I would say that our spirituality is not faith-based but something we can feel, touch, and see. Which is why the knowledge I learn from my elders, parents, siblings, and community is so valuable. This knowledge is directly woven into my narratives. That's what generational knowledge is, and I preserve it through story. By sharing my stories, I can ensure that this knowledge continues to guide my people, helping us navigate both historical and ongoing challenges.

I feel an overwhelming need to preserve and pass on knowledge through story because that is the only way my people will survive. Our stories, especially our creation stories, have always been told orally from generation to generation – we've always been storytellers. Our stories help us remember – they are powerful. I can enter a safe space with subjects, symbols, and niche jokes that only Native people would truly understand. But they are also an analysis, ethnographic research that we do within our communities to both document and push back against colonial subjugation, assimilation, and the dispossession of our land and knowledge. This dispossession – whether through forced relocation, the suppression of our languages, or the loss of food sovereignty – has severed the ties between our people and the land that sustains us, creating the need for healing through the restoration of those relationships. Storytelling is a way for me to address histories of enslavement, colonialism, genocide, and land dispossession, while offering a path forward.

Most of us would much rather create a story, poem, or piece of art to discuss the ongoing fight against colonization within our communities because these creative expressions allow us to capture our struggles in ways that are more immediate and honest. Art and storytelling give us the freedom to express our lived experiences, free from academic constraints, and to connect deeply with our communities. My fight for abolition can be portrayed through poetry and beadwork, giving me a sense of purpose in this fast-paced world. In these spaces, I feel listened to and understood without needing to follow a specific model or be "correct." I create art in the way I want for my people, declaring that our stories are not just records of the past but living testaments to our strength. These creative expressions are not only personal but also contribute to a larger movement that seeks to redefine and reclaim our identity and future. As we reclaim our voices through art and story, we also open doors for addressing pressing challenges like diabetes. By integrating Indigenous knowledge into research, we can ensure that our pathways forward are guided by our own stories and traditions, helping us envision a healthier and more resilient future.

In the following paragraphs, I describe the various elements that have led to the diabetes epidemic in Indigenous communities. I critique the limited views of this disease as understood by Western scientists, who, despite their expertise, fail to fully grasp the complexities of our struggle – complexities deeply rooted in the ongoing and pervasive processes of settler colonialism. The manifestations of colonization continue to disrupt our lives in profound ways, and Indigenous people, who live these realities every day, are best equipped to understand and address these disruptions. However, our voices are underrepresented in crucial spaces like academia, health care, and media. To truly disrupt the disease, and the colonial frameworks that sustain it, we need more Indigenous researchers, scientists, storytellers, and changemakers to bring forward our perspectives and knowledge. Important examples of this kind of work by Indigenous scholars include *Mark My Words: Native Women Mapping Our Nations* by Mishuana Goeman, *Braiding Sweetgrass* by Robin Wall Kimmerer, *Decolonizing Methodologies* by Linda Tuhiwai Smith, and the work of Kyle Whyte on Indigenizing futures and decolonizing the Anthropocene, among others (e.g., Sanderson et al. 2012). By reclaiming our voices and perspectives, we can address the root causes of diabetes in our communities with a depth of understanding that has been missing from mainstream research.

Diabetes research often focuses on genetic and lifestyle factors but frequently overlooks the broader socioeconomic and historical contexts of what our ancestors have endured. Many studies examine the prevalence of diabetes within Indigenous communities through a narrow lens, missing the critical influences of colonization, loss of land, and the forced transition to Western diets high in processed foods by way of commodity foods. These "commodity foods" refer to surplus foods distributed by the US government to Native tribes, which are often calorie-dense, processed foods that are low in nutritional value and unfamiliar to Indigenous diets. These factors have drastically altered our traditional food systems and contributed to the high rates of diabetes we see today. Additionally, the persistent lack of access to quality health care and culturally relevant medical advice exacerbates the problem. Effective diabetes research must consider these elements to develop interventions that are not only medically sound but also culturally appropriate and sustainable.

It is crucial to acknowledge that most of the time scientists enter communities where they hold no ties and engage in research with an extractive approach. As Indigenous people, we have historically been ignored and disregarded when it comes to research. Our narratives, which detail the struggles against settler colonialism, food apartheid, and food insecurity, illuminate both the harsh realities we face and the remarkable strength and adaptive strategies we have employed in the face of diabetes. Yet, without intentionally listening to the community, researchers overlook the complex forces shaping our experiences, leaving out critical perspectives. This exclusion is not just a matter of oversight – it results in interventions and policies that are misaligned with the cultural, social, and environmental realities of our people. How a problem is framed greatly influences the solutions that emerge. Without incorporating our perspectives, any proposed solutions will inevitably fail to meet the true needs of our communities. Until Indigenous voices and stories are fully integrated into diabetes research, any understanding of the disease will remain limited, and any interventions will continue to fall short of addressing the root causes of diabetes in my community.

Given this history of exclusion and the ongoing need for more inclusive research, if you are reading this and want to engage in a different kind of research in Indigenous communities, take my advice: be upfront about your intentions. Engage with us openly, build genuine relationships, and use theoretical frameworks that carefully embrace the contributions of both Indigenous and Western ways of knowing. Without these conversations and relationships, recovery becomes more challenging for our communities because we are left out of the dialogue and excluded from decisions that directly impact our well-being. While many scientists and researchers aim to create a better future, Indigenous scientists, researchers, and storytellers engage in this work for the survival of our people, carrying the weight of our history and the hopes for our future. Our stories, poems, and ethnographic research are plausible pathways for you to listen to and understand our experiences and strengths.

Due to our ancestors' survival, we possess thousands of years of inherited knowledge, including traditional ecological knowledge, but this knowledge is often systematically excluded and invalidated by Western science. While this knowledge continues to exist in our communities, it has been eroded by the manifestations of settler colonialism over generations. Before this disruption, my people, the Diné, lived in harmony with the land in prospering communities with well-established food systems that satisfied their nutritional needs and no health disparities.

During the Mission and Removal Period, the US weaponized our food. They destroyed supplies, animals, and the land we depended on for survival, forcing us to rely on the government to live. Even though we knew it wasn't in our best interest, we had no choice. The Long Walk of 1863 introduced my people to government food distribution, which included unfamiliar and oppressive foods like salt, sugar, lard, and flour. This shift in diet traumatized our digestive and immune systems. This forced relocation also killed hundreds of Diné through exposure, starvation, and disease. But we survived due to the stories our Holy People told us through ceremony, prayer, and our creation stories.

On the other side of this deeply rooted colonial pain, there is Indigenous joy and celebration because our ancestors fought for our survival and won. Despite the pervasive impact of diabetes and the historical traumas our community has faced, there is a deep and abiding sense of joy that fills our lives. A profound sense of community and hope that constantly surrounds me. A growing movement dedicated to Indigenous food sovereignty and protecting current and future generations is taking root. We are reconnecting with each other, using traditional ways of knowing to combat this epidemic that has plagued our community for over a hundred years. We are mobilizing once again, saving seeds, renewing ourselves through planting – a ceremony in itself.

Every Diné family is affected by the diabetes epidemic. In my family, both of my parents are type 2 diabetics; my dad was diagnosed in his midtwenties, and my mom was diagnosed in her late fifties. As my mother's diagnosis was more recent, it scared me and reminded me that I am just as susceptible to this disease. With its hereditary nature, along with the systematic inequalities we face, there seems to be no escape. As a result, fellow Diné individuals and I have adapted to coexist with diabetes and its persistent threats to our way of life. This adaptation includes integrating traditional practices, seeking culturally relevant health care, and creating supportive communities. Our collective efforts are crucial in managing this disease and striving for a healthier future.

In this new era of community care, I am surrounded by joy and solidarity. As we take care of one another and our knowledge systems, I find myself looking at my parents with a renewed perspective. I no longer see diabetes as a consuming force; instead, I see possibility. This sense of mothering each other – being thoughtful and caring – defines who we have always been as Indigenous people. Reaffirming what I've always known growing up in a Diné-centric community, we are the leaders of public health because we were raised to take care of one another. Our collective effort and the joy that comes from it give me hope for fostering a healthier future with Indigenous people in it.

In my beadwork, I express our collective effort to return and practice recovery. It's looking forward and looking back so we can envision a better food system untouched by the ravages of colonial foods. We look back because our original instructions show that engaging with the desert landscape as a whole evokes an entire ecosystem that is the ultimate teacher. We look forward to reincorporating ancestral principles and beliefs into our future traditional food systems along with new ideas for our recovery. Reestablishing our traditional food systems is imperative to the cultural restoration and health of all Native people.

This beadwork is intended for everyone because the disruption of Native food systems shifted all aspects of our well-being and not many know about this disruption. Ideas like Indigenous food futurisms set the stage for change – that is, envisioning the future of Indigenous food systems and culinary traditions. This concept encompasses a variety of

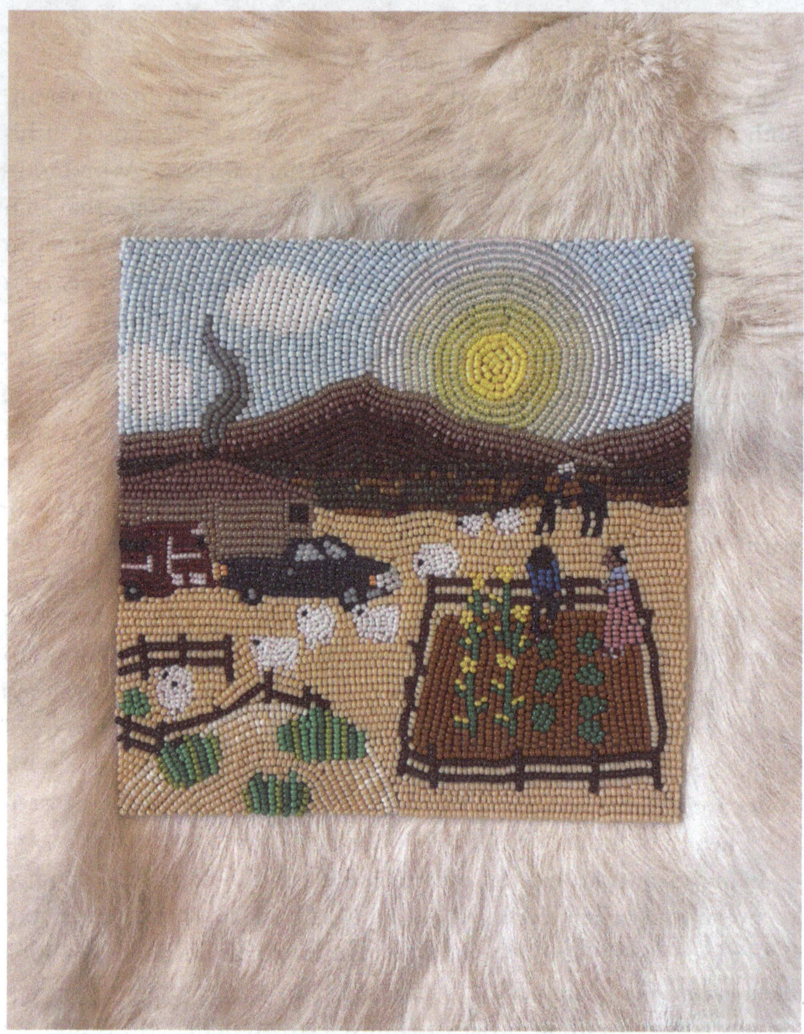

Figure 9.1: *I'm Going Home to Harvest* (Beadwork by Tommey Jodie).
This six-by-six-inch piece of handmade beadwork is an exploration of
Indigenous food futurisms. It displays the impacts of food sovereignty
on my home in Teesto, Arizona. Saddle Butte, a hill in the shape of a
saddle, looms in the distance. Closer, you can see a traditional hogan,
a horse trailer, a truck, a sheep corral, and my brother and me planting
and tending to the crops in the field. I intended for this piece to show
that Native people can rematriate, plant, cultivate, and harvest our own
foods again like we did consistently long ago, and in community.

perspectives, including those focused on the preservation and revitalization of traditional foods, sustainable agricultural practices, and the integration of Indigenous knowledge into contemporary food systems.

Native people can directly disrupt diabetes by providing ourselves with nutrient-rich diets, cultural reconnection, holistic health practices, and physical activity through traditional approaches. As Native youth, we hold the answers to the world's most pressing challenges. The emergence of diabetes can be combated through the influence of Native youth and our stories, as they are deeply rooted in joy and resilience, transcending the clinical understanding of the condition.

REMEMBERING WHAT WE'VE LOST IN ORDER TO REGAIN OUR FUTURE: JESSE'S STORY

Dreams of swollen feet that hold the absence of pain interrupts the slumber my body yearns for,

A dream negatively charged with a current known too well.

From the wave of the flag, absent of color, to a rapier drawn to my stomach containing the substance to make me well.

And the constant self-harm that remains so that I may see the level measurement, balance the solution contained in the living beaker, measure the economic value of choices made, bonds sold.

Good or bad, and "Will I regret this later?" is the question that stays afloat.

The hope to increase self-worth in the battle of supply and demand.

For I know without balance, blood stocks could rise or fall causing harm to the overall.

It is the signing of a loan in which 1x life is received with a collateral that is steep or a gamble on the life that remains with no safe points to be gained.

You can do this or that, but diabetes is what you have.

Open your eyes.

It was just a dream. Now what to do so that it does not become reality.

Diabetes. Native people know all too well what this disease can do to a family. I see myself succumbing to this disease; this dream (captured in the above poem) is a real and present threat. It is something that I have always feared, particularly after watching my grandparents battle the disease through the entirety of their adult lives. Their struggle was made harder by a lack of access to our traditional foods and, at the same time, an overabundance of high-calorie, "comfort" foods such as cookies and soda, and an overall lack of understanding of the disease and how to manage it effectively. I truly fear diabetes. I am trying to understand the causes behind this disease in my people and in my community, trying to save myself from the harsh truths that have become the realities for so many of us. It's always in the back of my mind. To confront diabetes, I want to understand why it has gotten this far and why there hasn't been a successful intervention to this epidemic for myself, my family, and my people.

At the beginning of my adulthood, I worked with youth in Native schools. The purpose of the program I worked with was to educate youth on the importance of cultural identity. We would go into classes and teach himadak (way of life). Within our first class, we asked "What is a traditional food?" to which the response would always be popovers (frybread), pinto beans, red chili, squash and cheese, and cemad (flour tortilla made from flour, lard, salt, and water). To hear this, over and over again, was soul crushing. The next generation of my people are ignorant to the culture shock that has befallen them. So many of these foods are adaptations from commodity foods, which are falsely identified now as traditional foods.

But what does this all have to do with diabetes? Let's review. This next generation sees foods that are not Indigenous as traditional. Foods that are cooked with greases such as lard or fatty oils, as well as loads of salt, sugar, and high-calorie ingredients. So, I ask again, how did people that had access to healthy foods become riddled with diabetes? The Tohono O'odham people have foods such as bawi (tepary beans), ha:d (drought-resistant squash), hu;n (sixty-day corn, which is the most drought-resistant corn in the world), mesquite beans, prickly pear, cholla buds, and saguaro fruit, to name a few. These are superfoods that have nourished my people for longer than I know or, to be honest, can even comprehend. So why? Why do I fear this disease? Why is it so pervasive? Why is it a common trait in my family? Why do the symptoms remain embedded in my mind? Symptoms such as limbs that are swollen and numb, headaches, stomachaches, nausea, and low or high blood sugar levels with little hope of regulating. Knowing that some must administer insulin through a shot in the stomach daily just to regulate blood sugar. Why?

The Tohono O'odham call the Sonoran Desert home; we historically thrived from the nourishment that this place provides. The knowledge of wild foods, as well as traditional domesticated Tohono O'odham crops, constituted what my people knew as himadak. To survive in the desert, my people knew that there was an order or cycle to the world. These lessons were passed down through generations by oral tradition. Historically, the Tohono O'odham people were known as farmers and runners, who nourished the body with crops native to the O'odham. These crops adapted and thrived in the desert, making some of them the most drought-resistant crops in the world. How, then, did a sovereign people that thrived in such an extreme environment as that of the Sonoran Desert fall victim to a disease like diabetes? How do people with access to such nourishing foods become a people suffering the highest rates of diabetes?

This fate started with the loss of our culture upon the arrival of non-Native people. When outside people came in, forcing their ways of life on the tribe, many disruptions began, forcing children, youth, and the next generation of Tohono O'odham culture to abandon our way of life and severing us from our traditional himadak. This led to a loss of culture and identity, resulting in a depletion in the production of foods that were crucial to Tohono O'odham survival. This also led to the acceptance of commodity foods that have become those traditional foods I mentioned earlier. We now know these lead to obesity and diabetes.

But as I contemplate this history, I can't help but wonder how much of this ongoing loss of our traditional diets was premeditated. During the boarding school era, there was a phrase that dominated the assimilation and reeducation of Native people. That phrase was "save the man, kill the Indian."[1] What a horrific combination of words. But does this sentiment remain?

Returning to the present time, how many Native tribes have lost their culture, land, and homes? So much of this loss ties to the loss of our Native foods. Without our identity, we lose our way of life. People become reliant and make do with what is provided.

Today, I grow traditional Tohono O'odham crops. These crops are known as the ha:l (squash), hu:n (corn), and bawi (tepary beans).

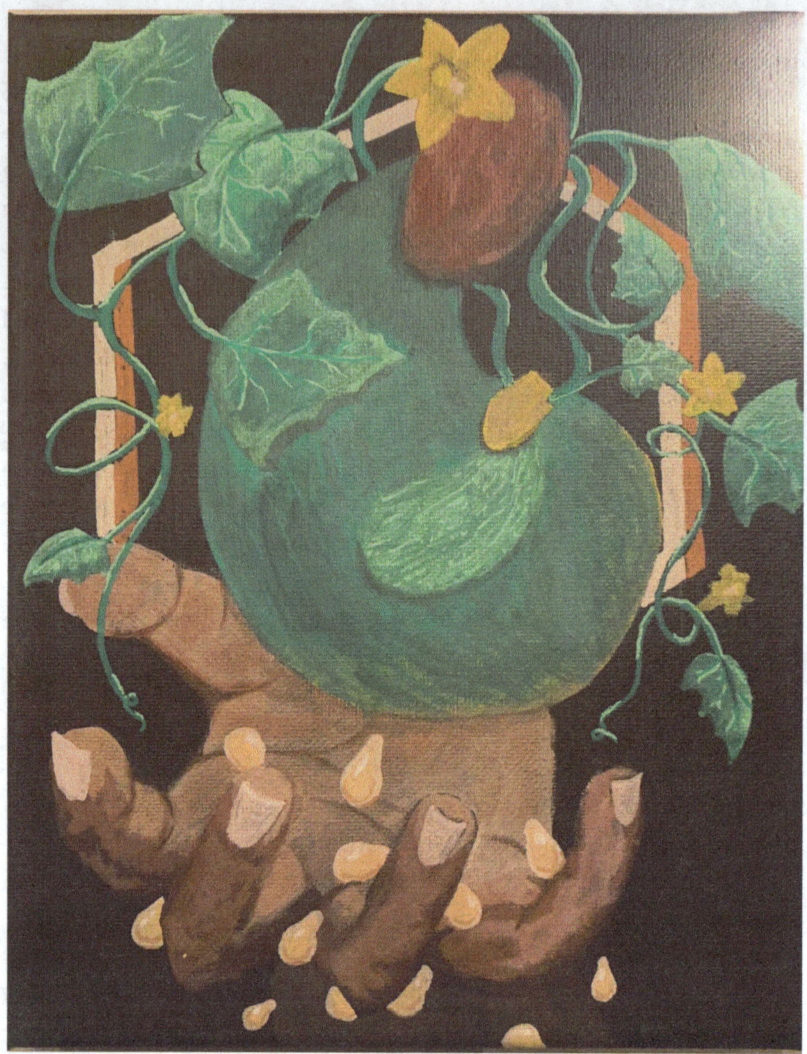

Figure 9.2: *Squash Mother* (Painting by Jesse Pablo)

Growing these plants makes me strong, resilient, and hardworking. They also give me a purpose. For a long time, I felt that I was missing something inside, that there was a piece of me that just seemed to be lost. Learning to farm gave me the ability to finally find the piece that was missing. This piece turned out to be my culture. As a Tohono O'odham youth, I knew that I was this person, but I never knew what that meant. I come from a strong heritage, but there are a lot of wounds

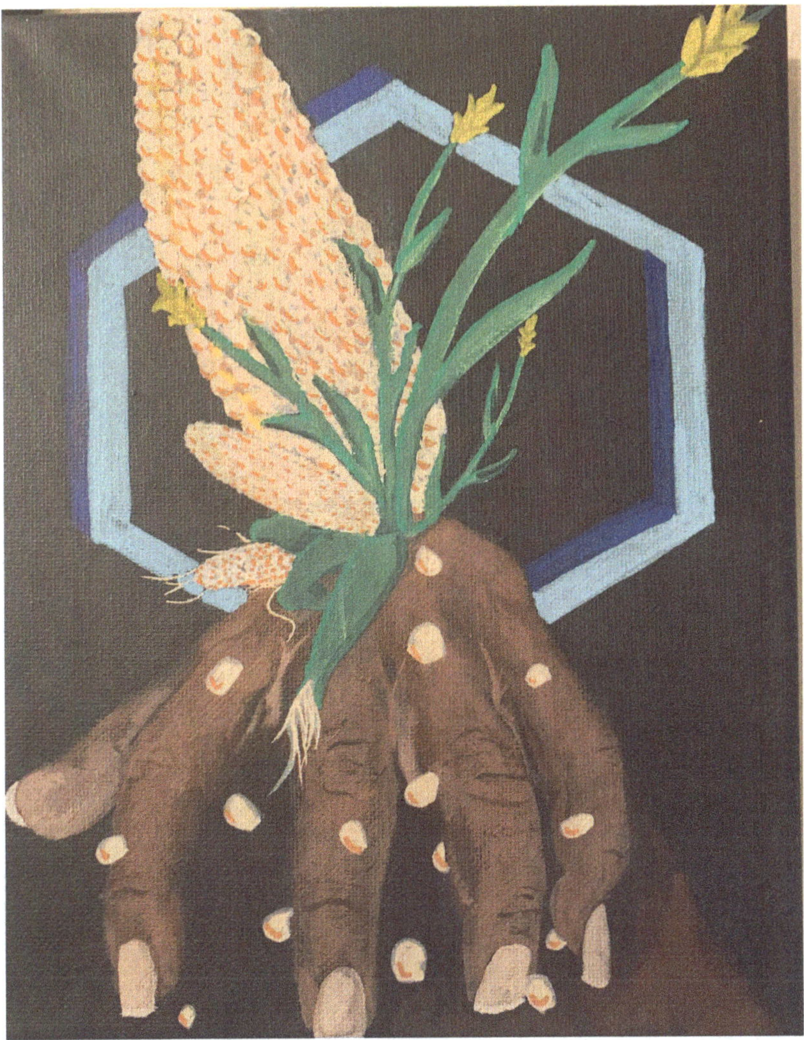

Figure 9.3: *Gift of Corn* (Painting by Jesse Pablo)

that need healing. Knowing that I am this person and being this person are two different things. I truly believe I am this person now: I am a teacher, student, caregiver, dependent. I am just another seed growing in this field we call earth. I am an Oidagem (farmer)! My people have been here since long before I existed, and they will be here long after I'm gone. I just hope that my presence will be known, and when I do go to whatever comes next, I will be able to say I lived, loved, spoke, taught,

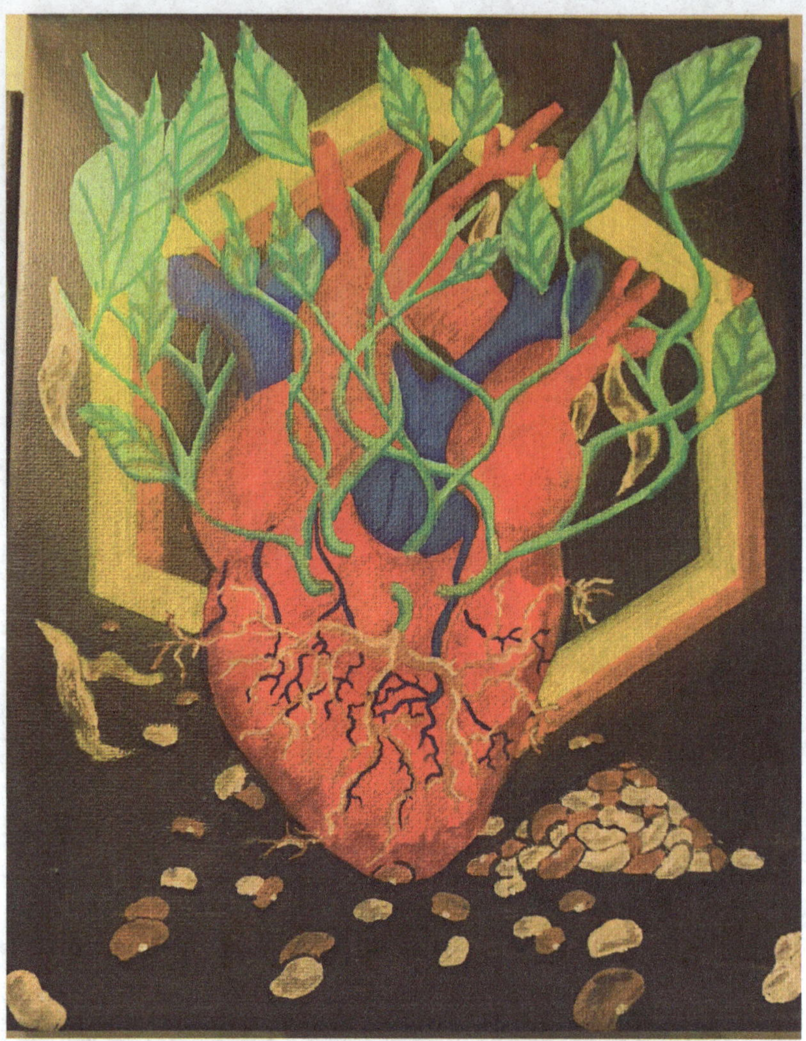

Figure 9.4: *Heart of the Desert* (Painting by Jesse Pablo)

and shared as much as I possibly could so the O'odham (people) would continue to thrive on this gift of a world we have. It was a seed that changed it all for me.

I will leave you with these words: Plant a seed, help it grow, and I hope you'll see that any hand can make a difference. One plant can become many; many plants can feed a people; and many people can preserve a world.

LIVING WELL, A COLLECTIVE ENDEAVOR

Type 2 diabetes is a pathology of settler colonialism. Within the United States, the prevalence of diagnosed diabetes is highest among American Indian and Alaska Native adults (16 per cent, compared with 7.6 per cent of non-Hispanic whites; CDC 2022). The disproportionate burden of illness presented not only by diabetes but also other health problems in Native communities, such as obesity and heart disease, is frequently framed by biomedical practitioners and researchers as the result of individual-level behaviors or deficits, such as poor diet, high BMI, lack of exercise, lack of knowledge, or yet-to-be-identified genetic factors (Benyshek, Martin, and Johnston 2010). Yet such framings overlook extensive evidence that the origins of the diabetes epidemic and other diet-sensitive health problems in Native communities trace back to the introduction of US government-subsidized food assistance during the 1940s (Coté 2016; Jernigan 2018; Young 1994). They also disregard the robust body of literature that demonstrates how ongoing environmental circumstances, such as food insecurity and the conditions of food apartheid introduced vis-a-vis land dispossession, forced removal, and circumscribing of reservations, have translated to negative health outcomes and lower life chances among Native people (Jernigan et al. 2016; Schulz et al. 2006; Sowerwine et al. 2019). Data suggest that food insecurity affects Native communities, specifically American Indians and Alaska Natives, at twice the rate compared to whites (Jernigan et al. 2016). Efforts to reintroduce Native foods and restore Native food systems, including efforts to build Native food sovereignty, have been declared essential to countering the embodied harms of settler colonialism, revitalizing culture, and nourishing community health and well-being (Coté 2016; Patchell and Edwards 2014; Sowerine et al. 2019).

In preparing to co-author this chapter, we embarked on a critical dialogue about present realities and aspirations toward living *well* with diabetes. It has become clear to us that any notion of living well with diabetes needs to be reframed as a collective endeavor. Yet, we identified many structural barriers to making this happen revolving around land, ancestral foods, diabetes awareness, tribal relations, and colonized subjectivities. Jesse alluded to the need for ancestral foods to be consistently available and affordable: "I want to be able to produce local sustainable foods, traditional foods, for a reasonable price, but have it constantly available." He also emphasized the need for educational initiatives that would reintroduce Native foods. Both Tommey and Jesse described a lack of diabetes education and support, and noted that the topic is even somewhat taboo, with Jesse saying, "We want to talk about it, but it just terrifies people." Relatedly, we discussed the ways in which diabetes is often discursively normalized and naturalized, contributing to symbolic violence within Native communities. As Tommey stated, "[Diabetes] is often talked about like 'It's just the way' or 'It's normal,' 'It just happens,' 'Everyone goes through it, so I'm not affected by it.' But it's not normal or natural. How can we come up with a solution to disrupt this way of thinking?"

By way of conclusion, we close with words from Tommey and Jesse as an example of the ongoing resistance of Native youth to the disruptive harms that they inherited and the alternative futures that they seek to seed and nourish.

> As I reflect on the journey shared in these pages, I'm reminded of the deep connections between disruption, diabetes, and storytelling. Each word captures the historical and ongoing impacts of settler colonialism on Indigenous communities, particularly in how it has disrupted our traditional ways of life and health. Diabetes isn't just a disease; it is a symptom of the larger disruptions that have altered our diets, eroded our food systems, and impacted our bodies in ways our ancestors never faced. Yet, our stories remain powerful tools of resilience and survival. Through storytelling, we reclaim our narratives, reaffirm our identity, and resist the forces that have tried to erase us. Our stories allow us to document our struggles, honor our past, and envision a future where we are not just surviving but thriving.
>
> We all share a responsibility to create healthy change and to honor our deep responsibility to the earth. But now, it's time for Indigenous people to reclaim our identity and rebuild our strength through nourishing foods and intergenerational collaboration. We must continue to connect with our elders by passing on their knowledge to younger generations. We are the vessels carrying this work forward, ensuring that our children grow up as healthy, empowered leaders. Our future is in our hands, and we

cannot wait for others to inspire us; we are already empowered by the strength of our ancestors. It is our time to lead with visionary change, creating environments of growth, stability, and sustainability. We must embrace this stewardship, caring for the earth as we care for each other, and be present for the future by being good ancestors today.

– Tommey

I have found myself lucky to be put in a place where I have been able to learn about traditional foods and how these superfoods have nourished us for generations. Currently, I am attending the University of Arizona to become certified in agricultural education so that I can return home to teach in my local high school and inspire youth to move forward with knowledge of our cultural identity and food practices. I only hope that one day these superfoods are available for all to enjoy and can serve as one way to help us to take back our health. Historically, cultural knowledge in O'odham culture was not hoarded or selfishly kept. As someone who wants to be an educator, my hope is to pass this knowledge on by any means, whether through education, ceremony, or even through art and storytelling as shared here. I understand that I am just one man, but with the help of others, even just one, two, three, or a hundred, we can begin to heal the wounds that one day will become scars. Over time, perhaps these scars will fade, becoming only memories, and will no longer be the nightmare that currently haunts me and disrupts the lives of so many of my people.

–Jesse

GLOSSARY

Diné Terms

ch'ééhjiyáán – Watermelon
hané – Story
Kinaaldá – Puberty ceremony
naadą́ą́' – Corn
naayízí – Squash

Tohono O'odham Terms

bawi – Tepary beans

cemad – Flour tortilla made from flour, lard, salt, and water

ha:d – Drought-resistant squash

himadak – Way of life

hu;n – Sixty-day corn, which is the most drought-resistant corn in the
   world

oidagem – Farmer

NOTE

1 Captain H. R. Pratt was the first to circulate this horrible phrase in a speech
   delivered in 1892. This and other of Pratt's ideas became foundational to
   assimilation programs, including boarding schools aimed at "civilizing" and
   "Americanizing" Native populations in the US. For more information, see
   Carlisle Indian School Digital Resource Center (n.d.).

REFERENCES

Benyshek, D. C., J.F. Martin, and C. S. Johnston. 2010. "A Reconsideration
   of the Origins of the Type 2 Diabetes Epidemic Among Native Americans
   and the Implications for Intervention Policy." *Medical Anthropology* 20 (1):
   25–64.

Carlisle Indian School Digital Resource Center. n.d. "Kill the Indian in him,
   and save the man": R. H. Pratt on the Education of Native Americans."
   Teaching Resources. Accessed July 7 2025. https://carlisleindian
   .dickinson.edu/teach/kill-indian-him-and-save-man-r-h-pratt-education
   -native-americans.

Carney, M. A. 2022. "Whiteness and Settler Colonial Logics in the Pacific Northwest
   Craft Beer and Hops Industries." *Food, Culture, and Society* 26 (1): 1–24.

Centers for Disease Control and Prevention (CDC). 2022. *National Diabetes
   Statistics Report.* https://www.cdc.gov/diabetes/data/statistics-report
   /index.html.

Coté, C. 2016. "'Indigenizing' Food Sovereignty: Revitalizing Indigenous Food
   Practices and Ecological Knowledges in Canada and the United States."
   Humanities 5 (3): 57. https://doi.org/10.3390/h5030057.

Elm-Hill, R., R. M. Webster, and A. Allen. 2023. *Serving Native Youth: A Dialogue
   on Native Food Sovereignty and Native Food Security.* First Nations Development
   Institute. https://www.firstnations.org/wp-content/uploads/2023/04
   /Serving-Native-Youth-04April2023.pdf.

Garth, H., and A. M. Reese, eds. 2020. *Black Food Matters: Racial Justice in the
   Wake of Food Justice.* Minneapolis: University of Minnesota Press.

Goeman, M. 2016. *Mark My Words: Native Women Mapping Our Nations.*
Minneapolis: University of Minnesota Press.

Guthman, J. 2011. "If They Only Knew: The Unbearable Whiteness of
Alternative Food." In *Cultivating Food Justice: Race, Class and Sustainability,*
edited by A.H. Alkon and J. Agyeman, 263–81.

Jernigan, K. A. 2018. *Embodied Heritage: Obesity, Cultural Identity, and
Food Distribution Programs in the Choctaw Nation of Oklahoma.* Doctoral
Dissertation. https://doi.org/10.7275/12340783.

Jernigan, V. B. B., K. R. Huyser, J. Valdes, and V. W. Simonds. 2017. "Food
Insecurity Among American Indians and Alaska Natives: A National Profile
Using the Current Population Survey–Food Security Supplement." *Journal
of Hunger & Environmental Nutrition* 12 (1): 1–10. https://doi.org/10.1080
/19320248.2016.1227750.

Kimmerer, Robin Wall. 2013. *Braiding Sweetgrass: Indigenous Wisdom, Scientific
Knowledge, and the Teachings of Plants.* Milkweed Editions.

Mohanty, Chandra Talpade. 2003. *Feminism Without Borders: Decolonizing Theory,
Practicing Solidarity.* Durham: Duke University Press.

Patchell, B., and K. Edwards. 2014. "The Role of Traditional Foods in Diabetes
Prevention and Management Among Native Americans." *Current Nutrition
Reports* 3: 340–44. https://doi.org/10.1007/s13668-014-0102-6.

Pine, A., and R. de Souza. 2022. "Hunger, Survivance, and Imaginative
Futures: A Racial Analysis of the 'Right to Food'." In *Organizing Food Justice:
Critical Organizational Communication Theory Meets the Food Movement,* edited
by S.E. Dempsey.

Reese, A. M. 2019. *Black Food Geographies: Race, Self-reliance, and Food Access in
Washington, D.C.* Chapel Hill, NC: University of North Carolina Press.

Sanderson, P. R., M. Little, M. M. Vasquez, B. Lomadafkie, M. Brings Him
Back-Janis, O.V. Trujillo, K. Jarratt-Snider, N.I. Teufel-Shone, B.C. Brown,
and R. Bounds. 2012. "A Perspective on Diabetes from Indigenous Views."
Fourth World Journal 11 (2): 57–78.

Schulz, L. O., P. H. Bennett, E. Ravussin, J. R. Kidd, K. K. Kidd, J. Esparza, and
M. E. Valencia. 2006. "Effects of Traditional and Western Environments
on Prevalence of Type 2 Diabetes in Pima Indians in Mexico and the U.S."
Diabetes Care 29 (8): 1866–71. https://doi.org/10.2337/dc06-0138.

Slocum, Rachel. 2007. "Whiteness, Space, and Alternative Food Practice."
Geoforum 38 (3): 520–33.

Sowerwine, J., M. Mucioki, D. Sarna-Wojcicki, et al. 2019. "Reframing Food
Security by and for Native American Communities: A Case Study Among
Tribes in the Klamath River Basin of Oregon and California." *Food Security*
11: 579–607. https://doi.org/10.1007/s12571-019-00925-y.

Smith, Linda Tuhiwai. 2021. *Decolonizing Methodologies: Research and Indigenous
Peoples.* London: Bloomsbury Publishing.

Whyte, K. 2017. "Indigenous Climate Change Studies: Indigenizing Futures,
Decolonizing the Anthropocene." *English Language Notes* 55 (1): 153–62.

Diabetes Is about *More than* Diet

Virginia receives a diabetes diagnosis shortly after giving birth to a fourth
child, marking the beginning of a challenging journey that ultimately
impacts family life and her sense of identity. Virginia, who once conjured
culinary magic, finds herself consuming more pills than tortillas as her
health spirals toward an untimely end.

Doña Teresa, a lively force from San Martín, expertly manages her diabetes
and high blood pressure while weaving a tapestry of community care that
underscores the vital role of social connections in health.

Emilia, an American anthropologist grappling with her own chronic health
issues, discovers through Doña Teresa the power of traditional remedies and
community support in navigating Mexico's rural health-care complexities.

Don Agustín, a dedicated weaver and village leader from Xaagá, grapples
with the intricacies of diabetes while honoring his family's weaving legacy,
illustrating how community support and traditional knowledge fuel his
resilience.

The stories thus far have introduced the ways that diabetes is both
a reflection of distinct social and cultural worlds and an illness that
shapes relational dynamics across the globe. You have read about the
endless everyday work people do to "manage" their diabetes, even in
instances where their numbers may not reflect their efforts. We have
also described the enduring impact of historical, social, political, and
economic patterns that shape life chances – what scholars refer to as

biopolitics. This section puts diet at the center of these approaches and considers how ideas, recipes, and practices around the world become central to diabetes stories.

Each year, significant resources are allocated to health education aimed at managing diabetes through simple behavior changes. Diabetes education classes encourage reducing fat, salt, and sugar and increasing physical activity. These efforts, though globally consistent, are delivered within profoundly different contexts, and scholars show this uniformity is not accidental, but influenced by cultural and political forces in nutritional science. Perhaps the most famous and influential expert in nutritional science and politics is Marion Nestle. She has dedicated her career to exploring how the ever-increasing complexity of nutritional science is more of a hindrance than help, and how the culture and politics around food may be more powerful in determining what you eat than individual psychology. In fact, the simplicity of the message that has remained the same for decades – "Eat less, move more, eat more fruits and vegetables, and don't eat too much junk food" – is made opaque by the role of capitalist forces in our food markets. Food industries provide enormous funding for nutritional research, revealing how corporate interests often distort scientific findings to promote unhealthy products.

Lines between food and medicine are often blurred, just as the connections between biomedical pharmaceuticals and clinical care and good health are hard to disentangle. The narratives of the chapters to come reveal that the management of diabetes is far more complex than merely adhering to dietary recommendations. The experiences of the people in these narratives illustrate the intricate interplay between cultural practices, economic constraints, and social relationships in shaping health outcomes. As we delve deeper into the relationship between food, health, and community, we must ask ourselves: How can we better integrate cultural understandings of food into public health strategies aimed at managing diabetes? In what ways do the social dynamics of food preparation and sharing enhance or complicate diabetes management for individuals and their communities? How might a more nuanced understanding of inherited chronic conditions inform future approaches to diabetes education and care?

CHAPTER TEN

Iatrochemistry: Recipes that Heal

Emily Yates-Doerr

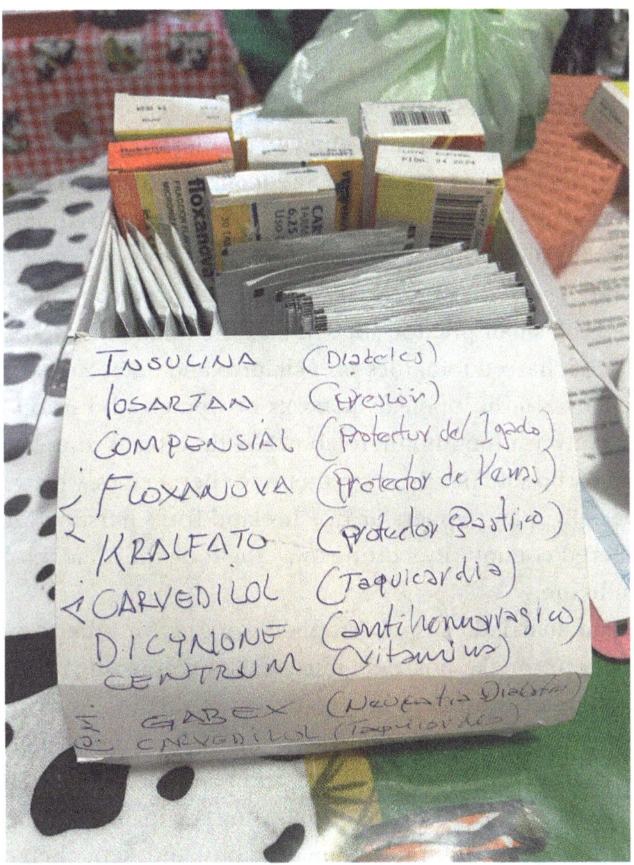

Figure 10.1: Pharmaceutical packets and a list of medications

A doctor diagnosed Virginia with diabetes shortly after the birth of her fourth child. Her head had been hurting, her vision was frequently blurry, and she found herself unstable on her feet. It was not a surprise. It seemed that everyone around her had diabetes. But her mother and grandmother had both died young, so in that sense the disease was unfamiliar – not known in her family, until then.

By the time I met Virginia she had lived under the diagnosis for more than a decade. In photographs of her youth, she appears strong, a large smile spreading across her full, dimpled cheeks. She had grown up on a farm on the low, hot plains of Guatemala among sorghum, tobacco, and ranchers. She described herself as a tomboy – always outside with the animals. But tomboy isn't much of a profession, so eventually she took a job as a housekeeper in Guatemala's capital. Trading farm life for a life in the metropolis, she stopped playing in the fields and instead learned to clean and cook. She had shrugged off school when she was younger and didn't feel confident reading and writing, but she began to decipher cookbooks. She liked learning their recommendations for mixing flavors and ingredients. One woman she worked for was from a Mexican family, and Virginia enjoyed the detective work required to cook Mexican food in Guatemala. She scoured markets to find vendors who sold the chipotle and ancho peppers or cloves and cinnamon used in recipes for mole. She also liked preparing foods from her ranching community: *churrascos* of thinly sliced beef with green onions blackened over the grill, small potatoes boiled and then pan seasoned, and *chirmol* sauce of charred tomatoes with cilantro and lime. Most produce in Guatemala is sold in open-air markets by women who sit on blankets and mix conversation into their labor. She developed connections with the people who sold her the ingredients for her recipes, who would save her especially spicy peppers or ripe lowland fruits bursting with flavor. They offered community, cutting away the loneliness she felt by being far from home.

After she married, Virginia stopped working for other women and instead began to take boarders into her home – mostly university students or travelers who slept in one of the two side rooms of her house. This was how we came to meet each other fifteen years ago. I was in Guatemala looking for a place to live, and I became a beneficiary of her care. I knew she did this work, in part, for the income. As with many Guatemalan families, Virginia and her husband kept their finances separate, and costs for her diabetes pill prescriptions and consultation were considerable. Still, I never heard Virginia offer a rate. The guests usually left folded bills on their pillowcases or in an envelope on the desk in the room, so there was an exchange, but this was not a clear-cut transaction since the give and take never lined up. She emphasized that people would pay what they could, and she, in turn, liked the activity of cooking.

Back then, when she was still busy in the kitchen, she piled our plates high with tortillas and eggs, and learned about our favorite foods so she could serve them when we stayed with her. Many of us were returning guests who benefitted over many years from her expertise. She grew the herbs she knew we liked in her windowsill garden, making us licorice or fig teas at night to stave off the evening cold. Black beans are an especially beloved food throughout Guatemala. Virginia bought hers from a woman in the market who cultivated them in nearby mountain soils for their taste. "They have three lives," Virginia told us. In their first life – their young life – they are cooked under pressure in tremendous heat with a touch of salt, where they become soft. These beans are eaten whole, each one a gift. In their second life, they are sauteed with onion and garlic and then mashed together in an electric blender, forming a thick, flavorful soup. Their third life is the richest and rarest: the soup is pan fried over low heat until the moisture disappears, leaving a black-bean recreation that is soft as butter and full of taste. She would marvel at the three phases of their life, pointing out to us how one recipe was recycled into another so none of the beans she cooked ever went to waste.

Her husband, looking at the food and the guests around the table, would shake his head, telling her to charge more – to charge *something*. When he wasn't in the room, she lifted her fist and tapped her forearm to signal that he was stingy. He worried about scarcity, complaining that their resources were finite, and, in this world of limited goods, their family would run out. She responded by piling more tortillas on the table so that the meal for whatever number of people would expand to be enough. Soups and stews worked especially well for sharing, so she served these often, placing bone broth with cabbage and carrots in the center of the table with a stack of tortillas next to our bowls. Additional guests or children or cousins would drop by, and the broth and tortillas would spread. We would eat, and after we finished, we would push

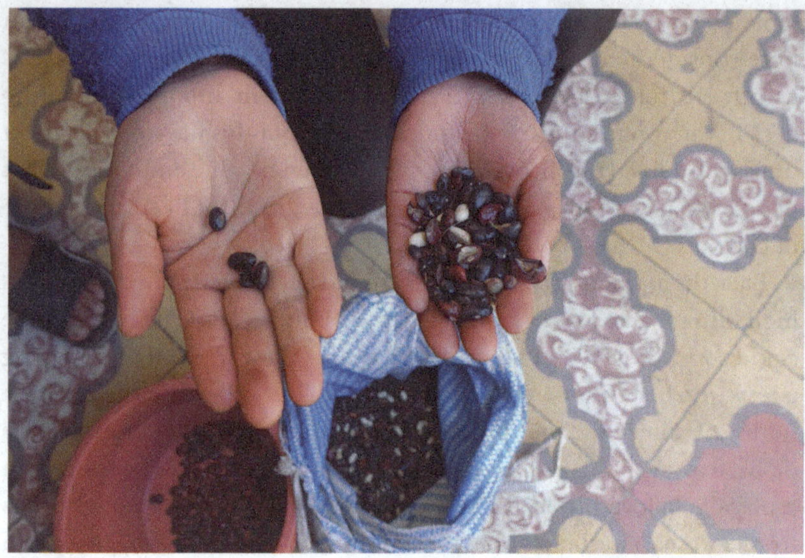

Figure 10.2: Expert cooks filter through beans, selecting ones with good taste and texture

back our chairs to talk about news and politics, the day behind us, our hopes for our futures, and other things that either barely mattered or mattered significantly in our lives. She would clear the dishes into the sink to wash later, boiling water for tea or coffee while looking over ingredients on her shelves as she began to plan what we would eat next.

The world she was working to make was one where her hospitality was not sold for a price. "I am lonely without company," she would explain when I asked her why she, who was poor, brought strangers into her home and cared for them. "You want to offer me something?" she would ask rhetorically, before providing her answer: "Come back." In her practice of nourishment, *use* did not lead to depletion – using was not *using up*. Instead, her meals were a practice of regeneration, a way of helping the communities around her to grow.

FÁRMACOS

In the last years of her life, Virginia suffered from the excruciating effects of liver failure – a side effect of diabetes, she said. The organ that

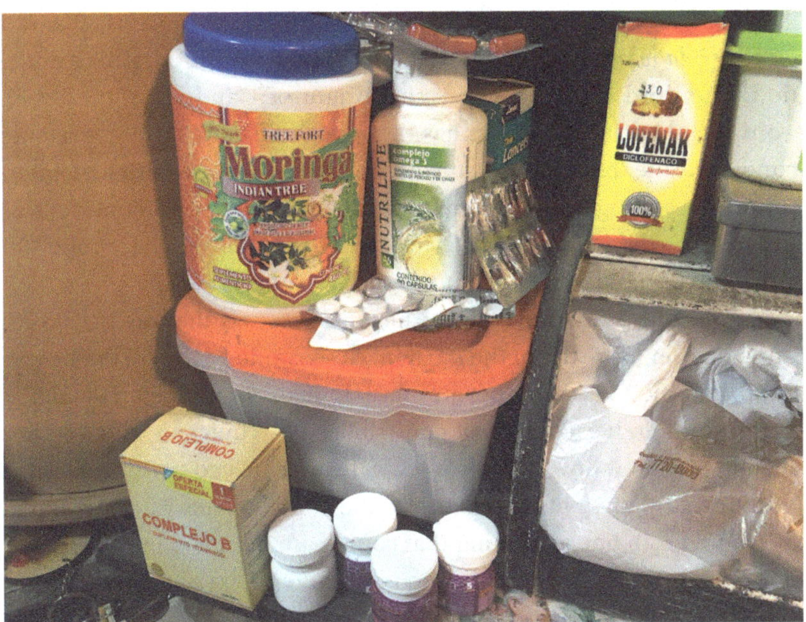

Figure 10.3: A bread box in Virginia's house was filled with diabetes-related medications she had collected over the years

filtered toxins from her blood had become swollen and scarred. Many associate liver failure with alcohol, but Virginia never drank. "My cocktail is drugs," she said with dark humor as the pills piled up. Her kitchen shelves were packed with *fármacos*, which began to overtake food. A bread box on her counter opened to reveal boxes and packages. The pills had brand names and off-brand names, and there were also satchels filled with concoctions of chemicals and herbs. One doctor would advise her one way. The pills might help for a while, but never for long. The medication might become too expensive, or the corner store pharmacy might run out of stock. Brands would change, and then the advice would change as new treatments entered her daily life. She'd meet with clinicians in the public hospital – in Guatemala the services at the national hospitals are free to everyone. She'd also save for private consultations, which is what anyone who can afford it does for care because of the long waits and high staff turnover in the national system. Although it didn't really matter whether the care was private or public since the advice was usually the same: "Avoid sugar, avoid fatty foods, change your behavior, change what you eat. If you want to feel better, take these drugs."

What do we call the fate of being poisoned by that which is meant to give life? *Iatrogenesis* is a good word for characterizing Virginia's affliction. The word comes from *genesis* – origin of – and *iatros*, the Greek word for physician (*pediatrics* has the *iatros* built into it). In iatrogenic conditions the treatment has furthered the disease, a health-care intervention operating not as remedy, but malady. Some might consider this the terrain of irony, but that term implies ignorance. Meanwhile, Virginia had known her treatment was shoddy since it began.

Among the many tragedies of her diabetes was the way the illness undercut her expertise in the kitchen. At sixty-odd years old, the hearth and mealtime table were her primary domains of mastery. Her skill – her position in her family – was destabilized by clinicians who told her she did not know how to cook or eat. She once hosted a visitor, Kevin, a nutrition student in his twenties from the United States. She had hoped he would teach her something that could ease her pain, but he offered her platitudes she had heard a thousand times: Less sugar, less oil. Did you know carrots are bad for you? Have you stopped eating beets? By then, she had tried every diet there was to try, contorting her appetite into knots. Still, none of the restrictions seemed to help, as her cells stopped responding to insulin and the pain in her liver remained strong. It is a banal, if terrifying story: Diets failed. Foods failed. Medications failed, too. Prescriptions for pills overtook her recipes. In Spanish the words for *prescription* and *recipe* are the same word, *receta*, but for Virginia there was no equivalence in this exchange.

As diabetes intensified, time began to move differently in her body. At the end of her life, she was frail – as if she were decades older than she was. The right side of her face drooped where she had lost muscle tone, leaving her eye half-closed even when it was open. She walked with an obvious limp. Her veins were swollen, but her skin was gaunt. She lived with pain everywhere – in her hands, her limbs, her heart. Hers was not typical aging. She was not grappling simply with the fate of death that will eventually overtake us all, but with the particular injustice of being robbed of her health by treatment pathways meant to make her well.

She should have been bouncing her plump grandchildren on her knees or singing them lullabies. Instead, her grandchildren spent their time at her house mostly in front of screens. Virginia's children would drop their children off with her in the morning – they had to go to work and could not afford day care. The ones in elementary school would make themselves breakfast in front of the television before leaving for school, the baby and toddler lying in cribs just outside Virginia's small room for hours on end with the phones they held in their chubby fingers to entertain them. Virginia could call a neighbor if she really needed help, but she was in too much pain to get out of bed. There is no shame in using mobile devices to help with the work of parenting – she had no other choice – but the hours a day her grandbabies spent watching videos on small screens was not what Virginia wanted for them or for herself. Along with the feeling of elevated blood sugar that plagued her, she felt the intergenerational loss of being a grandparent who cannot fully participate in the work of making kin.

CALCULUS OF SAVING

I'm uncertain of sharing some of these narrative details – of turning Virginia's suffering into spectacle – but I think it's important to spend time on her experiences because of forces that have worked to discount them from mattering, overriding her own strategies for living well. Not long after I started researching metabolic illnesses in Guatemala, I began to hear that middle-aged people with diabetes were not contained within the calculus of saving. Policymakers were reclassifying diabetes and similar metabolic illnesses as *epigenetic* and not clinical disorders, meaning that they were problems that should be treated by preventative health-care programs in early life. By the time people arrived at the health-care clinic with diabetes, it was already too late. One health expert, pointing to the expense and challenge of treating diabetes in adult bodies, told me that energy should not be wasted on the treatment of the already afflicted. It would be more efficient to consider diabetes as a problem of maternal nutrition, he explained. "Since the present was epigenetically programmed by the past, we cannot do anything for most health problems of today. It is only the future that can be saved," he said, making a plea to focus on improving metabolic pathways in early life and not on elder care.

The World Health Organization (2024) reports that global rates of diabetes rose from 108 million people with diabetes in 1980 to 422 million with diabetes in 2014. According to the International Diabetes Federation, 537 million people are living with diabetes today, with more than 4 million deaths from diabetes each year and the number of deaths steadily rising (2024). Drawing on data published in 2019, the Pan-American Health Organization (2024) points to Guatemala as having the sixth highest death rate from diabetes in the Americas, with 63.2 people dying for every 100,0000. The organization describes the burden of diabetes in terms of "years of lost life" (calculating this as 6.2 million years of lost life in the Americas in 2019) and "years of life lived with disability" (calculating this as 7.2 million years of life lived with disability in 2019).

Global health experts also frequently calculate the "burden" of diabetes in terms of lost economic productivity, with diabetics less able to contribute to economic growth. Health economists warn that the financial implications of the rise in diabetes in Latin America "represents one of the main challenges to health system financing and to the society as a whole" (Barcelo et al. 2017). Pregnant people are a regular point of concern in the conversations about economic potential, as previously demonstrated by my conversation with the health expert. Scientists describe poor nutrition and impaired metabolism in pregnancy as a conduit to future health and illness, with maternal malnutrition creating a burden that impairs subsequent generations.

As a group of scientists working in Guatemala report, feeding pregnant people a more nutritious diet during pregnancy and breastfeeding will result in a "substantial improvement in adult human capital and economic productivity" (Martorell 2017). The United States Agency for International Development writes that pregnancy is where they should be targeting their energy: "Undernutrition during pregnancy, affecting fetal growth, is a major determinant of stunting and can lead to consequences such as obesity and nutrition-related non-communicable diseases in adulthood" (2017). The agency emphasizes the importance of maternal nutrition investments, underscoring how good nutrition in pregnancy should be at the heart of the effort to reduce diabetes later in life. Eating well during pregnancy would help lessen the burden of chronic disease, which would in turn "improve an individual's educational achievement and earning potential; and increase a country's gross domestic product by at least 2–3 percent annually" (USAID 2017).

The attention paid to mothering may sound promising for Virginia, who had spent much of her life engaged in this labor. Yet Virginia long ago birthed her babies, and as a result, her body is excess in these calculations. Caring for it is inefficient, even "wasteful," given how much need there is. Instead, the care she received was hardly care at all. In 2020 she read me the list of all the medications and supplements she would take when she could afford them: insulin, losartan, Compensial, Floxanova, carvedilol, Dicynone, Centrum, Gabex, LevuSol, Glucerna. Much of the time she skipped doses. The list of medications was as long as the list of prohibited foods: no sugar (too sweet), no salt (sodium was risky), no starch (too sweet), no carrots (too sweet), no pumpkin (too sweet), no meat (too fatty), no eggs (bad cholesterol). One of the hardest pills to swallow was the advice to stay away from beans, which a doctor linked to the trouble she experienced with indigestion. Toward the end of her life, as her pain intensified, she found herself not eating so she could afford the drugs. She no longer shared in the meals – the food or all the conversation that came with it. She kept cooking for others for as long as she could, but she had all but stopped feeding herself.

THE ENERGETICS OF LABOR

In the early 2000s, I heard from doctors who worked in a diabetes clinic in Guatemala that their patients needed to find energetic balance. Their notion of metabolism was driven by the presumption of cleanly calculable exchange. They imagined the body as a machine running on calories, analogous to fuel in an engine: the body is a "human motor," in historian Anson Rabinbach's words (1992). The right metabolism would be achieved when input was equal to output – patients consuming what they "spent," through the calculations of their daily energy. There is a grand, total system, following rules and logic – an economy that can be calculated and known at a distance. This system of metabolic calculation says:

→ Money is finite; we must be careful with our investments. Forget diabetic grandmothers with their frail bodies and needy vascular systems, forget sons and fathers. The maternal body, the site of the future child – the site of the future – is what matters most.

→ Eating food here is taking from others; if you eat too much, you will run out.

Sociologist Hannah Landecker writes of how metabolism in the nineteenth and twentieth centuries became industrialized, describing the drive to maximize the biochemical process by which an organism metabolizes food and oxygen. She details how scientists learned to target fat synthesis or vitamin transfer to "scale up" chemical conversions happening within and between organisms (2023, 57). This is a version of metabolism that seeks profit, not balance. Bodies – whether those of animals used as human feed or of laborers and soldiers meant to produce and secure food as economic capital – are pushed toward efficiency, intensification, and mass production. What matters is their output, not anything like health or living well. In the animal realm, targeting metabolism through medicated feed would create higher-producing animals who could eat less and grow faster. In the realm of human labor, scientists have similarly medicated metabolism to serve financial ends.

Historian Dana Simmons also describes metabolic illnesses as *produced* through a historically and culturally contingent system of starvation technologies in which food and nourishment are "withheld in order to get people and animals to do things," such as working for minimal or no wages or purchasing medications that do not seem to help and which they cannot afford (2025). Simmons cites Liz Theoharis, from the Poor People's Campaign, who has forcefully argued that "scarcity is a myth" (Theoharis, quoted in Simmons 2025). This statement – well-supported by academic research – suggests that the idea that there is *not enough* has been socially produced (see Sen 2019; Hendrixson and Hartmann 2019; Garth 2020). The driver of "scarcity" is not a human universal or inherent truth, but its naturalization comes to have powerful cyclical effects. The belief that there is not enough incites a drive for ever more – resources, belongings, wealth, profits. In turn, this drive – not a basic fact of scarcity – will create the conditions of lack that compel the need for more.

I began with a discussion of iatrogenesis, the furthering of a disease via its treatment. A dictionary definition of iatrogenesis would describe it as the harm or *unintended* outcomes caused by a healer because of the health-care interventions they undertake. Sociologist Ivan Illich (1976) has worked to shift the focus of iatrogenesis away from a doctor's intentions and toward the broader system of medicine under capitalism, which so frequently has a disabling impact on people's lives. His point is that whether these outcomes are intended or unintended, they are part of the mechanics of capitalism, in which some bodies become expendable so that others can prosper (see also Parvin and Pollock 2020).

In the case of Virginia's diabetes, I am left thinking about the boxes of pills and stacks of prescriptions meant to treat her. In her final months of life, the effort to pay for her expensive medications left her without money for food, while the warnings that her staple foods were dangerous left her with nothing to eat. It is, of course, difficult to identify the cause of death of an elderly diabetic woman who had lived much of her life on the edges of poverty, but her death certificate said liver failure. Possibly the cause of this liver failure was unregulated blood sugar, but the liver can also fail through slow-onset poisoning that can be the result of incorrectly prescribed medication. I cannot know with any certainty, but I also cannot help but wonder if her irregular "drug cocktail" created conditions of toxicity that finally left her body damaged beyond repair.

Origins of harm and illness are difficult to decipher, but we can learn a lot from all the origin stories that are not told. Considerable professional energy went into telling Virginia to change what she was eating and to take more pills. Professionals tasked with her treatment rarely inquired into the broader social and environmental conditions shaping diabetic life. All the magic Virginia might be able to work with food would not change her history of having grown up on a farm where tremendous quantities of fertilizers and insecticides were used to grow commercial food. As anthropologist Vincanne Adams writes, glyphosate, a commonly used herbicide, will seep "into food and gardens but also into the soft tissues of humans, where it produce[s] a cascade of disruptions, undermining nutritional, digestive, pulmonary, neurological, and immune systems" (2023, 2; see also Agrad-Jones 2013; Guthman 2019). Many agrochemicals sold in Guatemala are banned in Europe and the United States for being hazardous to human development. Women selling and shopping for foods in the marketplace worry greatly about them, and yet agrochemicals are rarely part of medical conversations about the causes and treatments of diabetes.

Also absent from these conversations is a broader discussion of industrialized metabolism. Here, the issue is not only that food companies have targeted poor people with high-calorie, low-nutrient, highly processed foods (Monteiro et al. 2019). In fact, the dangers of industrialized diets have gotten considerable public health attention, with health professionals routinely advising patients to select low-sugar, low-fat "healthy" foods that are – not incidentally – often prohibitively expensive. While well intended, this overall emphasis on food and diet has come at the expense of concern for the broader landscape of industrialized labor in which diabetes is diagnosed and treated (Hite 2019; Carruth et al. 2019). Discussions of labor would connect diabetes care to concerns about shift work, sleep schedules, employment benefits, and minimum salary (Smith-Morris 2006; Landecker 2013). Are people paid a living wage for the work they do? Do they have the ability to rest when they need to rest? Discussions about labor would also reflect on the industrialization of diabetes diagnosis and treatment alike. While epidemiological research assesses the burden of diabetes-related *illnesses* globally (Ong et al. 2023), it rarely asks about the burden of *treatments* for diabetes.

The medical professionals who treated Virginia would typically write her prescriptions and send her on her way – not concerning themselves with how often these medications remained inaccessible and unaffordable, or whether the desperation she experienced when given yet another prescription might cause further harm. Meanwhile, Virginia's own recipes were based on marketplace conversations (What is in season? What is ripe?) and careful deliberations over appetites, preferences, and the taste of foods. Cooking and feeding others helped her to live well, and it helped those around her to live well. But since her recipes centered on relations – not profits – they found no place among the prescriptions that doctors who treated her would write.

Likewise, health professionals treating Virginia seldom considered how their act of giving advice about what to eat would disempower her primary domain of skill, burdening her with ever more responsibility and the exhaustion that comes with it. Focused on nutrients, doctors rarely discussed the interpersonal interactions of mealtimes. The famous Brazilian principle of healthy eating – "eat in community" – was not formally part of the dietary advice for diabetics in Guatemala (Ministry of Health 2015). Health professionals frequently overlooked or actively discounted what experts like Virginia knew about how to make good meals or how to make mealtimes good. They rarely made mention of a need to relish in the companionship of those with whom eating occurs. If anything, dieticians treated pleasure during eating as a source of harm (see also Vogel and Mol 2014).

IATROCHEMISTRY

In closing, I want to offer another Greek word, *iatrochemistry*, that we might use to consider living well with diabetes. Medieval medical alchemists called their practice *iatrochemistry*, or the chemistry of healing. Over time the experimental practices of chemical medicine have become the domain we look to for health care – the laboratory replacing the kitchen as a key site of chemistry, the scientists replacing the cook, and the male-dominated field of economics undercutting the earlier domestic space of the *oikos* or home.

Today, biochemistry is deeply tied to pharmaceuticals. As anthropologist Joseph Dumit (2012) writes, drugs today are "for life," with drug companies expanding prescription markets while also foreclosing

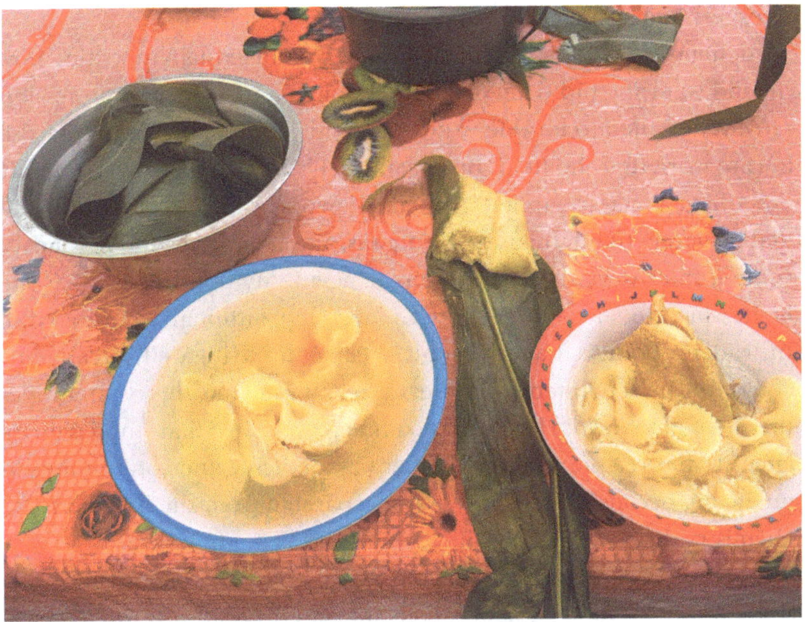

Figure 10.4: A meal of chicken noodle soup and corn tamales wrapped in banana leaves would spread to feed a large number of guests

other avenues for treatment by asking questions whose only answer is "more drugs." Yet there is also a critical opening for diabetes treatment and care to be found by looking at the chemistry of healing from the practices of the kitchen. It turns out that these so-called mundane activities of shopping, peeling vegetables, or simmering a pan of beans in their final phase of life hold within them powerful techniques of care that elude laboratory chemistry – or, rather, which are actively held to be outside of or in conflict with chemistry. Yet including cooking and feeding practices *within* the category of chemistry might make it possible to begin to articulate pathways for healing that we could not see before.

Data scientists tend to approach chemistry through stability and replicability. In their practice, energetic balance is equal to input minus output. One and one are two. But strange things will happen in an expert's kitchen. Foods can be expanded to feed unexpected guests, ingredients saved from one meal becoming the basis of another. Feasting produces abundance. Using is not always using up. Input may not correlate in any meaningful way to output; systems, much like bodies, leak and overflow in unexpected ways. Elderly women may not be waste or excess, but at the center of the world.

Alchemy was alive at Virginia's table. I cannot explain in writing how she did what she did – my years of schooling and academic profession are not designed to be able to attend to the kind of chemical expertise in care work that she held. But I could see what I am left insufficiently describing as magic happening there, as people came together with limited resources to fill their bellies, organs, and blood. Around her meals, communities were made and remade again. My point is not that she knew which foods could be used as medicine, although she often did. Instead, my point is that in Virginia's recipes for living well, "treatment" could not be separated from meals, mealtimes, and the communities they helped to form. Her work broadened the adage that "food is medicine." In her recipes, eating together was medicine and community was medicine, because "medicine" was inseparable from the interpersonal chemistry that happened while feeding and being fed.

Of course, there are tragic limits. Virginia died younger than she should have, in terrible pain, which she had lived with for many years. In the final months of her life, her skill in community-making all but fell apart as her affliction grew so extreme that she could not leave her bed, even as her grandchildren cried for her to pick them up. Yet up against these limits there are still openings. I can see her now slicing potatoes and squash, boiling bones for stock, and setting bowls of soup on the table. Her good eye would be accounting for everything, as her lopsided smile welcomed us to eat, insisting,

"Feast, enjoy it. There is enough."

REFERENCES

Adams, Vincanne. 2023. *Glyphosate and the Swirl: An Agroindustrial Chemical on the Move.* Critical Global Health: Evidence, Efficacy, Ethnography. Durham: Duke University Press.

Barcelo, Alberto, Armando Arredondo, Amparo Gordillo–Tobar, Johanna Segovia, and Anthony Qiang. 2024. "The Cost of Diabetes in Latin America and the Caribbean in 2015: Evidence for Decision and Policy Makers." *Journal of Global Health* 7 (2): 020410. doi:10.7189/jogh.07.020410.

Carruth, Lauren, Sarah Chard, Heather A. Howard, Lenore Manderson, Emily Mendenhall, Emily Vasquez, and Emily Yates-Doerr. 2019. "Disaggregating Diabetes." *Medicine Anthropology Theory* 6 (4). doi:10.17157/mat.6.4.730.

Dumit, Joseph. 2012. *Drugs for Life: How Pharmaceutical Companies Define Our Health.* Experimental Futures: Technological Lives, Scientific Arts, Anthropological Voices. Durham: Duke University Press.

Garth, Hanna. 2020. *Food in Cuba: The Pursuit of a Decent Meal.* Stanford: Stanford University Press.

Guthman, Julie. 2019. *Wilted: Pathogens, Chemicals, and the Fragile Future of the Strawberry Industry.* University of California Press. doi:10.2307/j.ctvp7d4bc.

Hendrixson, Anne and Betsy Hartmann. 2019. "Threats and Burdens: Challenging Scarcity-Driven Narratives of 'Overpopulation.'" *Geoforum* 101 (May): 250–59. doi:10.1016/j.geoforum.2018.08.009.

Hite, Adele H. 2019. "A Material-Discursive Exploration of 'Healthy Food' and the Dietary Guidelines for Americans." PhD diss., North Carolina State University.

International Diabetes Federation (IDF). 2024. "Guatemala Diabetes Report 2000–2045." *Diabetes Atlas.* https://diabetesatlas.org/data/.

Illich, Ivan. 1976. *Medical Nemesis: The Expropriation of Health.* Pantheon Books.

Landecker, Hannah. 2013. "Postindustrial Metabolism: Fat Knowledge." *Public Culture* 25, no. 3 (71): 495–522. doi:10.1215/08992363-2144625.

Landecker, Hannah. 2023. "The Food of Our Food." In *Eating beside Ourselves: Thresholds of Foods and Bodies,* edited by Heather Paxson, 56–85. Durham: Duke University Press.

Martorell, Reynaldo. 2017. "Improved Nutrition in the First 1000 Days and Adult Human Capital and Health." *American Journal of Human Biology* 29 (2): e22952. doi:10.1002/ajhb.22952.

Ministry of Health. 2015. *Dietary Guidelines for the Brasilian Population.* Brasilia: Ministry of Health of Brazil.

Monteiro, Carlos A. et al. 2019. "Ultra-Processed Foods: What They Are and How to Identify Them." *Public Health Nutrition* 22 (5): 936–941. doi:10.1017/S1368980018003762.

Ong, Kanyin Liane, et al. 2023. "Global, Regional, and National Burden of Diabetes from 1990 to 2021, with Projections of Prevalence to 2050: A Systematic Analysis for the Global Burden of Disease Study 2021." *The Lancet* 402 (10397): 203–34. doi:10.1016/S0140-6736(23)01301-6.

Pan American Health Organization (PAHO). 2024. "Burden of Disease from Diabetes – PAHO/WHO." https://www.paho.org/en/enlace/burden-disease-diabetes.

Parvin, Nassim and Anne Pollock. 2020. "Unintended by Design: On the Political Uses of 'Unintended Consequences.'" *Engaging Science, Technology, and Society* 6 (August 2020): 320–27. doi:10.17351/ests2020.497.

Sen, Amartya. 2019. "The Political Economy of Hunger." *Common Knowledge* 25 (1–3): 348–56. doi:10.1215/0961754x-7299462.

Simmons, Dana. 2025. *On Hunger: Violence and Craving in America, from Starvation to Ozempic.* Oakland, CA: University of California Press.

Smith-Morris, Carolyn. 2008. *Diabetes among the Pima: Stories of Survival.* University of Arizona Press.

USAID. 2017. "The 1,000-Day Window of Opportunity: Technical Guidance Brief." Archive – U.S. Agency for International Development. https://2012-2017.usaid.gov/what-we-do/global-health/nutrition/1000-day-window-opportunity.

Vogel, Else and Annemarie Mol. 2014. "Enjoy Your Food: On Losing Weight and Taking Pleasure." *Sociology of Health & Illness* 36 (2): 305–17. doi:10.1111/1467-9566.12116.

World Health Organization (WHO). 2024. "Diabetes." https://www.who.int/health-topics/diabetes.

CHAPTER ELEVEN

Connecting Care, Connecting Chronic Illness: Community, Rural Health, and Insecurity in Hidalgo, Mexico

Emilia Mercedes Guevara

I called Doña Teresa to let her know that I had arrived in Mexico. I had just boarded the six-hour bus ride to travel from Mexico City to see her in San Martín, Hidalgo. We had met a few years earlier on the Eastern Shore of Maryland, where Doña Teresa worked as a crab picker in a crab processing facility. She was *morena*, dark-skinned Mexican, like me. She had a small heart-shaped face, smooth skin, and a perpetually amused expression that was framed by a bit of blush and mascara. Doña Teresa was meticulous about her appearance, frequently wearing name-brand pastel-colored athleticwear and sneakers. But it wasn't her fashion that drew people in, it was her laughter and charisma. She would laugh, tease, and include me in the fun, introducing me to her coworkers, neighbors, and friends. She befriended me on Facebook within hours of meeting. When I eventually left Maryland's shores to return to Washington, DC, we continued to exchange memes, videos, pet pics, and family stories.

During my visit to San Martín, Doña Teresa insisted I stay with her in her guest house. "But first, you must make all your appointments in the city and ensure you care for yourself, too." Over the years, we shared our battles with our chronic illnesses. Doña Teresa had high blood pressure and type 2 diabetes that she had managed with various forms of biomedical and traditional Mexican medicine for over a decade. She had been in treatment at the larger clinic, a fifteen-minute shuttle ride away, and part of a diabetes and chronic disease support group sponsored by the largest social insurance institution, the Instituto Mexicano de Seguro Social (IMSS). In Mexico, the health-care system is divided into three analogous sectors: employment-based social insurance systems, public assistance to uninsured people, and the private sector, comprised of providers, insurers, and the pharmaceutical and medical-device industry (Block et al. 2020). Most people in rural Hidalgo went to the IMSS for public assistance or to the private sector.

My chronic illness stems from a titanium mechanical heart-valve replacement I received when I was in my twenties after my aortic valve disintegrated suddenly. I had a grueling six-hour open-heart surgery and six months of recovery. Since then, I have taken daily medication that must be monitored monthly by a cardiologist or general practitioner in an anticoagulation clinic to decrease the risk of adverse events like clots and strokes. I also suffered from fibromyalgia that came and went, and with it fatigue, musculoskeletal aches, and pain. My doctors in Washington, DC, were generally dismissive of my pain, offering nonsteroidal anti-inflammatory drugs and not much else. My primary-care physician once handed me an article about tai chi and suggested I try it to help ease my symptoms. She told me that this form of exercise showed more significant improvement in symptoms than aerobic exercise, the current most prescribed non-drug treatment for patients with fibromyalgia. I tried tai chi, yoga, meditation, water walking and stretching, and countless other forms of meditation and gentle movements that did not offer much relief. I was eager to join Doña Teresa in her home to understand her own experiences with diabetes, but worried about my health. What would happen if I experienced a pain flair or side effects from my medication? I had no idea what care would look and feel like in Hidalgo.

Doña Teresa was excited for me to experience her small community firsthand. She told me I could "learn more about *el campo* [the countryside] and how illness lives here with us in many ways." A year prior, Doña Teresa had broken her ankle in Mexico, which took many months to heal due to poor circulation related to her diabetes. Because of her injury that year, Doña Teresa could not travel to Maryland's Eastern Shore for work in the crab industry. She lost nine months of work and the additional income she made on the side, selling homemade breakfast sandwiches and hearty lunches to her coworkers. However, Doña Teresa's gait and mood improved after several months of rest, limited directed physical therapy, and her workout regimen. She told me that while her ankle felt more or less stable, she used a wooden cane for support during the rainy season because the concrete road and steps up to her house were very slippery. Even though her ankle felt much better, she was concerned that many months without her regular exercise routine had caused her to gain weight slightly, which led to elevated blood glucose and blood pressure that read higher than her target rate of 130/80 mm Hg. She confided that she did not want to turn out like other diabetes patients she knew – those who had had their feet amputated after minor wounds that were slow to heal and eventually turned gangrenous. Although her doctors reminded her frequently that she was responsible for her own health, I reminded Doña Teresa that living in an isolated, rural region with limited income and few medical resources created the conditions for a difficult time managing her diabetes. I reminded her that she was actively involved in taking care of herself and doing everything she could to stay healthy.

After landing in Mexico City, I visited with the maternal side of my family. Over the years I have occasionally visited a primary-care physician during my visits to Mexico City, and my family would take me to doctors affiliated with retail pharmacies that specialized in generic medications. I couldn't depend on this care, however, because medical records weren't kept, and I rarely saw the same doctor. I needed to establish care with a Mexican cardiologist who could monitor my health remotely while I was visiting with Doña Teresa. I contacted several cardiologists who were willing to accept US-based patients and US-based health insurance. The copayment was expensive, Mex$3,000, or US$150 – a cost likely unattainable for most Mexicans. A *médico particular* (private physician) charged approximately Mex$300 to Mex$500 per visit, and daily income in Mexico ranged from Mex$100 to Mex$300 per day. With a referral from a cardiologist in the United States, I quickly made an appointment to see the first available doctor. I took a taxi a few days later to Las Lomas de Chapultepec, an exclusive and expensive neighborhood in Mexico City. In the waiting room, fifteen stories up, I could see the city's panoramic skyline.

I sat on a comfortable chair surrounded by whiter, older, wealthier patients. Both the men and women wore expensive, fashionable suits and dresses covered in mounds of gold jewelry. I hadn't thought to dress up and felt underdressed in jeans, a T-shirt, and sneakers. I was called in to see the doctor and offered a seat in his plush office adorned with thick textbooks and framed diplomas from Mexico and the United States on the stark white walls. He looked at the intake form I filled out online a few days earlier and told me that he would monitor my warfarin medication, an anticoagulant used to thin my blood and prevent blood clots and strokes. Laughing, he said, "Well, you have a very complex chronic disease. By looking at these issues, you are lucky you are doing well. If you lived in Mexico, you would be dead already. As to your fibromyalgia, based on your responses to the intake, there's no indication that you have it. If you think you feel sore, take paracetamol twice a day." Stunned by his response and saddened by his callousness, I said nothing.

After leaving the office, I sent a voice message to Doña Teresa on WhatsApp, expressing my worries about finding adequate medical care in the region. Her response was immediate and comforting. "Take the doctor's advice to monitor your blood, and don't worry about the rest. We have many ways to stay healthy. There is a private laboratory that will not be too expensive for you, and you can send the results to your doctor from here. You can also go to my clinic here, too. You will be fine. *Tenemos poquito pero es bendito*," she assured me, meaning, "We have very little, but it is blessed and given with care."

I was uncomfortable when I first arrived in San Martín. People were interested in my life and family and questioned me intently. Culturally, I was familiar with Mexican life but only in an urban setting like Mexico City. I was used to getting up to the sounds of the city and the bustle of people and brief anonymous interactions. In Hidalgo, I had to acclimate to a slower pace of life. Doña Teresa could see my discomfort and asked me to join her on leisurely walks to visit friends and neighbors. She invited them over to get to know me in what I learned later were weekly gatherings at her home.

I ate whatever Doña Teresa suggested or had available for the family to eat that day. I thought I would be bored eating black beans and tortillas every day. However, I was in Hidalgo to conduct research, and after a long day of fieldwork, walking, errands, and gardening, I would look forward to soupy beans, fragrant tortillas, and savory avocados sprinkled with salt. Neighbors and friends stopped by to chat for hours and would bring items from their gardens (*milpas*).

Doña Teresa told me that "life in her rancho is healthy. It is the food from outside that we have to be wary of. We have fresh air and good water and work harder to stay healthy because medicine here is limited or we can't afford it … When I lived and worked in Mexico City many years ago, it was hard to take the time to prepare and cook food. I would buy *comida chatarra* [junk food] to get something in my stomach, and it made me sicker. What we eat is due to necessity … I buy and grow natural foods because they are healthier and expensive." I could see that Doña Teresa worked very hard to keep processed foods out of her household's diet; she limited her food intake, exercised, and cared for herself, her family, and her neighbors.

I was eager to help Doña Teresa with her daily chores. We took food shopping trips up and down the mountainside. I met her extended kin, neighbors, nearby store owners, and parishioners at their Catholic church. On days I walked alone through the community, people waved at me out windows and greeted me by name. It was clear that everyone looked out for everyone else in the community.

I would wake up early, assist in preparing coffee for potential guests, and aid in daily chores. I would sweep and mop floors, tend to her garden, learn about her favorite herbs and spices, and forage for flowers and buds from local plants. I would also wait happily for the young man on the moped who delivered kilos of tortillas daily. I accompanied Doña Teresa and her daughters on everyday errands to the daily *tianguis*, a pop-up open-air market one town over. We took the local *colectivo*, the cooperatively owned shuttle van, to different towns, searching for medicinal herbs, plants, and flowers at local markets or *naturistas* (natural foods shops). Doña Teresa took great care to answer the incessant questions about the usefulness of each plant and what their scientific, Spanish, and Indigenous names were. I would lean in or crush the plants to learn how they smelled.

Over time, I learned that *hoja santa* (Mexican pepper leaf) reduces fever and stomach pain. *Hierba de la Virgen* (*Loeselia scariosa*) assists with depression and anxiety. *Nopal* (cactus paddles) can be eaten to support a low-glycemic diet, as it helps regulate blood sugar and fills you with fiber. Doña Teresa showed me how to pickle nopales with vinegar and onions, and we would serve them as *botanas* (snacks) or add them to tacos or quesadillas. Doña Teresa was adamant that vinegar could aid in digestion and managing blood sugar – something that some scientific studies have also found (Siddiqui et al. 2018). Doña Teresa told me that *té de manzanilla* (chamomile tea) was taken for inflammation, to aid in digestion, and to calm the body and the spirit. *Flor de Jamaica* (dried hibiscus flower) was taken as a diuretic to help clean the kidneys. Doña Teresa gave me tea from the *flor de pasiflora* (passion flower), which was said to lower blood pressure and decrease fibromyalgia soreness. I found that drinking this tea instead of taking my usual pain medications would often bring me more relief.

Doña Teresa often took *quelites,* or a wide variety of edible leaves, stems, and flowers, to manage her weight and blood glucose. Doña Teresa's family had gathered them to supplement food stocks during leaner times throughout her childhood or purchased them from local markets to add to meals. I scribbled down at least a dozen types of quelites in my notebook. Still, some were more familiar to me, like an evergreen shrub called *romerito* (seepweed), *huauzontle* (Mexican broccoli), and *epazote* (Jesuit's tea), which were common in most regions of Mexico. Eating quelites for their tender leaf stems and flowers has been part of the Mexican diet since pre-Hispanic times, particularly among Indigenous groups like the Otomí (Basurto 2011; Linares and Aguirre 1992). Mexican scientists identify at least fifty types and note the potential of quelites as an example of underutilized traditional Indigenous knowledge that could aid in increasing dietary nutrition for all Mexicans but particularly for food insecure regions (Balcázar-Quiñones 2020; Mariscal and Peña Montes 2015).

After many months, I noticed that my clothing was much looser. When the technician weighed me after six months in Hidalgo, I was fourteen pounds lighter, just under 10 per cent of my weight. My warfarin levels were at the therapeutic level, my blood pressure was down a few points, and I had little to no fibromyalgia pain. Doña Teresa was not surprised I was feeling better; she explained, "Mother taught me the names for all these and how they cure diseases. It has taken years to learn because there are so many of them. These plants and remedies relieve or maintain physical, emotional, mental, or spiritual health. They improve our quality of life at a lower cost and even allow us to live longer, like my mother and grandmother. God rest her soul."

Many people in Doña Teresa's community used plants to relieve minor aches and pains. In addition to known traditional healers like herbalists, midwives, and *sobadores* (healers of muscle pain and sprains), who specialized in traditional medicine, most neighbors at once understood the importance of herbs and plants and showed interest in biomedical medicine. Lupe, Doña Teresa's neighbor whom I met at the local IMSS, served as a community health worker in charge of staffing the community-run clinic IMSS sponsored. Lupe's job involved visiting people at their homes who were living with chronic and acute illnesses such as type 2 diabetes, heart disease, osteoporosis, and acute viral respiratory infections and then reporting back to the IMSS with her findings. Lupe told me that these visits aimed to slightly improve chronic or acute conditions or stabilize them long enough to get people to their subsequent primary-care or specialist appointment, which could take weeks or months in larger cities. Lupe also dispensed first aid and essential medications like cough medicine, paracetamol, aspirin, and ibuprofen.

Lupe was also aware of the importance of nutrition and incorporated that understanding into her tamale business. Lupe's tamales were notable because they contained various quelites and vegetables. She would prepare and sell tamales to Doña Teresa and others who had chronic diseases like diabetes and hyperthyroidism. Lupe told me that Nurse Lola, the local nurse from the IMSS who helped manage Lupe's mother's diabetes, taught her that native and non-native vegetables contained important phytochemicals that could help manage her mother's chronic illness. She felt that offering these types of tamales was helping her mother and could, therefore, help her own neighbors.

Lupe provided many kinds of tamales, some vegetable-based or with no added sodium, some with traditional meat fillings made from free-range chicken, pork, and beef sourced from the local farmers in the community. Lupe noted that the black beans for the tamales were grown on the hill above Doña Teresa's house, the pork purchased from Doña Teresa's neighbor, beef from the local rancher one town over, and the traditional flowers and plants found on nearby trees. She heard from other neighbors that I often had muscle pain and began to make tamales with *flor de colorín* to help relax the muscles in my body. The tamales were tasty and filling and helped my pain dissipate. Doña Teresa often invited Lupe to sit with her friends, drink tea, gossip, and sell tamales. Lupe frequently drank flor de pasiflora tea, which she said relaxed her after being on her feet all day.

Doña Teresa's home was a sanctuary where family and community members would share sweet rolls, cookies, and *café de olla* – a strong, fragrant, cinnamon-laced coffee prepared in large earthenware pots. Doña Teresa always had treats for guests, symbolizing the warmth and hospitality that defined her household. "I occasionally take a nibble," she admitted to me. "But only a bite or two after eating a meal," she clarified, defending her disciplined approach to managing her diabetes. She tried to be careful to follow her prescribed diabetes diet and drank water and plain coffee. Coffee was essential to daily life, bringing people together, so there was a pot on her stove at all hours. "You never know when someone will show up, so you must be prepared," she would joke. She'd serve it piping hot throughout the day during the cold, wet winter and springtime. Spending time with Doña Teresa gave me a sense of routine, and I became known as *la sombra de Doña Teresa*, or Doña Teresa's shadow. She introduced me to many people (mostly women in her social circle) and rich Hidalgan coffee, and through these visits, we cemented our friendship.

One morning, Doña Teresa received a reminder text from Nurse Lola and then an immediate follow-up call. Nurse Lola insisted that Doña Teresa needed to drop everything to be at an earlier appointment because she had scheduled more appointments than could be accommodated. Doña Teresa quickly agreed, saying to me, "I don't want to disappoint Nurse Lola. If she gets annoyed, you might not get another appointment for weeks. The IMSS is the better clinic and has more technology." Doña Teresa wanted to know if her hypertension was improving, as she could feel tension headaches on occasion. She and I rushed to the imposing whitewashed concrete IMSS building at the highest point in the town.

The entrance door was made from thick, expensive frosted glass etched with the green IMSS logo – a simple, modernist design of a deconstructed Mexican eagle with outstretched wings gently carrying a mother holding a child. Underneath the eagle was an inscription that read *Seguridad y Solidaridad Social* (Security and Social Solidarity). Inside, the freshly painted white walls were adorned with a large map of Hidalgo and colorful and cheerful posters depicting proper hand-washing techniques, mosquito surveillance and breeding-prevention directives, and oral rehydration therapy instructions, a reflection of the seventy-year-old IMSS model that focused on acute illnesses. The two nurses chatting at the main reception area recognized Doña Teresa; one nurse gestured toward a room at the end of the hallway. It was a stark, white subway-tiled room with a small desk, a partition screen, a chair, and an examination table covered by a layer of waxed tissue paper. I stood in the corner while Doña Teresa hoisted herself onto the examination table and waited for her nurse. Nurse Lola was a slight, seventy-year-old white Mexican woman with a powdered face, long jet-black dyed hair arranged into a heavy low bun, and a no-nonsense attitude. Lola was notorious in the community for being curt and impatient with her patients. I had already had several encounters with Nurse Lola in this same clinic when I came in a few weeks earlier with a lingering chest cough.

Entering the room quickly, Lola reached out. She grabbed Doña Teresa's wrist and pricked her finger with a portable glucometer and then briefly checked her pulse, temperature, and blood pressure. Her glucose level was 138 mg/dL, higher than Nurse Lola wanted. She shook her head at Doña Teresa and told her it was time for her to rejoin the *grupo de crónicos*, the chronic illness support group she managed. The group was held at noon on Mondays, Wednesdays, and Fridays in the basement of the Catholic church a few blocks away. Doña Teresa asked for her blood pressure reading and attempted to protest, but Nurse Lola put her hand up to stop her and said, "If you want to get back on track, you will do this."

Nurse Lola told me I could also come along since she had already heard I had some chronic illness issues as well as an academic interest in health in general. "This will do you good, Emilia, to learn how we care for and educate ourselves in Mexico." I opened my mouth to speak, but she held a hand up at me while she continued to talk. "In fact," she told Doña Teresa and me, "you both can go later today. We will start in an hour." Nurse Lola reached into her desk and handed us each a 112-page glossy soft workbook entitled *Sobrepeso, Obesidad y Diabetes: Hacía Una Vida Saludable y en Armonia* (*Overweight, Obesity, and Diabetes: Towards a Healthy, Harmonious Life*). We agreed to go, and nurse Lola disappeared as quickly as she entered. I sat in the room dumbfounded and told Doña Teresa that I wanted to tell Nurse Lola that I had witnessed countless instances of her keeping tabs on her health and being what I would consider the perfect compliant diabetes patient. We sat in the room momentarily, leafing through the workbook before leaving.

Doña Teresa sighed and said, "I am fortunate to have Nurse Lola care for so many of us, and it is good that I have my blood glucose monitored often, but everything that comes from IMSS tends to be a directive, particularly if Nurse Lola is involved."

Doña Teresa and I took a short walk to the nearby church where the crónicos group met. We saw Nurse Lola walk across the courtyard, accompanied by several women, carrying a large tote bag full of patient charts. We stayed behind and watched them enter a building adjacent to the main church, and then we waited a few minutes and followed. Inside, we took a staircase down into a large empty classroom with a high ceiling. Nurse Lola sat at a large wooden desk at the end of the room, sifting through the files from her bag. It was humid, and filtered light streamed through small rectangular windows above us. Within minutes, fifteen women ranging from approximately twenty to sixty years of age began entering the room. The youngest woman had two preschool-aged children with her and directed them to sit in the corner with colored pencils, a notebook, and her cell phone to keep them busy. Nurse Lola directed each of us to take a plastic chair from a stack found against the wall, and we arranged them in the middle of the room into an oval.

Nurse Lola took roll call, added Doña Teresa and me to the roster, and excitedly welcomed us. She pointed at me and asked me to introduce myself. I quickly explained that I was an anthropology student from the United States and was here to understand how migrant women and their communities view chronic illness and how it affects their lives. Many women nodded in agreement. I asked if any women there were regularly migrating to the United States for work, had in the past, or knew of someone who had. All the women raised their hands.

Nurse Lola sat outside the circle and began lecturing on preventing chronic illness and the relationship between glucose levels, food, and diabetes. She emphasized the importance of waist size and how this support group would later involve a weigh-in every two months for each woman. This information would help her determine who would eventually be squarely in the chronically ill category and need further monitoring, and it would enable the clinic to identify the rate of obesity and indicators of possible chronic illness in the community. Nurse Lola told the group: "All of you are here because you have had or now have or will soon suffer from chronic illness. It is just a matter of time. The statistics do not lie. Seven out of ten Mexicans are overweight, and one in ten will have diabetes."

Nurse Lola then asked everyone to read chapter one on diabetes as homework to educate themselves on "what constitutes healthy and unhealthy habits" and then to turn to the inside cover of the workbook, where there was an exercise chart with figures, and pick out a few exercises. Several women raised their hands to ask questions, but Nurse Lola mostly ignored them. We all stood up from our seats and formed a circle. Each person took turns leading the exercise circle. Each leader stood at the center of the circle and offered their exercise for each of us to follow. Laughing because of the awkwardness of the physical movements, everyone diligently followed the person leading the exercises. The exercise routine ranged in difficulty from stretches to forward lunges. Some women had limited mobility, and a few had creaky joints. It was evident by the way some women winced that several of these exercises were difficult or painful. Almost all the women wore long skirts, making lunges difficult. Nurse Lola told us that we could each bring a towel to sit on in the future because the concrete floor was so hard.

I stood next to Liliana, a forty-five-year-old mother of three. She told me she had to be there, or else she and her family could lose benefits from a federally funded conditional cash transfer program called Prospera. She told me that she was a practitioner of traditional medicine, a *sobadera*, a skill she learned from her mother and grandmother, as they all had the gift of healing. Liliana could heal the body through musculoskeletal adjustments and massage. Doña Teresa told me that many people in the region sought her out for her ability to cure minor illnesses, like indigestion and infant colic, and more serious ailments, like severe pain, scarring, and former injuries. Liliana mentioned that diabetes, other chronic diseases, and pain could be better managed with general adjustments to both the body and spirit.

While we finished the last round of exercises, Nurse Lola took each person aside, pulled their charts, chatted with them about their weight and health goals for the next week, and had them verbally agree to follow the instructions she had written on a piece of IMSS letterhead and signed. By the end of the vigorous thirty-minute workout session, we were all out of breath and perspiring. After we did a cool down, Nurse Lola took pictures of us exercising and then asked me to take a photo of her with the group. I felt used by Nurse Lola and let down once again by a biomedical system that prioritized optics and statistics over actual patients.

After Nurse Lola let the support group out, the women sat outside on the benches by the church and chatted about what they said to Nurse Lola. Three women noted a lowering of their blood glucose; two others were pleased they had lost a few pounds since the previous check-in. Liliana was disappointed because despite losing several pounds, Nurse Lola was unhappy with her progress. Liliana said, "I do not think the numbers tell you everything about how your body is doing." I vehemently agreed and told her that people in this community put much work into keeping their bodies and minds healthy. I asked the women what the next week looked like for each of them. Several women had to care for their children after school, while others worked various jobs in restaurants, cleaned homes, and cared for elderly parents. Doña Teresa invited everyone to her house for coffee at the end of the week "to relax and enjoy the company of friends at least until the next session."

Stories like Doña Teresa's and Liliana's are not uncommon. In Mexico, type 2 diabetes mellitus is the second leading cause of death after heart disease (Arrieta-Canales et al. 2023). The lack of comprehensive health-service access and treatment in rural regions has much to do with Mexico's primarily work-based health system, which has long been problematic for migrant women like Doña Teresa and women in rural areas since migrant, informal, and minimum-wage labor do not qualify for work-based health care in Mexico (DiGirolamo and Salgado de Snyder 2008). Many migrant women return to rural areas with access to small health centers that may only be staffed by volunteer community-health workers or just one or two medical providers, typically a general practitioner or a nurse. These centers serve many surrounding communities in isolation and with limited resources. Patients must travel long distances to obtain more specialized secondary or tertiary care (Reich 2020).

Epidemiological data on disease prevalence provide strong evidence for broader trends in diabetes and chronic diseases in Mexico. These data are used by state, regional, and local health systems to prioritize clinical interventions that attempt to correct the "unhealthy lifestyles" of individual citizens. The experiences of Doña Teresa, Liliana, and the other women show us how Mexico's neoliberal public health policies decenter welfare from the state and place patients "within a frame of self-care and individual responsibility for themselves in a move toward 'shared responsibility' and 'co-management of risk'" (Gálvez 2018, 125). These broad national conversations also focus on the "uneducated" (generally implied to be Black), *mestizos* (a colonial term for those with mixed-race ancestry or brown phenotype), Indigenous people, and rural people. This focus on the "uneducated" and those without "health culture" reinforces what Moreno Figueroa (2010) calls "mestizaje logics." These "racist logics" are strategies of racial differentiation that are pervasive and normalized in the everyday and create the impression that racialized Mexicans are the ones who are unable to comply with public health directives, when in fact, health services are understaffed, undersupplied, and create economic barriers to treatment adherence, following up, and compliance (Calestani and Montesi 2020; Campos Navarro, Peña Sánchez, and Paulo Maya 2017; Moreno 2010, 3).

Reflecting on my time with Doña Teresa, the chronic illness support group, and the community of San Martín, I saw that she and others found communal solidarity, care, and connection in friendship and community, which helped them navigate the complexities of rurality, poverty, diabetes, and chronic illnesses together. Our chronic illness journey was not solely about managing physical ailments but also finding alternate nutritional and therapeutic options in constrained, tenuous health environments.

REFERENCES

Arrieta-Canales, Martha de Lourdes, Joia Mukherjee, Hannah Gilbert, Hugo Flores, Melania Muñoz, Zeus Aranda, Samuel DiChiara, and Carolina Noya. 2023. "Transforming Care for Patients Living with Diabetes in Rural Mexico: A Qualitative Study of Patient and Provider Experiences and Perceptions of Shared Medical Appointments." *Global Health Action* 16 (1): 2215004.

Balcázar-Quiñones, A., L. White-Olascoaga, C. Chávez-Mejía, and C. Zepeda-Gómez. 2020. "Los Quelites: Riqueza de Especies y Conocimiento Tradicional en la Comunidad Otomí de San Pedro Arriba, Temoaya, Estado de México." *Polibotánica* 49: 219–42.

Basurto, P. F. "Los Quelites de México: Especies de Uso Actual." 2011. In *Especies Vegetales Poco Valoradas: Una Alternativa Para la Seguridad Alimentaria*, edited by LM Mera O., D. Castro L., and RA Bye B., 23–46. Instituto de Biología, UNAM, México, DF.

Calestani, Melania, and Laura Montesi. 2020. "The Ethno-Racial Basis of Chronic Diseases: Rethinking Race and Ethnicity from a Critical Epidemiological Perspective." In *Critical Medical Anthropology: Perspectives in and from Latin America*, 170.

Campos Navarro, Roberto, Edith Yesenia Peña Sánchez, and Alfredo Paulo Maya. 2017. "Aproximación Crítica a las Políticas Públicas en Salud Indígena, Medicina Tradicional e Interculturalidad en México (1990–2016)." *Salud Colectiva* 13: 443–55.

DiGirolamo, Ann M., and Nelly Salgado de Snyder. 2008. "Women as Primary Caregivers in Mexico: Challenges to Well-Being." *Salud Pública de México* 50: 516–22.

Figueroa, Mónica G. Moreno. 2010. "Distributed Intensities: Whiteness, Mestizaje and the Logics of Mexican Racism." *Ethnicities* 10 (3): 387–401.

Gálvez, Alyshia. 2018. *Eating NAFTA: Trade, Food Policies, and the Destruction of Mexico.* University of California Press.

Gálvez, Maria Amanda and Carolina Peña Montes. 2015. "Revaloración de la Dieta Tradicional Mexicana: Una Visión Interdisciplinaria." *Revista Digital Universitaria UNAM* 16, no. 5 (May).

González Block, Miguel Á., Hortensia Reyes Morales, Lucero Cahuana Hurtado, Alejandra Balandrán, Edna Méndez, and the World Health Organization. 2020. "Mexico: Health System Review."

Reich, Michael R. 2020. "Restructuring Health Reform, Mexican Style." *Health Systems & Reform* 6 (1): e1763114.

Siddiqui, Fahad Javaid, Pryseley Nkouibert Assam, Nurun Nisa de Souza, Rehena Sultana, Rinkoo Dalan, and Edwin Shih-Yen Chan. 2018. "Diabetes Control: Is Vinegar a Promising Candidate to Help Achieve Targets?" *Journal of Evidence-Based Integrative Medicine* 23.

CHAPTER TWELVE

Don Agustín's Crafts: Patience, Skill, and Creativity in Weaving the Weft of Life

Laura Montesi
Spanish Translation by Michele A. Feder-Nadoff

Don Agustín's foot-pedal looms stood dusty and unused for two years below the tin roof of the patio. Don Agustín and his family stored many things of relevance to the past and of possible use in the future under the roof of the patio, including a diverse scattering of objects with wheels: a baby carriage possibly used when his grandchildren were newborns, a bench to sit on made of a tree trunk split in half with large wheels at its sides serving as feet, the rusted frame of an old bike supported upside down on a wooden stool with the rear wheel pulling a cotton thread, and a folded wheelchair whose fabric back announced its institutional benefactor, *Familia CONUNIDAD, DIF Oaxaca.*[1]

The ingenious and versatile use of these objects undoubtedly reflects the personality of Don Agustín, a man who has dedicated most of his life to physical labor – a weaver, farmer, brickmaker, taxi driver – according to the necessities of the moment and the conditions imposed by the fluctuating symptoms of his lifelong companion, diabetes. To understand Don Agustín's diabetes requires us to frame it within the history of his village, his craft, and his family.

When I proposed participating in this project to Don Agustín, he understood its significance immediately. And when I explained to him

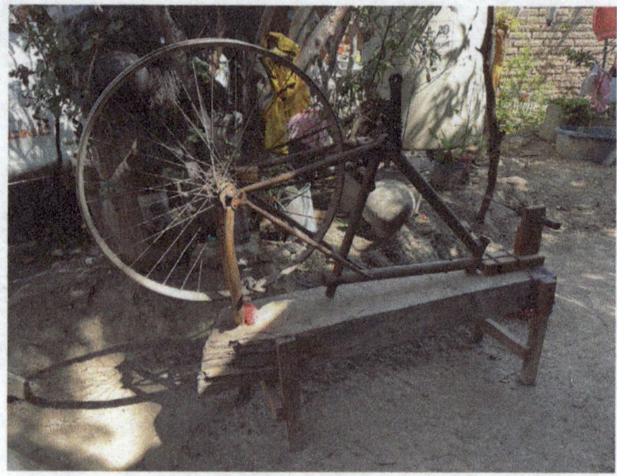

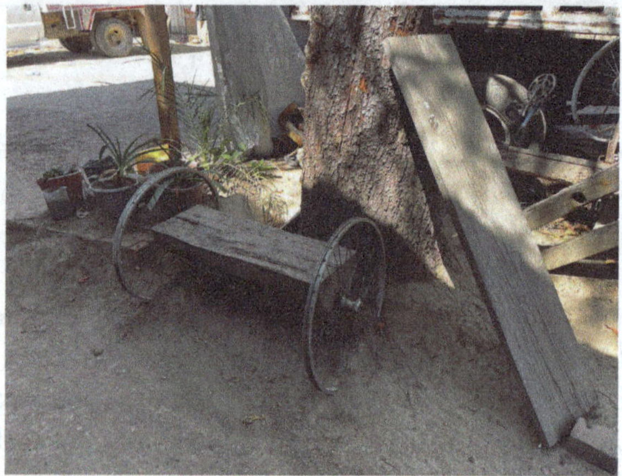

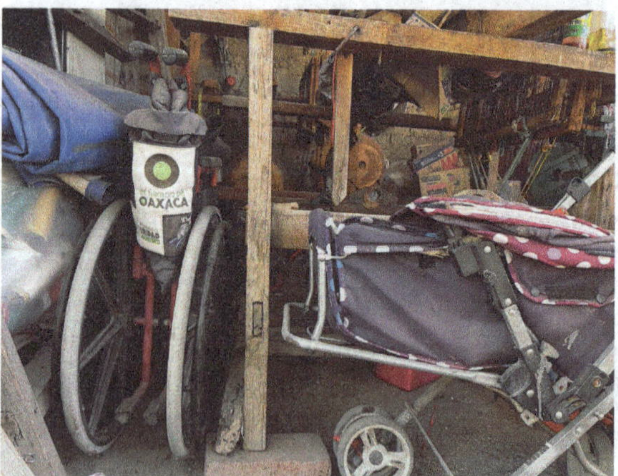

Figure 12.1: Don Agustín's wheels (Photos by Juan Mayorga)

that writing would take time and would involve revisions and subsequent follow-up visits to make the text more precise and to refine various details, he said there was no problem: "We can change, recut, and move different parts of the text so that the final version will come out well." I believe that he understood the "patchwork" involved in creating a written text because it resonated with his work as a weaver and textile artisan. The composition of this text was based on dialogue and exchange, in a manner similar to the comings and goings of the shuttle whose passing from one side of the loom to the other makes the weaving possible.

One autumn day I got into the taxi that Don Agustín was driving, and we passed through many roads until we finally made it to a hill where we could make out a view of Xaagá, his native *pueblo*. As we sat on some rocks underneath the shade of a tree overlooking the village below, which was blooming green from the rains of the recent summer, Don Agustín began telling me: "Our grandparents told us that many years ago the first loom arrived at the *hacienda* of Xaagá.[2] Here the hacienda landowner created *rebozos*, traditional shawls of cotton thread." While he talked, I noticed below us, between the rocks, the paths of determined and laborious ants and the heads of the barrel cactus breaking through the earth spontaneously. "Later on, when the enterprise was in decline here, a *Señor* from Mitla[3] bought the loom and took it back to his own pueblo. There they began to weave with wool thread, and from then on Mitla realized this activity was successful. Why? Because there was an archeological site nearby to Mitla that drew many visitors. But in reality, the tradition of weaving began here in the hacienda of Xaagá," continued Don Agustín.

Foot-pedal looms are common in the Zapotec villages in the Oaxaca Valley. They were introduced by Spaniards during the Conquest and readily adopted by the Indigenous artisans who already had established their own extensive textile traditions. Historical records indicate that the Bishop of Oaxaca, López de Zárate, was the one who introduced sheep and pedal looms to this region in the sixteenth century (Stephen 2005, 141). This made a lasting mark on the histories and identities of many villages, including Xaagá, which today is a pueblo of 1500 inhabitants. These looms, predominantly worked by men, weave wool and cotton threads that are organized vertically on the "warp" and horizontally on the "weft" to form rugs, blankets, rebozos, and other textiles. In the past century, with the consolidation of the tourist sector and the increased consumption of ethnic and folk art, the looms and their artistic production have gained renewed interest. But this has also been woven into an unequal commercial network in which producer communities, such as Xaagá, are not favored in comparison to the communities that not only produce, but also market and sell their products directly, such as San Pablo Villa de Mitla and Teotitlán del Valle. These economic dynamics create rivalry between the villages, and it is common for each to claim to be the oldest and most authentic producer of this craft.

Don Agustín, now fifty-seven years old, inherited the textile craft from his family and his village. At the entrance of Xaagá, there is an archway framing the view to the mountains, giving a welcome to visitors with its colorful murals. "Welcome to Xaagá, land of liberty and artisans," it declares. On the right pillar an artisan is spinning thread on his wooden spinning wheel. On the pillar to the left, another artisanal scene associated with Xaagá appears, the production of red bricks. Flying out from the two pillars, toward the arch, are two birds with nests of leaves that they have entangled with the cotton thread, clutching rebozos with their talons. At the apex, around the *Virgen morena*, a few patterns adorn the arch, the same ones that are now renowned due to their association with the pre-Hispanic buildings of Mitla, which are also represented nowadays in the local textiles. These glyph patterns have been interpreted in many ways: Do they represent waves of the sea? A shell? Quetzalcoatl, the feathered serpent (Markens 2017)?

In Xaagá very few people speak Zapotec. Yet the community identifies as Indigenous by their *usos y costumbres*, through which its traditions are transmitted and inherited within the intimacy of the village and home.[4] Yet the word *inheritance* – which in its common usage is usually associated with property, tangible or intangible, that is received from our ancestors – in recent years has also become associated with new and more sinister connotations. The rise of diabetes in the rural zones of Mexico has made this illness an unwanted, increasingly common family inheritance. Don Agustín mentions this with serenity and acceptance: "This surged because it descends from the family. We carry this infirmity. My father told me that my mother died very young, at the age of twenty-five. But then they didn't identify this disease. By the symptoms that they told us she had, we now understand that she suffered from *el azúcar*, diabetes. For this reason, it has become an inheritance in this

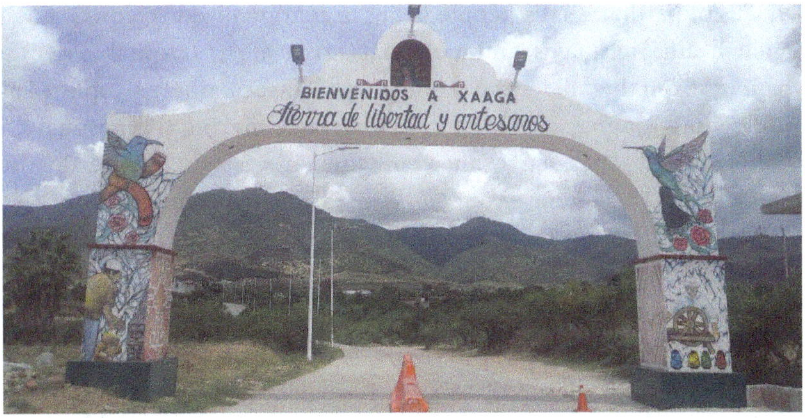

Figure 12.2: Entrance to Xaagá (Photo by Laura Montesi)

family. Seven years ago, my brother died, also of this infirmity. Afterwards, three years later, another brother died. We are five brothers and four have this sugar problem. Only one brother doesn't."

Don Agustín is concerned with diabetes in part because, for many, this diagnosis is a trauma: he knows people who thought of dying by suicide. Scientific studies have demonstrated how suicidal ideation or attempts at suicide increase in people with diabetes, as does depression (Mendenhall 2014; Alzoubi et al. 2018), especially when dealing with financial precarity. Social support, feeling like one is part of a community, and having a group of friends are crucial to being able to live well with this disease (Sharif et al. 2023). "I don't want to place myself as an example; nonetheless, I have lived fifteen years with diabetes, and I hope to be able to tell people that the diagnosis is not a life sentence," Don Agustín told me.

Over the span of the twentieth century, diabetes soared dramatically: "No disease has ever suffered an increase of this magnitude in Mexico's history" (Rodríguez Saldaña, Sosa Espinosa, and García Martínez 1994, 18). In recent decades, diabetes escalated in rural areas to match the diabetes cases in urban ones (Soto-Estrada et al. 2018, 285). Don Agustín was diagnosed with diabetes fifteen years ago, and he accepted his diagnosis without much surprise.

Don Agustín completed primary school and has worked in the informal sector most of his life, so he doesn't have social security.[5] Instead, he travels twenty kilometers from Xaagá to a rural government hospital in Tlacolula that serves people living in marginalized regions. Under a harsh sun, vans, taxis, and moto taxis arrive at the hospital to deliver patients from the valleys and mountains of Oaxaca, where people speak Indigenous languages and Spanish dialects. Entering the hospital for emergencies or regular exam visits, they are asked: "Where do you come from? Do you have your *carnet*, medical appointment book?"

Many Indigenous languages echo through the hallways, while most of the medical staff speak exclusively Spanish. Timid glimpses of the politics of intercultural health peek through in the medicinal plants planted on one side of the fencing that divides the hospital area from the noisy avenue. These plants are residual testaments to an institutional initiative that once promoted traditional medicine within hospital settings. Today, this hospital offers Agustín internal exams and his metformin pills, which he needs to manage his sugar. When there is money, Don Agustín uses private medical services because he can quickly get an appointment as well as the most up-to-date care. The government hospital, however, is just fine for those in-between times when he needs metformin refills.

In the first year of the COVID-19 pandemic, when everything was shuttered, Don Agustín had a serious wound on his right foot. He tried herbal medicines, but it wouldn't heal. Usually, when he has had small wounds, Don Agustín would use ointments as poultices: "With many wounds this functioned marvelously," he explained. "We have tried this; we are witnesses that this really works." But on this occasion, something went wrong. Don Agustín explained that he didn't observe the necessary precautions and ate food contraindicated for his condition. This dietary breach contributed to the growing infection in his wound, confessed Don Agustín, and for this reason the medicinal plants were not effective. "*Papá*, we don't see your foot improving. Let's go to the doctor. It will cost what it will cost!" his children told him. Don Agustín sought help from a private doctor that he trusted.

Initially, the doctor scolded him for waiting too long: "What were you thinking? Why didn't you come in earlier?" The doctor sent him to a clinic specialized in diabetes complications in Oaxaca de Juárez, the state capital, about fifty kilometers away. This began a long and expensive path of therapies for Don Agustín that involved forced rest from work, constant travel to the city to receive these therapies, emotional exhaustion, and tremendous economic cost. His foot-pedal loom sat idle, too.

Many scholars have explained the financial costs and impediments to productivity due to diabetes, not only in personal terms but also collectively (Breton et al. 2013). For men, whose identities are very much tied to the value of their work, the loss of employment or the reduced ability to contribute financially to the family can cause a profound existential crisis and trigger conflicts and tensions (Valdez Flores and Castro Saucedo 2021), especially when there is a lack of a social support network involved in the care.

Yet this was not the case with Don Agustín, who nurtured hope that he would get better and fostered healing through the support of his family, his friends, and his Seventh-day Adventist Church community. "I say that *gracias* to God I have been able to associate myself with these people. This is how I am. I enjoy talking and creating friendships. At times when I go to the market with my wife, the whole world says hello to me. Ha ha! This is how I am, very connected to people. I enjoy being like this!"

New and old threads were woven into this dense network of relationships. Don Agustín engaged in an ancient custom, where he received the assistance of his fellow villagers. "What is beautiful about my village is that the entire community visits the person if they are sick or dying. They bring help, a little money, bread, or flowers. The beautiful thing that I like about my village is that they never leave one alone – *solo*. With the illness that I had, many people came to visit me and brought me money, assistance in food. They even brought me … *hijoles* … beans and many other things."

It was this camaraderie that also characterized the new threads of his network within the Seventh-day Adventist Church. Many people from his church visited him, and this helped him regain strength. His uncles and grandfathers were the first to join the church and had taught him about the faith, and he considered his ties there to be intergenerational. Some scholars have found that people who live well with diabetes do so with the mutual support dynamics that are evident in Don Agustín's life, as opposed to doing this care work on their own (Juárez-Ramírez et al. 2015).

Care is always relational, even when it is personal, because it is based on learning. Don Agustín inherited and perfected many lessons from working the loom, not only related to his skills at weaving rebozos and other textiles but also qualities that were vital to handling his diabetes:

patience, skill, and creativity. His loom remained silent for two years while he regained his health and healed his wound, but its lessons endured. He shared with me some of these lessons by inviting me to his home and showing me his weaving workstation.

PATIENCE

Weaving is a cycle characterized by various steps, requiring great patience, to process, develop, and integrate multiple materials. For example, natural dyes for wool must be prepared with cochineal insects, marigold flowers, or pomegranates. In contrast, cotton threads, the material Don Agustín uses, are prepared this way:

> We purchase the thread in colored cones, first the warp thread, and then we gather it into a bag. Afterwards we fill the spool using little pieces of wood to wind up the thread. We place this in the loom, and then, thread by thread, it is passed into the meshes of the loom. Each thread goes into one mesh, and later it is placed in the slits of the comb. Each tooth of the comb takes two threads, two, two, and two. This all is a process. According to the size of the rebozo, we measure out the quantity of thread necessary: it is possible to be 400, 500, or more.

The material and the loom impose careful processes, periods of waiting, and specific qualities that establish the limits and possibilities of the work. This mutual relationship between organisms and environments, and hence between people and objects, has been defined as "affordance" (Gibson 1979) and refers to "the diverse opportunities for action in accordance with the perception of the welcomed object" (López-Silva 2020). Every object presents specific qualities and properties that permit its particular uses and discard others, although a person who is an expert and very familiar with these can successfully imagine many possibilities. An artisan knows their materials extremely well. Yet their mastery does not arise from dominating or imposing upon the materials. Rather, mastery is found in collaboration with them, to enhance their final refined state or resonance in order to bring out the best of each material.

Artisanal work requires patience. And patience, in the field of health, is related to accepting times of illness and the process of healing. Over

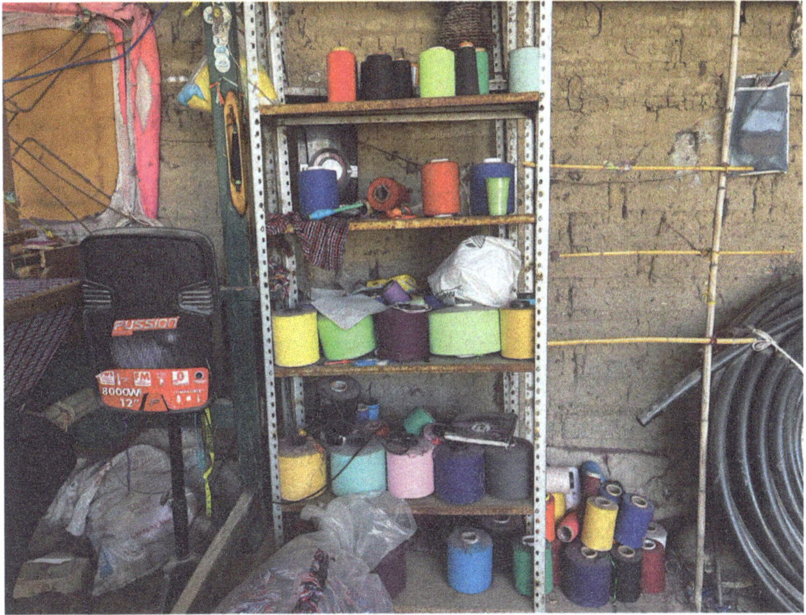

Figure 12.3: The cones of colors (Photo by Juan Mayorga)

the course of two years of treatment, Don Agustín experienced healing to the wound on his foot. During this time, Don Agustín sometimes went to appointments in Mitla and other times to Oaxaca de Juárez. He took his antibiotics, applied his topical ointments, and confronted surgeries – the amputation of his little toe, the removal of all the necrotic tissue – and finally in the end they were able to save his foot. Don Agustín carefully, as if planning to show his weaving, took his phone out of his pocket and quite naturally showed me the crude images of his foot before, during, and after the treatment. As he did, Don Agustín explained,

> They had me stop weaving entirely because the infection was entering my foot. It was a case of total putrefaction of my foot, like a peach that began to rot. If they didn't stop this decomposition, the infection could advance further and destroy my entire leg. Thank God, nowadays the doctors can restore a foot, and now my foot has regenerated substantially. Now we are content and conscious that we have advanced each day a little more in the healing of my foot.

> But it has been an enormous experience: one needs to take great
> care with this illness.

Healing and the recovery of the foot's tissues required much more time than the surgery itself. This required rest, constant cleaning, and chronic care on a grand scale. Every area of tissue responded in a different way to the treatment, and the cells regenerated slowly. Don Agustín became stronger with the assistance of medical specialists as well as with that of his children, wife, fellow countrymen, and "brothers" from the Seventh-day Adventist Church. Don Agustín was able to acquire his "social security" through this combination of social relationships and networks, each woven throughout the course of his life and obtained as a result of hard work, affection, community service, and reciprocity.

Don Agustín served his village over the course of his life by taking on civil and political responsibilities. He served on committees for schools, health, celebrations, potable water, the cemetery. This is customary in Indigenous communities like the one Don Agustín resides in. In 2017 he was named an agent of the community, the highest responsibility: "We served with great enthusiasm and satisfaction because to be elected to this position means that people trust you." This requires a lot of patience as well as deep networks with others. The *guelaguetzas*[6] constitute a community network of support that protects, cares for, and sustains one's existence and can inspire a patient's recovery. Don Agustín today chooses to check his glucose levels with his fellow villager Abundia, the nurse of the village, who checks him privately in her home with a glucose monitor: "The cost of the monitor has gone down so that I can afford it now; nonetheless, I prefer to go to Abu. We have such close friendships it is better to go to these people."

SKILL

> Once we have the threads ready, the spindle keeps going until the
> cloth is complete. We call this *rollo*, this *julio*, this *puente*, this *cuadro*,
> these *mallas*, and turning to the *peine*.[7] We call this piece of wood
> *cajín*, and when we pass the thread, we enter using the *lanzadera*,
> shuttle, and this lifts the *canilla* that we thread over here. It is gath-
> ered in the *casquillos*, and it stays like this. It is passed here, and

then it is passed there. This is the movement of the feet, the hands, and now the fabric is created. If you want to create a design, it is the hands that know how to design it and to locate the various colors.

Don Agustín lifted his entire body over the four pedals of the loom and, with coordinated gestures, moved his hands, arms, feet, and thighs to work with an agility that generated patterns in the rebozo. His movements flowed here and there along the frame of the loom, and his flaming-red tennis shoes danced on the pedals.

Artisanal work shares a material and practical dimension with care from a medical professional or community health worker. In fact, it has been stated that, "Since the western Antiquity, the status of medicine has been swinging between that of a science and that of an art" (Rosa and Parodi 2011, 14). The practice of medicine (and caregiving) is founded on various characteristics amply debated in practical philosophy since Aristotle, such as prudence (*phrónesis*), ingenuity (*métis*), and skill (*téchne*): "Métis, as we have seen, is a sort of cunning possibly bordering on trick, while phrónesis is always aimed at the good. On

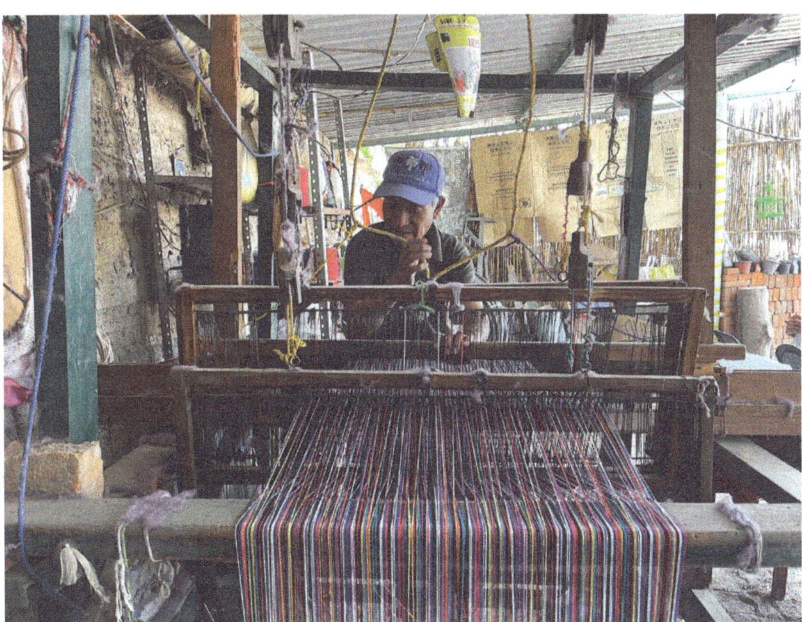

Figure 12.4: Don Agustín works at the loom (Photo by Juan Mayorga)

the other hand, téchne is a set of general and particular knowledge, of manual skills and experience in a specific field" (Rosa and Parodi 2011, 28). These qualities actualize interactions between caregivers and patients, each from their own affects and embodiments. And bodies are not docile, rather they present their own *affordances*. Present-day philosophers Mol, Moser, and Pols remind us that in health and illness, "people look for care in the first place: their bodies happen to not submit to their wishes, let alone their commands. They are unruly ... [Care] involves living with the erratic" (2010, 10).

Each intervention realized in the threads of cotton used to weave a rebozo, or the soft and bony tissues of the diabetic's foot, requires a combination of ingenuity and skill oriented toward the "good" through prudent yet decisive acts (carefulness). To intervene means to "be there," to situate oneself, to evaluate and understand the body of another through one's own senses. Don Agustín, an expert weaver, handed over his trust to a physician, Dr. Torres, who specialized in the comprehensive treatment of wounds, and his medical team. "Each lesion is different, just like each medical chart," Dr. Torres told me after receiving me in his clinic following a full day's work.

> To begin, there are three types of neuropathy: autonomic, motor, and sensory. In addition, there can be an involvement in the arteries as well. When these pathologies combine, we are talking about neuroischemic ulcer. In this case, we need to combine treatments. Depending on the type of wound, something topical, an antibiotic or something less interventionist, can be applied. When we are dealing with a moderate situation, we would have to determine whether the arterial disease or neuropathy is more predominant or whether it is infection. When it is infection, what we have to do is to remove the infected tissue. If it is not removed, no matter how many antibiotics you give it, it is not going to work.

The infection is rebellious; *no se deja*, it does not lend itself to treatment easily. This makes the removal of the infected tissue necessary. To counteract the infection, it is necessary to proactively treat the healthy tissue with antimicrobials or other treatments. Dr. Torres explains, "There are various treatments, including hyperbaric oxygen therapy, chelation, ozone, and larval therapy."

Each clinical case requires that medical theory be adapted to the material conditions of the patient's particular body, their history, and their living environment. This is not unlike craftsmanship, where skilled and knowledgeable practices are repeated over and over again, almost by instinct and by *métis*. However, each time they must adapt to the character of the material and to the environmental conditions that make it express itself differently. It is for these reasons that every artisanal piece, even as it involves well-established knowledge and skills, becomes unique and unrepeatable.

Each diabetes experience is different. The diagnosis can occur by observing ants, attracted by the sweetness of urine, swarming where urine has passed or by the needle of a glucometer on the finger. The news of the diagnosis of diabetes can create a great shadow of incredulity, or it can be expected, as in the case of Don Agustín. Eating more vegetables may be impossible if they are not available at the local market. Oral medicines are successful for some, but for others they generate nausea and other unbearable side effects. Medical information can be communicated effectively, or it can be incomprehensible because there is no interpreter to translate Spanish to Zapotec. For some, the family is a site of care, for others it is a site of violence, fear, emotional volatility, and stress. In this way, each story must be seen as singular, distinct, like *artesanía*, or craftwork. Both are thoroughly cultural, as craftwork has the particularity of varying depending on the social context, its material circumstances, and the history of the place where it is produced.

CREATIVITY

> We learned the designs we make from our grandparents; this is our inheritance. Once you know how to work, then you are able to be creative. You can weave looking for different kinds of designs. We search imaginatively for the designs in the *mallas*. And for this reason, we search with our feet, moving them over the pedals. Certainly, we already have an idea of what type of design it is; then we go searching. We have completed one half, and now we are going to complete the other half. You are sorting in your head, and your feet are down there searching. It is pure creativity; it is imaginary. Look, I just made the little diamond shape that comes out of the archeological ruins.

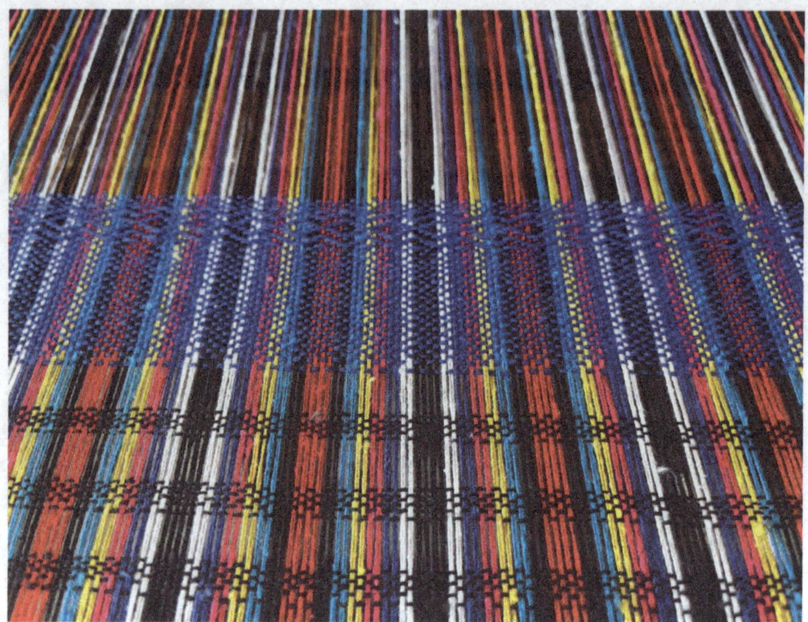

Figure 12.5: The little diamond glyph of the archeological ruins (Photo by Juan Mayorga)

Contrary to the triumphant, individualistic idea that regards creativity as an innate capacity for "genius," Don Agustín explains that people are only creative because of skills that are learned and passed on, innovating within tradition. To create, to innovate, and to encounter solutions that are adopted in the moment presuppose having a consolidated reservoir of knowledge that is adjusted and that, in the process, is capable of creating new situations or re-signifying them by giving them an unexpected twist.

For Don Agustín, working at the loom before these diabetes complications was a productive activity. Now, after his partial amputation, working at the loom has become a form of "exercise" (responding to the biomedical call for self-care and good health) that he took up little by little, according to how the healing of his foot progressed: "It is work that makes you exercise a lot because you need to use your feet, your hands, and mostly your sight. You have to move all of your body. I still have dexterity in my feet. And the doctor told me, 'It is going well because you are exercising. It's good, the activity you are doing in the shade. You can work there at the loom.'"

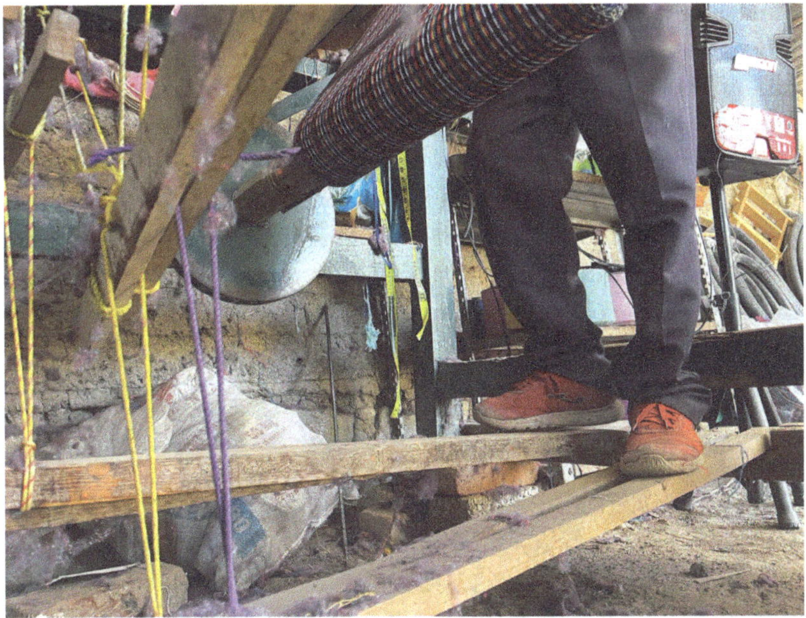

Figure 12.6: Dancing on the pedals (Photo by Juan Mayorga)

Imagination is set in motion when he treasures the diabetes-care expertise that he has consolidated over the expanse of many years and uses it to adjust his treatment. Weaving together the diabetes stories of his family members, along with information provided by health workers and the ancestral medical knowledge passed down to him by grandparents, he seeks to heal the weft of life. Don Agustín drinks his *cacahuatón* tea, a bitter plant whose flavor reminds him of pills, to accompany his metformin, adding traditional plants to biomedical pills. Cacahuatón is a wild plant that his grandparents taught him to harvest in August, when the plant "has all of its strength, *fuerza*." Like a bricoleur, he combines taking his medicines with cacahuatón tea, a diet based in vegetables, and the monthly check of his glucose levels with Abundia. These healing strategies demonstrate the creative and committed actions he devotes to his health.

Moreover, these actions contradict a recurrent medical trope that patients are "negligent" and "careless," i.e. noncompliant, when they take traditional herbs to manage their diabetes. Jim Trostle explains it this way: "When physicians label their patients 'non-compliant' they often distance themselves from their patients' actions, judging and labelling rather than analyzing and understanding." He goes on to question this, however: "Yet thinking about patient behavior in terms of 'compliance' constrains communication by substituting a simple epithet for *a complex act or series of acts over time*. We know that a non-compliant patient has not followed a clinical prescription, but we do not know what that patient has done instead" (1988, 1305; emphasis added). In this way, Trostle emphasizes how clinicians might misinterpret Don Agustín's self-care or his collective community care – which is based on inter-generational knowledge and relationships – because biomedicine is so individualized. Yet Don Agustín's healing is truly communal.

Leaving his house, Don Agustín flipped the handle of his car door and almost as an afterthought said, "I believe that this is something fundamental: When I work, I forget my illness. When I get up, I give thanks to God who has let me live another day and who has saved me. I go out with a grateful heart."

NOTES

1 "Familia CONUNIDAD, DIF Oaxaca" translates to "Family with Unity of DIF, Oaxaca." The acronym DIF stands for Integral Family Development, which is a decentralized public body in charge of coordinating the National System of Public and Private Social Assistance. It runs several programs, including, in the past, CONUNIDAD.

2 The term *hacienda* refers to a rural worksite owned by a *latifundista*, large landowner. According to Porras Allende: "The origins of the Hacienda de Xaagá, located in the region of Mitla, date back to the allotment of cattle ranch sites in Mictlan or Miquitla, to Spaniards living in Oaxaca half a century after the settlement of Oaxaca. The 'Casa grande' of the hacienda of Xaagá was later placed literally on top of the pre-Hispanic tomb located in the indigenous community called, in the Zapotec language, Xaaga lobella" (2022, 3; author's translation).

3 Mitla, shortened version of San Pablo Villa de Mitla, is a 13,587 inhabitant Zapotec town, renowned for its archeological site featuring pre-Hispanic buildings with richly decorated walls of limestone mosaics in fretwork patterns. For more information, see Gobierno de México (n.d.).

4 Colloquially, the set of laws, rules, and habits that regulate and organize the social and political life of Indigenous communities are called *usos y costum-*

bres. In Oaxaca, the state constitution recognizes and grants autonomy to Indigenous communities, who can run themselves according to their Indigenous normative systems. Currently, among the 570 municipalities that form the state of Oaxaca, 417 elect their political representatives according to customary law.

5 The Mexican health-care system is tripartite, comprised of social security public institutions (for formal employees), public assistance, and the private medical sector. The system is highly fragmented, and people without social security usually face the greatest obstacles accessing medical care.

6 The Zapotec term *guelaguetza* refers to a variety of practices that entail free and reciprocal labor, or mutual aid. It is the basis of conviviality, morality, and social organization.

7 Each of these are the specific parts of the foot-pedal loom. Don Agustín named and signaled them with the intention to explain to me how the loom works and how he masters his craft. I am unable to translate these technical terms and prefer to leave them as they were spelled originally by Don Agustín.

REFERENCES

Alzoubi, A. R., Abunaser, A. Khassawneh, M. Alfaqih, A. Khasawneh, and N. Abdo. 2018. "The Bidirectional Relationship Between Diabetes and Depression: A Literature Review." *Korean Journal of Family Medicine* 39 (3): 137–46. https://doi.org/10.4082/kjfm.2018.39.3.137.

Breton, M. C., L. Guénette, M. A. Amiche, J. F. Kayibanda, J. P. Grégoire, and J. Moisan. 2013. "Burden of Diabetes on the Ability to Work: A Systematic Review." *Diabetes Care* 36 (3): 740–49. https://doi.org/10.2337/dc12-0354.

Gibson, James. 1979. *The Ecological Approach to Visual Perception*. Hillsdale, NJ: Lawrence Erlbaum Associates.

Instituto Nacional de Antropología e Historia. 2025."Zona Arqueológica de Mitla." INAH. Accessed July 7, 2025. https://www.inah.gob.mx/zonas/zona-arqueologica-de-mitla.

Juárez-Ramírez, C., F. L. Théodore, A. Villalobos, A. Jiménez-Corona, S. Lerin, G. Nigenda, and S. Lewis. 2015. "Social Support of Patients with Type 2 Diabetes in Marginalized Contexts in Mexico and Its Relation to Compliance with Treatment: A Sociocultural Approach." *PLOS ONE* 10 (11): e0141766. https://doi.org/10.1371/journal.pone.0141766.

Markens, R. 2017. "Los Significados Prehispánicos de la Greca Escalonada en los Palacios de Mitla." Instituto de Matemáticas de la UNAM. https://www.youtube.com/watch?v=9qdEVrLEJQw&t=2589s.

Mendenhall, E., S. A. Norris, R. Shidhaye, and D. Prabhakaran. 2014. "Depression and Type 2 Diabetes in Low- and Middle-Income Countries: A Systematic Review." *Diabetes Research and Clinical Practice* 103 (2): 276–85. https://doi.org/10.1016/j.diabres.2014.01.001.

Mol, A., I. Moser, and J. Pols, eds. 2010. *Care in Practice: On Tinkering in Clinics, Homes and Farms.* Transcript Publishing.

Porras Allende, Jorge Alberto. 2022. "Narrativa Histórica de la Ex Hacienda de Xaagá, la Transferencia del Poder entre Propietarios de Tierras en el Valle de Oaxaca." *International Journal of Human Sciences Research* 2 (9): 1–17.

Rodríguez Saldaña, J., P. V. Sosa Espinosa, and M. A. García Martínez. 1994. "Epidemiología de la Diabetes Mellitus en México: Pasado, Presente y Futuro." *Revista Facultad Medicina UNAM* 37 (1): 15–28.

Rosa, F., and A. Parodi. 2011. "Medicine among Métis, Phrónesis and Téchne." *Medicina y Ética. Revista Internacional de Bioética, Deontología y Ética Médica* 22 (1): 13–32.

Sharif, H., S. Jan, S. Sharif, T. Seemi, H. Naeem, and Z. Jawed. 2023. "Depression and Suicidal Ideation among Individuals with Type-2 Diabetes Mellitus: A Cross-Sectional Study from an Urban Slum Area of Karachi, Pakistan." *Frontiers in Public Health* 11: 1,135964. doi:10.3389/fpubh.2023.1135964.

Soto-Estrada, G. A., L. Moreno Altamirano, J. J. García-García, I. Ochoa Moreno, and M. Silbermane. 2018. "Trends in Frequency of Type 2 Diabetes in Mexico and Its Relationship to Dietary Patterns and Contextual Factors." *Gaceta Sanitaria* 32 (3): 283–90.

Stephen, L. 2005. *Zapotec Women: Gender, Class, and Ethnicity in Globalized Oaxaca.* Durham: Duke University Press. Second edition.

Trostle, J. 1988. "Medical Compliance as an Ideology." *Social Science & Medicine* 27 (12): 1299–1308.

Valdez Flores, G. A., and L. K. Castro Saucedo. 2021. "Cuando los Varones Enferman: Apuntes desde el Socioconstruccionismo y las Masculinidades para el Diseño de una Intervención con Hombres que Padecen Diabetes." In *Redes Temáticas: Género, Migración y Trabajo Social,* edited by C. Reyna Tejada, N. Macedonio Toledo, and G. Hernández Ríos, 32–58. Hidalgo, México: Acanits y Universidad Veracruzana.

Diabetes Is *More than* Numbers

Amma, amid the pressures of managing her diabetes, transforms her relationship with food, defying societal norms while reclaiming joy in her culinary traditions.

Gurpreet, a dynamic tiffin caterer in New Delhi, navigates the challenges of diabetes and family life, using her entrepreneurial spirit to defy the odds stacked against her.

Sarita, despite the comforts of her affluent lifestyle, grapples with the emotional turmoil of her husband's near-fatal health crisis and distance from her beloved children, all while managing her own diabetes with unwavering resolve.

Genesis battles chronic pain and a traumatic past while achieving remarkable success in managing her diabetes, revealing the hidden burdens behind her clinical triumphs.

Mothers, sisters, daughters, and grandmothers weave together in the juggling of demands, pains, and pleasures of life with diabetes. In many ways, conventional knowledge about diabetes doesn't capture the realities of managing sugar day-to-day. This requires us to look beyond narrow definitions of diet to understand the myriad ways that people seek healing through food, and to look beyond the metrics-based understanding through which a "good patient" is evaluated. Whether using a finger prick, a continuous glucose monitor, or an HbA1C test, diabetes control is almost always reduced to successfully producing laboratory values deemed to be appropriate. While we are not contesting that these tools can be useful, we show how diabetes management, or living well with diabetes, exceeds these metrics.

Social science approaches to enumeration, metrics, and other forms of quantification reveal the role of numbers in creating systems of surveillance and governance that manage everything from periods (in cycle-tracking apps) to funding determinations in evidence-based interventions in public health. Scholarship on obesity is useful here as scholars have explored the social life of metrics like BMI and weight and how they fuel moral panic. Obesity, typically measured by body mass index, is a measure derived of averages that centers weight as the epicenter of disease despite unsettled scientific studies about the cause of obesity and the problems obesity is thought to cause. In other words, metrics frame the way we think about ourselves and others, and when such metrics get it wrong, it causes more harm than good (medically and socially). Demands for evidence-based interventions and cost-effective rubrics are ever increasing in the global health landscape, relying upon specific kinds of quantitative metrics to address the world's most complex health problems. Yet, metrics are anything but neutral. They carry with them meaning and often conceal complex realities of trauma, suffering, and inequality.

As you read, you will bear witness to narratives of mothers managing diabetes that highlight how they strive to flourish despite the challenges posed by the condition. The stories illuminate how conventional knowledge and metrics can provide important insights while also falling short in capturing the nuanced realities of daily life with diabetes. These mothers demonstrate that living well involves more than just achieving favorable laboratory values; it encompasses resilience, emotional strength, and the ability to cultivate joy and meaning amid adversity. Their experiences underscore the need for a more holistic understanding of health that prioritizes flourishing over survival. Consider reflecting on these questions: How can health-care providers foster an environment that empowers patients to define what it means to flourish while living with diabetes, rather than focusing solely on metrics? In what ways can integrating emotional and social support into diabetes care help patients not only manage their condition but also enhance their overall well-being and quality of life?

CHAPTER THIRTEEN

Embodied Measuring

Pallavi Laxmikanth

My mother's name is Radhika. I call her Amma, which is the Tamil word for mother. In 2018, she was diagnosed with type 2 diabetes, with an HbA1c of 12.[1] She was fifty then, living in Hyderabad – the city in India with the highest rate of diabetes. Given the high value, the doctor prescribed an injectable insulin to take until her blood sugar levels (BSLs) were under control. That was the beginning of this experiment. When the measuring, reporting, and contestation about her body began.

Appu,[2] my father, is a software programmer who believes that almost any problem is solvable with the right kind of quantitative data mapping. On a green chalkboard in our kitchen, he had noted the dietician's recommended meal plan – he made it his mission to ensure she ate accordingly. There was a column noting the things she could eat five times a day with a corresponding column noting her blood glucose levels. On days when Amma's blood sugars were 160 mg/dL instead of 140 mg/dL, my father would ask her: *did you eat something that's not on the list?* If not, he went back to the drawing board for more dietary tinkering.

Amma had no respite from this schedule and began to resent the pressure he put on her and the form of control he and the dietician cultivated through her illness. This was harder still because she already had a propensity to feel guilty for minor indulgences such as popping a sweet on a difficult day (see Weaver 2019). On our walks on the apartment track, she would voice her frustration to me, rhetorically asking, "Is this a body, or is this math?"

After several months, Amma revolted. No matter how much she tried to adhere to the doctor's orders, her blood glucose levels would not equate to the mathematical equation of inputs (foods) and outputs (exercise). Even so, she resisted the idea of becoming "dependent" on insulin or other medication, which Lesley Jo Weaver (2019) has also observed among Indian mothers of a similar age, class, and caste in Delhi. Instead of taking insulin, Amma consumed multiple books and watched videos on how to "reverse" diabetes (see for example Shah 2017). She decided to try a vegetarian version of a low-carbohydrate, almost ketogenic[3] diet to keep her BSLs around 120 mg/dL without the help of medication.

On an average day on this diet, Amma would ask Pranita who was our domestic worker, to pulse two medium heads of cauliflower in a blender and steam it on the stovetop. Rice was our staple food, and this was her keto version. She would store this in a large box in the fridge and have it replenished every few days. She would eat this with dry curries, like okra and raw banana sauteed in oil and finished with chili and coriander powder, or *poriyals* – steamed vegetables with tempered spices and grated coconut. She mixed her rice with tangy vegetable chutneys, *sambar* (cooked pigeon peas in a tamarind broth, with spices and vegetables), *rasam* (a spicy tamarind soup with tomatoes and tempering), or boiled, mashed greens. She loved to cook and would make these by herself. She would finish her meal with a cup of yogurt. On days when she felt like eating rotis, she would make them with flaxseed meal and almond flour, and pair them with a North Indian style *paneer butter masala*, which is cottage cheese in a creamy, cashew, onion, and tomato gravy, or *baingan bharta*, a fire-roasted eggplant fried with spices, onions, tomatoes, and roasted garlic.

She was also practicing "intermittent fasting" (IF), which for her involved eating no or few calories for sixteen hours, between 8:00 p.m. and 12:00 p.m. the next day, and consuming two meals in the remaining eight hours. Within three months of her starting this diet, her HbA1c came down from 12 to 8; she was incredibly pleased. As my father witnessed this transformation, he grew to respect her process and began to fast along with her. He shifted to eating millet instead of rice. Together, they would spend evenings in front of the television watching various dietary influencers talk about keto, fasting, insulin, and diabetes.

A SLIP

In March 2020, Amma attended a religious gathering with my father at the home of family friends who were known for their delectable food. The spread that night was savory. They had prepared *chole bhature*, deep-fried flour rotis with buttery chickpea curry, and *dahi papdi*, deep-fried crunchy flour discs combined with boiled yellow peas, yogurt, sweet-and-sour tamarind sauce, and mint chutney. Finally, they served a sweet: *rabri*, a thick, spongy sweet made from simmered, thickened milk, drenched in a cardamom-and-pistachio flavored sauce. When she returned from the event, my mother hurried into the house and went to the cupboard to find the glucometer pen.

These devices come in many shapes, sizes, and brands, with promises of accuracy and improved blood glucose management. They function by taking a blood sample – usually by pricking the skin using a pin and letting the blood drop onto a strip that is inserted into the monitoring device. The device then presents a reading. This reading is then assumed to depict how this person ate, what they did, and how they are "taking care" of their body, both in an individualistic frame and, especially, through the prism of the household (Weaver 2014, 2019; Mendenhall 2019) and class (Laxmikanth 2023). Numbers are crucial to a biomedical diagnosis of diabetes and its "management" and, as my mother shows, the experience of the illness and its care.

Amma pricked herself and the screen showed 270 mg/dL. The tension in the room was palpable, and my sister and I prepared to witness extended hours of Amma pacing along the corridors of the house or an angry outburst. She was visibly upset. She paced for a bit and then busied herself in the kitchen, preparing dinner for us. I sidled in and poured myself a cup of tea. While I made space for her to feel comforted, she turned toward me and said, "I couldn't control myself. I had two spoonfuls. They offered *dahi papdi*. And I had just two spoonfuls of it. And my number is 270."

I braced myself. This wasn't looking good. Her frustration mounted in intensity.

"How can this be? I don't eat anything. I starve myself every day. How can it show 270 when I ate just two spoonfuls?"

My mother calmed down shortly, and I went back to watching our favorite TV program with my sister. However, the next moment, we heard her scurrying. She entered the bedroom where my father sat, her hand raised above her head, in a position one would use to stab someone – she had the glucometer ready with a shiny, sharp tip. She rushed into the room and demanded my father's attention: "I want to check your numbers."

"Absolutely not," he replied.

My mother insisted, "I want to check it. How can it be normal? You ate so much. I want to check."

"Amma don't," I said. "It will only make you feel worse."

As my sister and I tried to calm her down, her mind entered into a series of numerical calculations: "He is eight years older than me. He ate a whole plate of chole bhature, a cup of rabri, and a whole dahi papdi. I want to check his numbers. How can mine be 270 and his be normal?" She was murderous. "I want to check his numbers" she repeated, holding her hand high with the glucometer, ready to stab.

She wanted her husband's body and blood glucose levels to react to the food; especially since she had a small bite, and he ate generously. My sister and I convinced her slowly to leave the room. "It's not worth it," we told her.

She collapsed onto the living room sofa and burst into tears. When her eyes were dry, she almost involuntarily sprung up from the chair and began pacing up and down the corridor. We were familiar with the pacing: she knew it would burn her blood sugars down to 130 in exactly thirty minutes. She would stop the pacing intuitively and go about her other work. As I watched her pace through the hallway, I realized that she perceived the glucometer to be a weapon: it exposed her, quantifying a feeling that was invisible and hard to grasp. It was constantly plotting a numerical narrative of where she was and where she had to go – a type of storytelling over which she lacked control. In the hands of the biomedical patient, the glucometer is perceived to enable better choices and better control, but as numbers become visible, people with diabetes become vulnerable. Numbers chart successes and failures, "good" choices and wrongdoings. Despite my father's growing empathy toward her illness and eating, she knew he did not understand. She wanted him to feel as exposed and vulnerable as her. She wanted to catch him, pin him down to a number.

EMBODIED MEASURING

Amma's story demonstrates her resentment toward the numerical orientation to life. Yet, she also embodied aspects of it in ways that would help her manage her illness. She used her senses and felt experience to reconcile not just blood glucose levels and foods but various life experiences and everyday actions. In many ways, this metabolic intuition framed the messy complexity through which she lived and managed her illness; she demonstrated how managing her symptoms was not as simplistic as my father wanted to map out. In contrast to the helpful technology he imagined it to be, Amma came to view the glucometer as a weapon, producing numerical bullets and stab wounds that could threaten and hurt her sense of self. Through the discrete numbers, the glucometer was a tool that established the dynamics of power and biomedical authority over her own will.

More than 74 million people have been diagnosed with type 2 diabetes in India, and epidemiologists estimate another 53.1 million are undiagnosed but living with insulin dysregulation (International Diabetes Federation 2021). This means around one in ten people are estimated to have diabetes. I conducted two years of fieldwork during the COVID-19 pandemic in Hyderabad, where the prevalence of diabetes is one in six (Kaveeshwar 2014). This prevalence is attributed to the changing spatiotemporal rhythms and stress of urban living accompanying the establishment of the offshore IT services industry. Throughout the pandemic, I resided with my parents in Hyderabad to quarantine as well as conduct research. The people with diabetes who I spent time with belonged to educated, privileged, middle-class households, much like mine. They either worked in or resided in the city's IT district. They, like my mother, were encouraged by private biomedical health providers to monitor their blood glucose levels regularly using a glucometer.

People diagnosed with diabetes, however, understand these numbers and indices in drastic contrast to biomedical authorities and carers. These numbers are not just abstractions or representations of parts or processes of the body; they are deeply embodied and entangled with sociocultural practices and household contexts. Numbers are meaningful actors contributing to the embodiment of measuring or what I conceptualize as *embodied measuring* (Laxmikanth 2023).

Embodied measuring is a conscious ability to compare and reconcile the felt sense of diabetes (through a dry throat or nausea, for instance) and blood glucose levels in the body, with everyday experiences and life events. It is a sense that people with diabetes like my mother cultivate in order to know, for instance, that a thirty-minute walk would bring her blood sugar levels to 130 mg/dL. As this sensitivity becomes part of their bodies and way of living, it provides them with opportunities to decide on their own terms how to manage their health. In this sense, embodied measuring entails sensing much more than a "value" or number as a separate entity that acts *upon* the body. Instead, embodied measuring speaks to the ways in which numbers are felt, sensed, folded *into* the flesh of the body, and become socioculturally significant through it.

During my time in Hyderabad, I discovered how significant taking a blood glucose measurement was in Amma's life, something you can only understand when you live with diabetes or care for someone living through it. Through this experience and research with others in Hyderabad living with diabetes, I focused on the sights, smells, emotions, people, and most importantly, the foods that rendered specific glucose readings significant to her and those around her. We just encountered dahi papdi, and going forward, we will meet her other favorites – *Banganapalli*, a variety of mango endemic to the Telugu-speaking region, and some simple, sweet jaggery.

I place each of these events on a linear timeline. Over the course of illness, Amma's relationship to the glucose monitor and the reading shapeshifted in relation to her food, the folds of her body, and the ways in which she perceived the illness at that time. I show the messy and proximate relationships that people with diabetes share with biochemical indices and blood glucose readings, and how numbers become intimately familiar to the body and social contexts over time, which becomes instrumental to how well people live with and outwit their diabetes.

EATING BANGANAPALLI MANGO

"I shouldn't eat mangoes again," Amma said with an air of disappointment. A few months into the pandemic, in May 2020 – three months after the dahi papdi incident – a fruit vendor arrived at the community gate. It had been one of the coolest summers we had experienced in Hyderabad in a long time. On Fridays, fruit vendors stopped by as part of the weekly arrangement that our residential community had during the COVID-19 lockdown and set up a little stand for residents to shop from.

She reminded me of their arrival three times while I drank my morning tea. And I knew why. It was because they had mangoes. She asked me if I wanted any repeatedly, as if to portray that she was caring for my needs. I knew she wanted them as much as I did. I could see her excitement as she paced about the kitchen, waiting for me to finish my tea and pick up the shopping bag. I grabbed Rs.1100 cash and stuffed it into the dark blue cloth bag, following her out the door and toward the fruit stall stationed near the basketball court close to the gate. There were two men, covering their faces with handkerchiefs as face masks, with crates of different varieties of mangoes as well as other fruits. There was *Banganapalli*, a famous local variety named after a place in Kurnool, also called *benishaan*, which translates to "without blemishes" (in our opinion it was indeed flawless). There was also *Himayat*, sometimes called *Imam Pasand*, a name that suggests it was favored by the erstwhile royalty. The fruit seller also had watermelon, chikoo, muskmelon, banana, and apple.

Despite the tempting array, we both knew what we wanted. "Let's just take mangoes!" We paid the store owner exactly Rs.1,100, and the man placed them in the bag I held in my hands. I carried the eight-to-nine-odd kilograms of fragrance back home; three kilograms of Himayat (because they looked green and soon to be ripe) and five kilograms of Banganapalli (because they looked ripe, golden yellow, and ready to eat). I washed my hands and filled a large steel bowl with water, vinegar, and salt. I took the bowl to the table where I had placed the bag. One by one I delicately removed the mangoes, immersed them in the bowl, and took them out. I used a white cloth with small pink flowers to dry them individually, resting one on top of the other in a pyramid shape, such that they glistened collectively. Each mango felt personal. My family members all visited the dining table to take in the sight and smell of the mangoes.

In the afternoon, my mother went into preparation mode. She was making *jowar rotis* for us with *kaal* (a lentil curry with mild spices). While on her keto diet, my mother would not take her prescribed diabetes

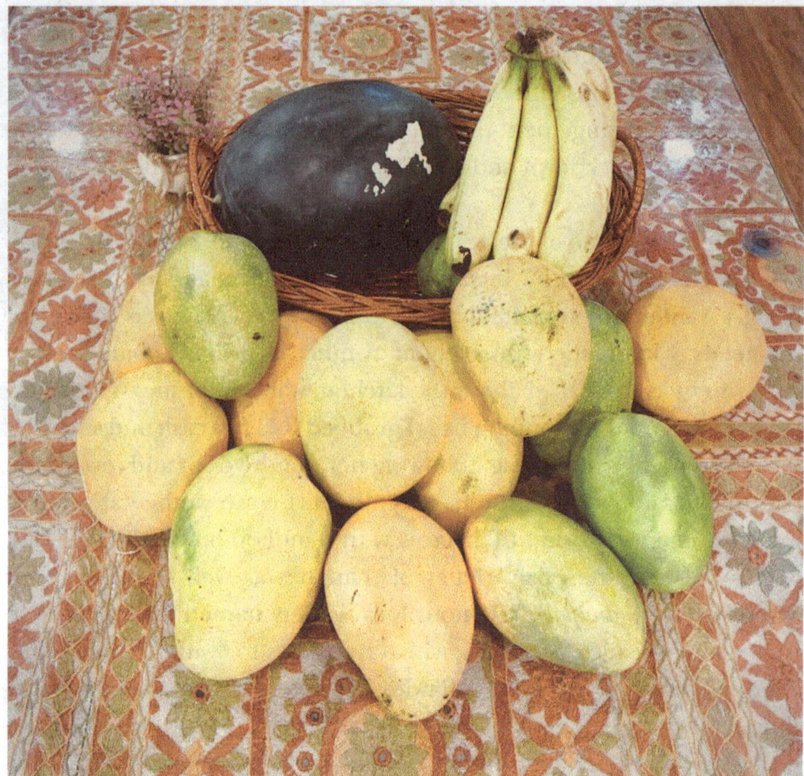

Figure 13.1: The mangoes

medication, which was a 1 mg tablet of Amaryl, and would eat her usual cauliflower rice or flaxseed roti. On days when she was going to eat carbohydrates, she would calculate the amount of medicine she would require to keep her blood glucose levels in check. On this day, she took Amaryl in preparation to eat the roti, kaal, as well as mango. There was both excitement and tension in the air. At 12:30 p.m., she ate three rotis and one Banganapalli. Sitting at the table, in anticipative meditation, she gingerly poked at the fleshy chunks of yellow with a fork and finished off the mango by holding on to the seed with her right hand and slowly sucking on the last bits of flesh stuck to it.

We retired to our rooms for an afternoon nap after this delicious meal. At about 2:30 p.m., I walked to the kitchen to get some coffee and found my mother sitting on the balcony fiddling with her glucometer. "I checked my numbers. My glucose is at 220," she said, sounding worried.

I was surprised that her blood glucose levels had spiked despite taking the medicine. I was also surprised that I had trained myself to interpret the number according to the food she ate and the dosage of medicine she took. "It's not possible," I said.

To my amusement, her tone changed, and rather matter-of-factly she said, "Well this glucometer is sometimes wonky." Given the incident in March, I hadn't expected her to change her tone so quickly. It was a brand called Beato, marketed as a "high-tech" glucometer, which meant it sent unwanted texts to my bemused father (who was her emergency contact) each time her blood sugars were elevated. She returned to the medicine cabinet and removed another glucometer; this time it was a brand called Dr. Morepen, recommended by the go-to physician. She took the kit, came back onto the balcony, and opened it. She pricked her finger, put the thin black glucometer strip on the blood that was oozing out of the puncture. She did all this deftly, with quick, swift movements. Within seconds, the meter showed 120.

"I thought so … but not sure which one is right," she said.

She laughed hastily and put the glucometer back in the cupboard. She told me later that after her 220 reading, she had paced up and down the hallway for twenty minutes.

"Something is maybe off with the glucometer, and we should get a new one," I replied.

"Or maybe I pricked the most sugary part of me."

We both laughed. She related the incident to Appu and said, "That one finger had so much sugar. Now I have to calculate which body part to prick." Crestfallen, she walked back to the dining table, where the mangoes were kept. Gazing at them longingly, she said, "I shouldn't eat mangoes again."

This is an exemplar of embodied measuring. Despite her concern with her "sugary finger" and the risks of pursuing her love affair with mangoes, the tenor of her voice suggested that she knew the glucometer's pronouncements were not absolute. She questioned the accuracy of the glucometer, and along with that, even which part of the body could represent her better numerically. She had a sense of what was "wonky" about the whole process. Her familiarity with her body, the number, and the capacities of the glucometer was growing as she began to experiment with eating fruit and incorporating these various actors into the process. Every time I would cut mangoes, she would eat a few pieces and check her sugar levels after a meal. She was training her body to attune to mangoes, blood sugar levels, and the ways in which they related to each other through her body. When she realized a few pieces weren't affecting her numbers, she would have half a mango. "I ate half a mango today; my number was still 116 after lunch," she said to me proudly. She started telling all houseguests and relatives about this discovery. And this was not all that she had found.

In late May 2020, my mother and I visited the home of family friends and participants Deepa and Pradeep, carrying some medicines they needed. Having tutored Pradeep on the mechanics of the keto diet for the past year, enabling him to reduce his HbA1c, she was keen to share her trial-and-error data on the mango and encourage him to eat Himayat. Seated at their dining table, with our masks on, she began excitedly, "You can eat thick mangoes with a lot of flesh. Like Himayat … I am eating half a mango after my meals. Nothing is happening. It's not spiking." Since Pradeep had been on the keto diet for more than eight months, she insisted his fasting BSLs would have come down considerably by now, which would enable him to eat mangoes.

Deepa, however, was concerned: how would they check if his BSLs were spiking or not? She feared having an episode where she had to wade through the unsanitary and dangerous conditions in hospitals due to COVID-19, which had also prevented them from getting a laboratory-based diagnostic test. The value provided by the glucometer, she said, was always very different compared to the tests from the diagnostic center. My mother, who had had her own incident with a "wonky" glucometer a month before, quipped excitedly to explain why: "That's because they are taking it from here," she said, pointing to the crick inside her left elbow where the laboratory sample was often taken.

"HbA1c, because they take it from here, it will be different. The glucometer shows ten to twenty points higher because we take it from here." She pointed to the tip of her left index finger.

"When you take it from the vein, it will be lesser." She had outwitted the glucometer and figured out its inaccuracy! Amma had moved from viewing the glucometer as a weapon that could act to control her every move. She found that enacting a relationship situated in negotiability and adaptability could bring the device and her body into a plane where they could be made intelligible to each other. This embodied measuring then enabled her to re-introduce foods back into the diet that she loved.

EATING JAGGERY AND BANANAS

Seven months after the mango debacle, Amma procured a continuous glucose monitor (CGM). A CGM is a device that measures your blood sugar throughout the day, taking stock of small fluctuations and providing data in real time. She was prompted to buy it following another incident after eating sweet potatoes at the funeral of my grandfather, who had passed away due to COVID-19. Before the incident, she worried that she would feel controlled by such a device. She didn't want it to fuel a preoccupation with keeping her BSLs regulated and therefore affect her mood and well-being. Yet, she was indignant and sure that sweet potatoes would not cause her BSLs to spike.

After the funeral, Amma and I stopped by the home of our neighbor, Naveen, who was also a participant in my research study. Naveen had contracted a steady supply of CGMs from a local vendor to help manage his father's severe diabetes. After a heated discussion, Naveen agreed that sweet potatoes were not supposed to read at 260 mg/dL. The next morning, he came over to place the CGM device on my mother's arm, which would stay there at all times to consistently measure her blood sugar. He helped install an app on her phone and showed her how to hold her phone against the sensor until she heard a beep. Her phone would then display the reading.

She was ready for fifteen days of measuring and being measured. Thrilled and satisfied at her conspiratorial skills, my mother walked around the house with a smirk. Every half an hour, she would hold up her phone to her arm, and I would hear a beep. At times we would be engrossed in a show on the TV, and I would hear a beep. When I turned toward her, I would notice a tiny smile on her face. The reading was often 120mg/dL or less. She would walk up to me after meals to show me how her blood sugar levels remained stable, relishing in the little victories, which suggested that she was getting away with managing her blood sugar levels without medication and a doctor's intrusive questions.

I tracked my mother's diet over the next few days and was curious as she turned into a cyborg of sorts (Haraway 1991), with a piece of technology that was embedded into her arm and constantly monitoring her blood. The experiment with the CGM revealed that foods she loved, like jaggery and bananas, did not spike her blood sugar levels. Since observing this data, Amma has allowed herself to pop a little chunk of jaggery when she goes into the kitchen and even make jaggery sweets. She continues to eat bananas.

It was the transformation of her relationship with the glucometer that has affected her way of thinking about living with her illness. Instead of the glucometer being perceived as a "weapon" or threat for which she would be punished or shamed, it became a liberating tool through which she could choose to eat certain foods that gave her joy. Even though she had sought out a low-carbohydrate diet to escape biomedical dietary dictums, she continued to push at its limits, to assert her body as unique.

Anthropological scholarship has rightly critiqued biochemical measurements and numerical representations of the body such as calories or BMI as simplistic reductions of more interconnected processes and embodied ecologies (see for example Guthman 2011; Yates-Doerr 2015). This is echoed in scholarly work on "self-tracking" of physiological indicators, which emphasizes how numbers are used to "normalize" a body and exert authority and power over it (Lupton 2017). However, in embodied measuring, numbers are enacted differently. They are not just discrete entities acting upon bodies; people cultivate the ability to sense how numbers feel. And this experience is not just an individual sense but a collective one.

When Amma took a glucose reading, there was tension in the air as her family surrounded her. Her anticipation, anxiety, relief, or disappointment was deeply palpable. The logistics of pricking and recording the reading, the sweat on our brows in the scorching Hyderabadi summer, and, significantly, her experience of dry throat, thirst, irritability, or stress – all contributed to the phenomenological and social dynamics of the illness. Diabetes is an (inter)subjective experience that is distributed across family (Mendenhall 2019), the city (Solomon 2016), and other illnesses and social structures (Weaver and Mendenhall 2014). Similarly, metrics and their meanings cannot be divorced from this (inter)subjective experience (Yates-Doerr 2012; Hardin and Mccullough 2013) – doing so furthers a legacy of demarcating the qualitative and quantitative, subjective and objective, through false boundary making (Law 2016). Amma felt her numbers, and these feelings strengthened as the glucometer became embedded into her life and surroundings. She was not merely learning or internalizing the number, she was actively merging with it (Mol and Law 2004, 51), folding the experience into her body in a way that made both her and her family attuned to how it felt.

Embodied measuring represents a fleshy space where Amma need not stop eating mangoes but could eat a few pieces. These small changes encouraged her to watch out for other sugar-spiking foods and enjoy jaggery and bananas, reclaiming her body and cultural practices in ways that external forms of control would not have allowed. Inspired by the "measuring body" (Carusi and Hoel 2014; Hoel and Carusi 2015, 2018), based on Merleau-Ponty's (1968) concept of flesh – an indeterminate extension and meeting point of subject and object that is experientially located – embodied measuring treats the body as a site, a tool, a standard, that "brings bodies, symbolic systems, and technologies into a new constellation that reconfigures agency and materiality" (Hoel and Carusi 2018, 46). Embodied measuring provides a lens to consider the environment, her body, our bodies, affective exchanges, and sensibilities, along with the glucometer, its display, and the numbers shown, as part of an intertwined constellation.

Amma's measuring reveals how diabetes can produce values that are not distanced objectively from the body but extend the self's experience of the world. In a world inundated with biochemical indices like calories, nutrients, and blood sugar markers, it is crucial to pay attention to the experience of numbers. This doesn't imply that numbers seamlessly fold into the body, but their idiosyncratic incorporation influences how the body experiences them. Through this, bodies, foods, and glucometer readings occupy an "inter-world" where each element becomes intelligible in relation to the others and is, consequently, contextualized into the larger sociocultural fabric of life in middle-class, urban India.

Living well with diabetes, in this context, involves tinkering and attentive experimentation (Mol, Moser, and Pols 2010) with restricted foods, glucometers, and insulin-based medication toward embodied measuring and outwitting diabetes. This approach allowed my participants to push at the limits of their diagnoses and illness. For my mother, it was a way of outwitting the glucometer – not by erasing and uprooting the structures that designed the management of illness, but by contending with "the multiple overlapping normative orders that constitute people's lives" and "navigating their sometimes discrepant demands" (Purcell 2017, 138). For Amma, this emerged from a clash in thoughts, a dissonance between what is, what should be, and what could be, prompting her to take the risk and change this course. Mangoes, jaggery, and forms of pleasure must find a place within this continued processual negotiation of what gets eaten. With the glucometer in hand and her tinkering, she can work toward a fleshy incorporation of numbers and foods into her body, adhering to the normative orders of diets while breaking them apart.

NOTES

1 HbA1c, or glycated hemoglobin, is the average measure of a person's blood glucose levels over three months, assessed by the percentage of glucose attached to the hemoglobin molecules in the blood. The scale measures in single-digit numbers, from 5.7 onward. A diagnosis of diabetes is at 7 and above.
2 The Tamil word for father is *Appa*. We affectionately call him Appu.
3 The ketogenic diet, developed in the 1920s for epilepsy treatment, emphasizes high-fat, low-carbohydrate, and adequate-protein foods. In its classic form, the ratio of fat to carbohydrates and protein is 4:1. Widely known as "keto," this diet has also been used to manage conditions like type 2 diabetes, obesity, cardiovascular diseases, and PCOS. By reducing carbohydrate intake, the body shifts to burning fats for fuel, producing ketone bodies as an alternative energy source for the brain and body (Fenton and Fenton 2016; Fung 2016).

REFERENCES

Anton, S. D., et al. 2018. "Flipping the Metabolic Switch: Understanding and Applying the Health Benefits of Fasting." *Obesity* 26 (2): 254–68.

Carusi, A., and A. S. Hoel. 2014. "Toward a New Ontology of Scientific Vision." In *Representation in Scientific Practice Revisited*, 201–222. Cambridge: MIT Press.

Fenton, C. J., and T. R. Fenton. 2016. "Dietary Carbohydrate Restriction: Compelling Theory for Further Research." *Nutrition* 32 (1): 153.

Fung, D. J. 2016. The Obesity Code: Unlocking the Secrets of Weight Loss. Vancouver: Greystone Books.

Guthman, J. 2011. Weighing In: Obesity, Food Justice, and the Limits of Capitalism. Berkeley: University of California Press.

Haraway, D. J. 1991. *Simians, Cyborgs, and Women: The Reinvention of Nature*. New York: Routledge.

Hardin, J. A., and M. B. McCullough, eds. 2013. Reconstructing Obesity: The Meanings of Measures and the Measure of Meanings. New York: Berghahn Books.

Hoel, A. S., and A. Carusi. 2015. "Thinking Technology with Merleau-Ponty." In *Postphenomenological Investigations: Essays on Human-Technology Relations*, edited by R. J. Rosenberger and P. P. Verbeek, 27–45. New York: Lexington Books.

Hoel, A. S., and A. Carusi. 2018. "Merleau-Ponty and the Measuring Body." *Theory, Culture & Society* 35 (1): 45–70.

International Diabetes Federation. 2021. *IDF Diabetes Atlas.* 10th ed. Brussels, Belgium.

Law, J. 2016. "STS as Method." In *The Handbook of Science and Technology Studies*, 3rd ed., edited by Ulrike Felt, Rayvon Fouché, Clark A Miller, and Laurel Smith-Doerr, 31–57. Cambridge, MA: MIT Press.

Laxmikanth, P. 2023. Embodied Measuring: Outwitting Type 2 Diabetes in Middle-Class Urban India. New York: Routledge.

Lupton, D. 2017. "Self-Tracking, Health and Medicine." *Health Sociology Review* 26 (1): 1–5.

Mendenhall, E. 2019. Rethinking Diabetes: Entanglements with Poverty, Trauma, and HIV. Ithaca: Cornell University Press.

Merleau-Ponty, M. 1968. *The Visible and the Invisible: Followed by Working Notes.* Edited by A. Lingis and C. Lefort. Evanston: Northwestern University Press.

Mol, A., and J. Law. 2004. "Embodied Action, Enacted Bodies: The Example of Hypoglycaemia." *Body & Society* 10 (2–3): 43–62.

Mol, A., I. Moser, and J. Pols, eds. 2010. *Care in Practice: On Tinkering in Clinics, Homes and Farms.* Bielefeld: Transcript Verlag.

Purcell, B. 2017. "Rebellious Matter." In *Unfinished: The Anthropology of Becoming*, edited by João Biehl and Peter Locke, 125–44. Durham: Duke University Press.

Shah, N. 2017. *Reversing Diabetes in 21 Days.* London: Ebury Press.

Solomon, H. 2016. Metabolic Living: Food, Fat and the Absorption of Illness in India. Durham: Duke University Press.

Weaver, L. J. 2014. When Family Comes First: Diabetes, Social Roles, and Coping among Women in Urban North India. PhD diss., University of California.

Weaver, L. J. 2019. *Sugar and Tension: Diabetes and Gender in Modern India.* New Brunswick: Rutgers University Press.

Weaver, L. J., and E. Mendenhall. 2014. "Applying Syndemics and Chronicity: Interpretations from Studies of Poverty, Depression, and Diabetes." *Medical Anthropology: Cross-Cultural Studies in Health and Illness* 33 (2): 92–108.

Yates-Doerr, E. 2012. "The Mismeasure of Obesity." In *Reconstructing Obesity: The Meaning of Measures and the Measure of Meanings*, edited by J. A. Hardin and M. B. McCullough, 113–28. New York: Berghahn Books.

Yates-Doerr, E. 2015. The Weight of Obesity: Hunger and Global Health in Postwar Guatemala. Berkeley: University of California Press.

CHAPTER FOURTEEN

Thriving while Struggling to Access Care in India

Lesley Jo Weaver

Gurpreet was one of the most industrious women I had ever met. I would visit her kitchen, squeezed into a dark and musty apartment rental in New Delhi, where she ran her tiffin catering business. Tiffins are hot lunches packed into stainless-steel bowls that get latched together in a little portable stack. Gurpreet prepared and delivered these to her clients all over the city, mostly single men and women working in offices, five days a week. She was like a small force of nature, gesturing animatedly and practically jogging around the tiny apartment in her red-and-green chiffon salwar-kameez, her long braid trailing down her back. Sharp, garlicky cooking smells emanated from giant stainless-steel vats that bubbled on propane-run stovetops. The scale of food preparation in her kitchen was almost unbelievable, especially given that the whole space was only about sixty square feet.

Gurpreet's family faced their share of health and financial challenges. Gurpreet grew up in a poor family in a rural part of Punjab state, the daughter of a farmer. She moved to New Delhi shortly after her marriage when she was eighteen in hopes of finding steady work. Gurpreet's husband was the main breadwinner for many years, working in home internet sales. A few years ago he sustained a spinal injury in a vehicle accident that made it impossible for him to continue riding around the city for work on a motorcycle, which was their main mode of transportation since they could not afford a car. Gurpreet, meanwhile, was diagnosed with gestational diabetes when they were expecting their son, causing worry; however, her health improved after his birth. More than a decade later, she was again diagnosed with type 2 diabetes, after a period of feeling exhausted and thirsty all the time.

Gurpreet struggled to change her diet based on what the doctors told her she should do to manage her sugar. Punjabi cooking was both her identity and her livelihood, and many Punjabi dishes feature heavy starches like potatoes and lots of oil and *ghee* (clarified butter). The day I was visiting, she was preparing a deluxe lunch menu consisting of traditional Punjabi fare meant to mark the upcoming Sikh holiday commemorating the birth of Guru Nanak, the founder of Sikhism: *dal makhani* (lentils cooked with cream, tomatoes, and butter), *aloo pyaz* (potatoes fried with onions and spices), an optional chicken or *paneer* (fried cheese) dish for those willing to pay a bit more, and accompaniments including *roti* (buttered flatbread made from whole wheat flour), white rice, and a small side salad of fresh tomatoes, cucumbers, and onion.

I arrived very early in the morning just as she was making the dal – my favorite dish. Gurpreet had already cleaned and soaked the black lentils overnight to prepare them for today, and I watched as she dumped heaps of glistening lentils into a giant pressure cooker with generous helpings of oil, salt, and water. Soon the pressure cooker was hissing and whistling, giving off bursts of steam that made the already oppressive kitchen feel like an oven. While the cooker whistled at her elbow, Gurpreet processed ginger and garlic into a fine paste with an appliance that looked like a coffee grinder. When she eventually opened the cooker, the heavy lid suctioned away from the body with a loud *thunk* and in went the ginger-garlic paste, followed by chili powder and finely diced tomatoes. This time she didn't replace the lid but let the mixture simmer with an open top. We chatted for the next hour as the mixture bubbled beside us. Later, as a finishing touch, she would add hunks of butter and generous splashes of cream. And this was just one of several dishes she would cook today for her customers' lunch.

Gurpreet's cooking was her family's saving grace once her husband became disabled and could no longer work. Her cooking career took off, however, by chance. One day, neighbors smelled her delicious cooking coming out of her flat. A single man living down the hall asked her to pack a tiffins for him to eat at work. What started as a favor turned into a business (even if the pay was nominal). She became beloved and sought-after by the community, rising at five every morning to prepare fresh hot lunches accompanied by freshly made rotis for over 120 working people. The lunches weren't always as fancy as the dishes she made today, but they were still very labor-intensive. When she described her demanding orders, she laughed and her bangles clinked: "That's 360 rotis I roll every day!" The work had become not only hers but her family's: her husband carefully folded napkins into the top of each lunch box from a padded chair that accommodated his sore back. "Home cooking, away from home" read the slogan on the paper napkins. Then, her son and an employee would zip around town all morning, delivering these meals to shiny office buildings and humble auto repair shops. The business was lucrative enough to sustain Gurpreet's entire family, and even to fund her son's ongoing post-graduate correspondence education. The tiffin business success made Gurpreet feel exceedingly proud.

In between cooking and feeding her neighbors, Gurpreet struggled with several approaches to managing her diabetes and, eventually, used the entrepreneurial spirit she gained from her business to improve her health. At first, she tried taking oral hypoglycemic drugs such as metformin, but she found their side effects intolerable. "English medicines are harmful for me," she told me over hot, sweet chai. "They made my insides burn and my urine smell bad; they're too hot," she told me. I nodded and wrote down her mention of temperature in my journal: the concept of temperature balance is crucial for overall health in the Ayurvedic medical system. After exploring several treatments, Gurpreet stopped taking Western medications and relied entirely on Ayurvedic plant-derived medications to control her blood sugar.

As we sat next to an open window, the delicious aromas of the morning's cooking dissipating into the foggy autumnal air, Gurpreet passed me a plastic jar of powder she took every morning. I peered closely at the label and saw several familiar ingredients. There were *neem* leaves from a tree in the mahogany family. There was *karela*, which is a bitter gourd. There was also an extract of *jamun*, a tree fruit. The final ingredient was ashwagandha, a form of Indian ginseng that has received increasing attention from holistic health groups in the West for its use as an adaptogen – an herb that helps with stress. There were also ingredients I'd never seen before, despite the decades I'd spent in kitchens not unlike Gurpreet's as a medical anthropologist studying the interplay of gender, mental health, and diabetes. It was this Ayurvedic therapy that enabled Gurpreet to feel that she managed her diabetes well, though her metrics suggested that her blood sugar often fluctuated. She reported no disabilities or symptoms that would typically be associated with elevated sugar levels, despite having had diabetes for over a decade. Gurpreet bought her Ayurvedic medication from a charitable trust working out of the complementary and alternative medicine wing of a major national hospital chain. She rarely went there for checkups though – only when she felt sick, she told me. Regular preventative checkups were too expensive, and besides, she quipped, "What's the point of going to the doctor if you're not sick?"

One weekend in December, when the winter fog seeped into every nook and cranny of Delhi's concrete buildings, Gurpreet and her husband took me to see Gurpreet's favorite faith healer. We crammed into a hired car and drove across state lines to a small, dirt-road town in Haryana that had only one large house, painted neon green and pink. A sign printed on a tarp over the door read, "Sugar normalizing treatment," followed by, "Neither any medicine, nor insulin, nor any herbal medicine." During normal hours, Gurpreet told me, a line might form around the entire block, but we arrived on an off day.

After hearing how far we had come, a small, dignified man dressed in white welcomed us inside and offered us treatment even though it was a clinic holiday. Gurpreet lay down on a narrow cot first. The room was darkened by brown floral curtains, and the pink concrete walls had peeling spots where monsoon rains had loosened the paint over the years. Gurpreet's husband and I watched silently as the healer started by gently touching Gurpreet's stomach, eyes closed, as if he were listening or feeling for something. Then he bent one of Gurpreet's legs at the knee and, again closing his eyes, gently but firmly pinched the back of her hamstring with a large set of brass tongs wrapped in many layers of medical tape to create cushioned handles. He held this for a moment, did the other leg, then did the same to other fleshy parts of her body, such as her upper arms. He finished by standing back-to-back with her, linking arms, and impressively lifting her into the air as he bent forward, cracking her back audibly.

I was up next. Slightly nervous, I lay down in my long, loose clothing as Gurpreet and her husband watched. At the healer's direction, I bent

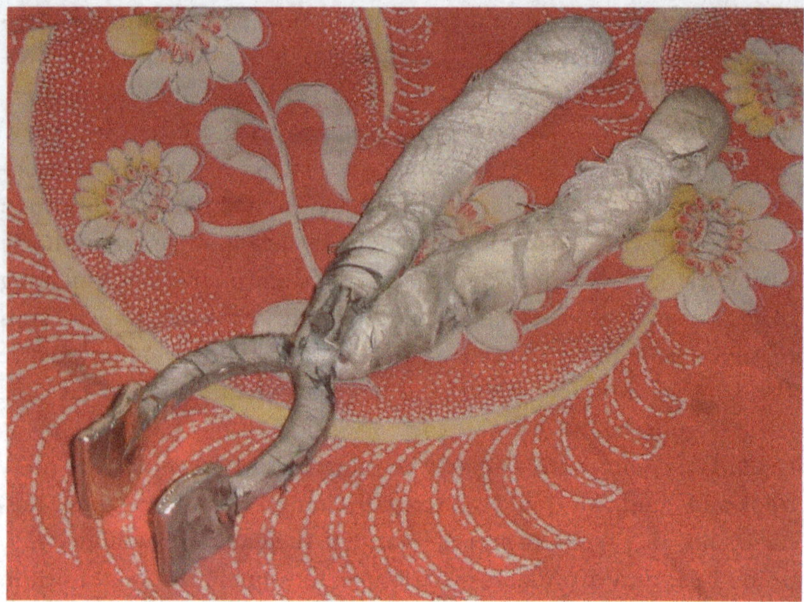

Figure 14.1: The faith healer's nerve-opening instrument

my right leg as Gurpreet had done and rested my foot flat on the cot. He reached to the back of my leg with one hand, and with the other, placed the instrument around my hamstring muscle. Since I am a runner, I always have tight hamstrings. The healer clamped and held the muscle with firm pressure for about ten seconds, then released. This felt like a firm, almost painful massage. Next, he moved on to my other leg. He pinched my triceps in a similar way, then my forearms. This spot was a little tender due to the carpel tunnel syndrome I was developing from too much typing, but he held the pressure just to the point where I felt I could not take it anymore, then released. Finally, he pinched the trapezius muscles in my upper shoulders. This felt like a Swedish massage. The healer left my entire trunk untouched. He ended my treatment as he had done with Gurpreet, linking arms with me as we stood back-to-back and bending forward so that my back arched over his and cracked in two places, even though I was about four inches taller than him. He set me down gently, and I breathed out a long breath, feeling a sense of relaxation and relief.

This procedure, the healer explained, had provided me and Gurpreet (and countless others) relief because it opened the nerve pathways. When nerve paths are clogged, this can create harmful blockages that prevent the humors from maintaining a healthy balance in the body. Here he was obliquely referencing the Ayurvedic *doshas* (humors) of *vata, pita,* and *kapha,* which each person has in varying amounts. Vata represents the air and space elements of the body, and those with dominant vata tend to be slim, irritable, fast learners, and on-the-go multitaskers. Pita-dominant people have an abundance of fire and water and are known for having tenacity, internal heat, muscular builds, athleticism, and a competitive and aggressive spirit. Finally, kapha dosha comprises earth and water elements. Kapha-dominant people are thick-boned, caring, laconic, and may be prone to weight gain and oversleeping. Though each person has different mixtures of these doshas, they should be balanced for ultimate health. Blockages in the nerve pathways might cause some humors to build up and others to be cut off. The treatment, he explained, coaxed those pathways open to restore balance.

Gurpreet prided herself on doing things differently than others, both in her family life and with her diabetes. "See the lady over there?" she said, gesturing to an apartment several doors down from her own once we returned from the faith healer. "She has diabetes, too, and she's always moping around and acting sick. 'Oh, I'm this, I'm that …' Not me. The other day, I had a fever and could barely get out of bed. I just drank some water and rested for a bit, and before I knew it, I was up doing the cleaning and cooking." When I asked what allowed her to be so successful in life, she said, "It's all in the mind. It's your thinking that can make you sick or well." Plus, she explained, the business kept her sharp. "My customers rely on me. If I just decide not to cook lunch one day, what will they do? Do you think they'll say, 'Oh, Gurpreet, no problem that we had nothing to eat today; we understand that you weren't feeling well.' No! They'll quit my business and find another one."

I was struck by Gurpreet's strong sense of purpose and status as the family's sole breadwinner. It was clear that this played a role in her motivation to manage her diabetes along with her very demanding work schedule. So did her gratitude for the fact that her family was now able to live relatively comfortably. "I've seen poverty," she said, "and my son deserves chances in life." Finally, Gurpreet's entrepreneurial spirit gave her avenues to take action on her health that felt meaningful to her and, according to her lived experience, made her feel good, such as the Ayurvedic and faith healing treatments. Although her family was barely clinging to the lower rungs of the middle class compared to many of the city's wealthier residents (some of whom were her customers), Gurpreet was content with their station in life, and it was clear that the whole family was aiming toward a more prosperous future.

SARITA

Sarita greeted me at the door. Her house, in a wealthy suburb of New Delhi, was one of the most elegant spaces I had ever stepped into. The scent of jasmine wafted from the fresh blossoms floating in a decorative urn by the entrance on this lovely spring day. French doors opened onto a tiny backyard boasting an immaculate patch of grassy turf. Long curtains billowed in the warm breeze.

Sarita herself was, like her surroundings, the picture of poise and elegance. The wife of a retired diplomat, she was a high-caste, high-class woman who wore an understated but elegant *kurti* (short tunic) in a traditional block print with jeans. Her salt-and-pepper hair was cut into a fashionable bob, and funky glasses framed her face. Her feet were bare, and she spoke fluent English with a British-sounding accent. She was highly educated and had traveled the world with her husband before his retirement. A life-size portrait of Sarita and her husband, she seated and he standing with his hand resting on the back of her chair, accompanied by a large black dog, hung on a far wall. Sarita came across as remarkably humble and down-to-earth, despite all the extravagance. A servant dressed in a beautiful *sari* brought me *nimbu pani* (a sweet-and-salty lemonade), her anklets jingling musically as she walked through the room with a tray. Sarita thanked her graciously.

Though Sarita's life might sound idyllic, and she was indeed grateful for her "life of leisure," as she described it, it also had its challenges. For starters, Sarita had type 2 diabetes. She had been diagnosed fourteen years prior in her late forties. Her diagnosis came as a shock, in part because she had always been relatively thin and never had any health problems. However, she had struggled a great deal with her family. Her beloved adult children all lived abroad with her grandchildren, and she missed them dearly. Most pressingly, her husband had nearly died from what she described as a case of medical malpractice just five months prior. He had miraculously survived cardiac shock followed by multiple organ failure and remained in the hospital for two-and-a-half months. He was still recovering at home when I visited Sarita, who was serving as his primary caretaker.

Sarita was attentive about managing her diabetes, and she had been doing it for so long that it felt like it was practically an afterthought for her. Her approach was, by all measures, matter-of-fact. When I asked how she found it so easy to adhere to the diet, exercise, medication, and medical checkup regimens that so many other women I knew struggled with, she told me about her uncle and about a close family friend, both of whom she had watched suffer with – and eventually die of – diabetes complications. "I mean – I would never ..." she said, trailing off. I took this to mean that she would never want to emulate these individuals, and once she told me about their lives, I understood why. Her uncle had developed diabetic retinopathy and neuropathy that eventually led to a foot injury and the amputation of one leg. Her family friend, meanwhile, ended up in a diabetic coma multiple times (meaning her blood sugar had dropped so low that she lost consciousness) because, according to Sarita, she would delay eating lunch until her grandchildren came home from school. "What nonsense!" she scoffed, though I found it rather touching (if clearly ill-advised) that this woman was so devoted to her grandchildren.

At the time, insulin pumps were not available in India. Sarita managed her diabetes with daily insulin injections and glucose monitoring. She described how she also ate primarily "continental food" (meaning Western food, such as soups and sandwiches) instead of Indian food because she felt it was "lighter." I didn't ask where she had gotten the idea that Western food was healthier than Indian food, but this was something I heard from others as well. She walked daily. When her husband was hospitalized, Sarita described how she felt tempted to let go of her self-care routines. "I had some palpitations, but my diabetes was under control. I'm [usually] the first one to faint, but in all this time – I'm so proud of myself – I didn't faint, and I ate well because I felt that I needed to conserve my energy; I needed to feel strong. So instead of somebody telling me [to take care of myself], I took the pains to do it myself." Sarita stayed in touch with her endocrinologist by phone throughout her husband's ordeal, and she did increase her insulin dosage one time after her blood sugar began creeping upward. When she went for a checkup after he had stabilized, her doctor was surprised by her metrics, which showed her blood sugar had largely remained within a healthy range for the duration of her husband's crisis.

What factors allowed Sarita to persevere? She described herself as an active socialite whose friends and family called so often during her husband's hospitalization that she eventually had to give up answering the phone. Her children and grandchildren rotated visiting throughout this time so that she was never alone at home. As she described above, she made a conscious choice to prioritize her own health so that she could be strong. And she actively cultivated a sense of gratitude for the small steps her husband was making toward full recovery. "It was a very tough time, a very tough time," she reflected. "But you can see I am smiling again. I took him to see a movie yesterday, and today I am taking him out for lunch."

Sarita was brave, and this no doubt contributed to her resilience. But it was also clear that Sarita had plenty of money to afford the best quality medical care and an uninterrupted supply of insulin. She had a direct line to her endocrinologist and could call her anytime she wished if she felt unwell. She could afford to move her husband to the city's best hospital, a world-class private institution. And she could afford servants to manage things like cooking and cleaning. Rather than having to fight "uphill" with family members who might not appreciate having to change their diets to accommodate someone with diabetes, she was able to request specially catered items because her full-time cook had the time to make those foods.

Women like Gurpreet and Sarita occupy two very different points in the wide (and growing) wealth disparity in India today. India is home to some of the world's richest and poorest people, who may live, sometimes literally, right alongside one another in big cities like New Delhi (Oxfam International 2022). Gurpreet's lower-class family was engaged in the struggle for upward mobility through entrepreneurship and education. Sarita, by contrast, was already part of India's intelligentsia – a world-traveling, English-speaking elite. These differing social statuses mapped onto their differing approaches to managing diabetes, but these two women had one very important thing in common: if you asked them, both would say they are thriving with their diabetes. And, as I explain here, there are lessons to be learned from each of their experiences.

These two women's stories, and the diverse stories of the many other women who participated in my research, beg the question: what does it mean to "thrive" with diabetes?

For Gurpreet, we might consider what constitutes "thriving" with diabetes when one's blood sugar is not as tightly regulated as a health-care provider might wish. Gurpreet was a self-made woman who took an entrepreneurial approach to her livelihood and her diabetes management alike. She placed little importance on the diabetes control metrics most physicians use to assess overall diabetes health and rarely, if ever, checked her blood sugar. She rejected biomedical medications in favor of Ayurvedic ones, and although she had been living with diabetes for over a decade, she was doing quite well physically and mentally.

Gurpreet was one of the many women in my study who rejected conventional biomedical diabetes treatment and did not suffer from complications usually associated with fluctuating blood sugar. Around the world, there are many medical and spiritual systems from which people draw to take care of their diabetes health (Hardin 2019). In places like India, where medical syncretism is common, people draw from multiple healing traditions at once to manage illnesses, and in many cases, this can be effective. Gurpreet was living with diabetes on her own terms and defining for herself what "thriving" looked like.

Gurpreet's thriving was also reflected in her body. Gurpreet reported almost no disability in daily life. However, when I measured short- and medium-term blood sugar stability[1] alongside other markers of immune health and overall inflammation,[2] her blood sugar appeared to have been fluctuating a lot. Even so, her other markers were well within healthy ranges.

Most physicians I worked with would view women like Gurpreet as reckless – one referred to it as "playing dice with your health." They'd pointed out that if she had not yet developed debilitating health consequences from her fluctuating blood sugar, then she surely would develop them eventually. And they might be right. Yet women like Gurpreet were surprisingly common in my study, and some had been thriving with diabetes for more than three decades without developing the complications we typically see in people with diabetes whose blood sugar fluctuates a lot (Harding et al. 2019). Nor did she have any of the mental health problems that are often associated with fluctuating sugar (Weaver et al. 2015; Roy and Lloyd 2012). In fact, only those who had been recently diagnosed with diabetes reported higher levels of mental health symptoms, not those who had been living with it for longer (Weaver and Madhu 2015). What could be causing this unusual pattern?

I've found that for women like Gurpreet, being socially engaged – with work, with family, with community – is a powerful health-promoting force that could attenuate some of the negative impacts we would normally expect with diabetes (Weaver 2019). We have long known that a sense of social belonging is crucial for human thriving and health across the life course (Diener and Seligman 2002; Cornwell and Waite 2009). Women in India, on a population level, are at an important moment in terms of changing social (and especially gendered) roles. Where the cultural ideal was once that women would function primarily as self-sacrificing homemakers (and many still do so), women have been entering the workforce and engaging in public discourse in new ways over the last thirty years (Radhakrishnan 2011; Loomba and Lukose 2012).

The sense of purpose, social respect, and belonging that Gurpreet derived from her business was part of what allowed her to thrive with diabetes, even when her blood sugar was not within the recommended range. If she had taken a different approach that involved strict adherence to a diabetic diet, medications, and exercise, would she have experienced greater thriving than she was when we met? She most likely would have avoided complications related to diabetes for a longer time, but for her, the tradeoff – compromising her quality of life now for ambiguous future gains – was probably not worth it. From that perspective, then, Gurpreet was thriving on her own terms.

Sarita's story illuminates how socioeconomic status and access to health care shape people's ability to thrive with diabetes. Sarita's access to resources was evident in her everyday talk: her routine doctor's visits, dependence on a reliable source and flow of insulin, purchasing and consuming the "right" foods her servants would prepare for her, and ensuring that her husband was well cared for after his life-threatening illness. Sarita relied on regular blood sugar monitoring, insulin, diet, exercise, and preventative care to ensure her metrics remained within healthy ranges. Compared with Gurpreet, this approach to diabetes management adhered much more closely to what physicians would recommend in this setting. For Sarita, those management techniques were not overly burdensome, and she, too, had been thriving with diabetes for over a decade.

Overwhelming evidence demonstrates that, around the world, people with higher socioeconomic status experience better overall health and fewer complications with chronic diseases like diabetes, especially in societies like India with larger inequality between the rich and the poor (Nelson et al. 2019; Roy 2004; Jotkowitz et al. 2006; Williams et al. 2018). This is partly because higher socioeconomic status means more resources. For instance, Sarita had both the time and the money to accommodate her diabetes with minimal inconvenience to herself and others in her life. Sarita's household employed both a servant and a full-time cook, who could make separate food for everyone in the household if they wished to eat different things.

Gurpreet was an exception; generally, I found that the lower-income women in my study experienced more stress and health complications related to a lack of resources (Mendenhall et al. 2012). Most women (who were lower income) could not afford a full-time cook; instead, they might be preparing two or three multiple-dish hot meals every day for their extended families and simply would not have the ability to prepare separate diabetes-friendly foods for themselves. For many, the act of cooking was important care-work aimed at meeting the needs and preferences of senior male family members, such as husbands and fathers-in-law. "When the husband has diabetes, everyone changes [their diet]," explained one female diabetes physician. "But when the wife has it, nobody changes."

Moreover, taking time away from domestic work to exercise or attend diabetes checkups could be viewed as excessively self-centered; several women complained that their male family members, who controlled family finances, refused to pay for regular consultations their doctors wanted them to attend. For others, low socioeconomic status created barriers to necessary medical care, such as not being able to afford diabetes medications or glucose test strips. "When I have money, I take my medicines. If not, I don't," explained one low-income woman who worked as a domestic servant. Sarita's thriving, therefore, cannot be understood separately from the many advantages that made it easier for her to manage diabetes than most Indian women.

The experiences of Gurpreet, Sarita, and others show us that thriving with diabetes can mean many different things. They demonstrate how women who lead lives in harmony with their culturally shaped family and social roles have more resilience to life's challenges – including diabetes. "Resilience" in this case might not mean having optimal blood sugar levels, but rather finding ways to thrive with diabetes. One might do this by prioritizing other elements of life over diabetes health and choosing non-biomedical treatment modalities, as Gurpreet did. This might or might not lead to a quicker onset of other health complications, but even if it did, that tradeoff might be worthwhile. Or one might do this by carefully monitoring one's blood sugar fluctuations and taking medication daily, as Sarita did. This might or might not lead to a slower onset, or even prevention, of health complications. Some women had little ability to choose their own path because of a lack of money, autonomy, or both.

The key challenge for women like Gurpreet was that the people treating diabetes – physicians, nurses, and dieticians, primarily – recognized only one narrow path toward living well with diabetes. This path involved strict behavioral management, expensive medications and other equipment, and regular checkups that were out of reach for many women either because of competing life demands or a lack of resources. Gurpreet's and Sarita's stories demonstrate this juxtaposition, and suggest that alternative routes to thriving with diabetes may or may not be captured by the strictly medical guidelines that regulate most diabetes management plans.

NOTES

1 Measured via instantaneous glucose and HbA1c (glycated hemoglobin), respectively.
2 Measured via Epstein-Barr antibodies and C-reactive protein levels in the blood, respectively.

REFERENCES

Cornwell, Erin York, and Linda J. Waite. 2009. "Social Disconnectedness, Perceived Isolation, and Health among Older Adults." *Journal of Health and Social Behavior* 50 (1): 31–48.

Diener, Ed, and Martin E. P. Seligman. 2002. "Very Happy People." *Psychological Science* 13 (1): 81–84.

Hardin, Jessica. 2019. *Faith and the Pursuit of Health.* New Brunswick, NJ: Rutgers University Press.

Harding, Jessica L., Meda E. Pavkov, Dianna J. Magliano, Jonathan E. Shaw, and Edward W. Gregg. 2019. "Global Trends in Diabetes Complications: A Review of Current Evidence." *Diabetologia* 62 (1): 3–16.

Jotkowitz, Alan B., Gad Rabinowitz, Anat Raskin Segal, Ron Weitzman, Leon Epstein, and Avi Porath. 2006. "Do Patients with Diabetes and Low Socioeconomic Status Receive Less Care and Have Worse Outcomes? A National Study." *The American Journal of Medicine* 119 (8): 665–69.

Loomba, Ania, and Ritty A. Lukose. 2012. *South Asian Feminisms.* Durham, NC: Duke University Press.

Mendenhall, Emily, Roopa Shivashankar, Nikhil Tandon, Mohammed K. Ali, K. M. Venkat Narayan, and Dorairaj Prabhakaran. 2012. "Stress and Diabetes in Socioeconomic Context: A Qualitative Study of Urban Indians." *Social Science & Medicine* 75 (12): 2522–29.

Nelson, Lyndsay A., Michael T. Ackerman, Robert A. Greevy, Kenneth A. Wallston, and Lindsay S. Mayberry. 2019. "Beyond Race Disparities: Accounting for Socioeconomic Status in Diabetes Self-Care." *American Journal of Preventive Medicine* 57 (1): 111–16.

Oxfam International. 2022. "India: Extreme Inequality in Numbers." Oxfam International, September 9, 2022.

Radhakrishnan, Smitha. 2011. *Appropriately Indian: Gender and Culture in a New Transnational Class.* Durham, NC: Duke University Press.

Roy, Jean-Pierre. 2004. "Socioeconomic Status and Health: A Neurobiological Perspective." *Medical Hypotheses* 62 (2): 222–27.

Roy, Tapasha, and Cathy E. Lloyd. 2012. Supplement, "Epidemiology of Depression and Diabetes: A Systematic Review." *Journal of Affective Disorders* 142.

Weaver, Lesley Jo. 2019. *Sugar and Tension: Diabetes and Gender in Modern India.* New Brunswick, NJ: Rutgers University Press.

Weaver, Lesley Jo, and S. V. Madhu. 2015. "Type 2 Diabetes and Anxiety Symptoms Among Women in New Delhi, India." *American Journal of Public Health* 105 (11): 2335–40.

Weaver, Lesley Jo, Carol M. Worthman, Jason A. DeCaro, and S. V. Madhu. 2015. "The Signs of Stress: Embodiments of Biosocial Stress among Type 2 Diabetic Women in New Delhi, India." *Social Science & Medicine* 131 (April): 122–30.

Williams, Julianne, Luke Allen, Kremlin Wickramasinghe, Bente Mikkelsen, Nia Roberts, and Nick Townsend. 2018. "A Systematic Review of Associations between Non-Communicable Diseases and Socioeconomic Status within Low- and Lower-Middle-Income Countries." *Journal of Global Health* 8 (2): 020409.

CHAPTER FIFTEEN

Confianza and Collaborative Care: The Value of Patient-Physician Partnerships

Jessica P. Cerdeña and Genesis Santos

"Ah, but Doctor, it *hurts!*" *Ay, pero doctora, ¡me* duele*!* Genesis Santos grasps her legs, digging her nails deep into her calf muscles. She shares that pain in her legs has kept her from sleeping and has become unbearable. "I'm doing everything you said, but it still *hurts!*"

Genesis is a star patient, well known to the practice for her perfect attendance, sharp sense of humor, and insistence on others speaking her native language (*¡Yo no speak English!*). In quarterly reviews of diabetes metrics across the clinic's patient panel, Genesis also stands out: Her hemoglobin A1C is perfectly at goal, having dropped from 10 to 6.8 over the course of three years. She also checks all the boxes of regular screenings, with her vision, kidney function, and cholesterol meeting their targets every year. These are the numbers that Jes has observed as her doctor for several years now. However, as they discuss Genesis's story, the complex factors – of biological success in spite of social distress – become entangled and demonstrate an imperative resilience (see Cerdeña 2023). When Jes asks her about the source of her success, she says, "It's because I have a great doctor!" followed by a hearty laugh suffused with tobacco smoke.

By all metrics, Genesis is living well with diabetes. She successfully transitioned from an insulin-based medication regimen to a combination of tablets and weekly injections, dramatically improving her glycemic load and her overall risk of cardiometabolic disease. She arrives to all her appointments early, with her blood work and specialist appointments completed. Her numbers show a poster portrait of health, but her medication list and progress notes tell a different story. Genesis fights against chronic pain, loneliness, and the haunting of her past traumas as a child and young woman.

"My life hasn't been easy at all." *No ha sido nada fácil*, Genesis says. "It's been hard. I feel it inside my bones."

"Oh my childhood … my childhood was *horrible*," Genesis tells Jes with a heavy sigh, swiping a strand of hair back from her face and into her bun. "I came from a family that treated us with beatings, bad words … my father abandoned us … and my mother, well, she left us alone most of the time. And it was my sister Liliana and me, the oldest ones, who took care of the others. For more than thirty years, I've avoided going back to Puerto Rico because if I go back there, I will remember all the terrible things."

Genesis struggles to recount the details of her childhood, having repressed many memories as a method of coping with her trauma. In her rearview, childhood is a blur of physical and emotional abuse, punctuated by sparks of happiness that were rapidly extinguished.

"I was the ugly duckling of the family, I say. They treated me so badly. My mom would see that I was happy at my aunt's house and then drag me back home for a beating. She couldn't stand to see me happy, so I learned not to be."

Genesis moved to the mainland United States from Arecibo, Puerto Rico at age fifteen with a friend from school. Her aunt paid her way and told her to find her estranged father in New York. She settled in with her father and stepmother, finding herself fleeing one form of abuse then trapped in another.

"I was like a slave, like a fairy tale Cinderella. She made me wash clothes, clean; I could never leave the house. She never helped me get health insurance, so one time when my belly hurt so badly and they said they needed to operate, my stepmom dragged me out of the hospital and wouldn't let them do it. Thank God I survived."

As a young woman in an unfamiliar city, without a formal job or health insurance, Genesis had few options for improving her situation. So when the man who became her first husband offered her a way out, she took it.

"I said to my sister, 'Look, the first crazy who asks, I'm going with him.'" And she did.

Her husband, Mexican by origin, moved them to the Chiapas region of Mexico, where Genesis was cut off from family.

"At first it was great. We went out together all the time; I learned to dance to Mexican music." Genesis laughs and hums a few measures of a Mexican country song. "But then I became pregnant, and we came back to the States for the birth, and God, it was awful. Him, drunk all the time, the baby crying, crying, crying. It's only by God's hand that I'm still here."

The marital issues only worsened as their family grew. Genesis soon found herself the sole caretaker for three children, fighting back an abusive, alcoholic husband and father.

"He wouldn't let me work, spoke nastily about me to other people, got drunk all the time … I couldn't take it anymore."

For the third time in her life, Genesis fled. "I called my sister and said I was coming to Connecticut." But the arrangement failed because her sister grew jealous, suspecting her husband was attracted to Genesis. "She kicked me out – to the street, with three kids! – because she thought her husband was after me, because I was skinny and *trigueñita* [light brown in coloring] and pretty."

Again, Genesis strategically sought the support of a man, her second husband, who she believed would rescue her from single motherhood and homelessness.

"But it only got worse. He threw knives at me, locked me up, broke my phone, called me a whore in front of my kids. He used drugs, and when I caught him with a little baggy, asking, 'And what is this?' he left, screaming at me. It's been a battle."

Genesis ultimately raised her two sons and daughter by herself. She balanced working in restaurants and grocery stores with her obligations as a mother, supporting them through adulthood. With somber sobriety, Genesis admits that she struggled to be the mother she wanted for her children.

"I won't tell you that I was a good mother, but I wasn't a bad mother, either. The beatings that they [my parents] gave me, I gave to my kids. And I remember one time my kids were whining to me, 'You smacked my bottom. You hit me,' and I was just so ignorant because I was treating them the way that I had been treated. Sometimes I would ask myself, why? Why do I act that way with my kids? I still think about it. Because that's how I lost my daughter."

Genesis's daughter died by suicide at twenty-five years old after a long battle with depression. Following a lethal mix of alcohol, crack cocaine, and fentanyl, Genesis's daughter passed away before the emergency medical team could revive her.

"I moved to be with her … I was just two blocks away. I had never been away from her. I was so good with her. But she was awful with me. She would come home drunk and call me a bitch. One time, we fought so hard we were each pulling the other's hair. I said, 'Just let the state, let DCF [the Department of Children and Families] take her.' God forgive me, but I just wanted to kill her for what she did to me after all I had done for her. God forgive me for saying that."

Genesis winces before continuing.

"I kept needing to take her to the hospital. She tried to drown herself, she tried so many times until she finally did it."

Abuse, instability, and the profound grief that comes with losing a child cost Genesis her health. She believes she had been perfectly healthy until her daughter's death.

"I was never sick. I never suffered from anything," she says. "As a kid, if I had anything, my grandmother had a quick remedy … a little bit of raw onion or honey or who knows what. And I would be fine. All the depression, all the illnesses – the sugar, the blood pressure – they only came around now."

Genesis's illness narrative speaks to anthropological characterizations of somatic issues as embodiments of social suffering and politico-economic oppression (Scheper-Hughes and Lock 1987; Csordas 1990; Lock 2017). Specifically with respect to diabetes and hypertension, medical and biocultural anthropologists and epidemiologists have traced the ways psychosocial trauma and racial discrimination influence glycemic regulation and vascular tension to induce disease states (Geronimus et al. 2006; Gravlee 2009; Kuzawa and Sweet 2009; Worthman and Costello 2009; Thayer and Non 2015). An emerging consensus in diabetes research attributes the development of diabetes to the accumulation of environmental insults, likely mediated by epigenetic modifications, and aging on a background of genetic risk (Kwak and Park 2016; Beulens et al. 2022). On a theoretical level, anthropologists, biomedical scientists, and people living with diabetes agree on the model of diabetes pathogenesis, though clinical medicine has yet to keep pace. Overemphasis on genetics and problematic notions of racialized risk continue to divert attention toward pharmacological interventions and away from policy reforms that would support people like Genesis. As such, Genesis remains forced to contend with failing health in a persistently harmful sociopolitical environment. Her need to rely on her personal cognitive and social faculties to endure those harms compounds the breakdown of her body.

THE LIVED REALITY OF DIABETES DISTRESS

Genesis and Jes agreed to share her story together to highlight how even the "best" diabetes patients grapple with biosocial sequelae despite optimal laboratory values. The two have co-narrated an account of living with diabetes beyond the numbers and brief clinic visits. Genesis and Jes trouble the concept of "diabetes distress," emphasizing the burden of strict adherence to medication regimens that earn patients recognition for "adherence" and meeting "target goals" but cost them on the day-to-day. Deploying the medical anthropologist Emily Mendenhall's model of diabetes as a syndemic that co-occurs with the social oppressions of poverty and trauma, Genesis and Jes emphasize how diabetes not only emerges from these conditions but also constitutively produces them (Mendenhall 2012). However, in doing so, they illuminate a concept of "imperative resilience," or cognitive and social strategies used by migrant women to overcome racial, economic, and gender-based oppression (Cerdeña 2023), to offer insight into the physical toll of supposedly "thriving."

Diabetes distress generally refers to the negative emotional impact of living with diabetes (Dennick, Sturt, and Speight 2017), which has been proposed as a barrier to self-managing diabetes as well as a concomitant condition of living with the disease (Skinner, Joensen, and Parkin 2020). This construct measures constructs of fear, discouragement, deprivation, worry, burnout, frustration, and medical neglect; however, no practice guidelines exist for screening for diabetes distress even though the American Diabetes Association encourages providers to ensure that each appointment "includes opportunities for the person to express how they are feeling about life with diabetes" (Hermanns, Bremmer, and Snoek 2018). Yet this rarely happens.

There are many barriers to addressing diabetes distress. First, medical appointments generally address multiple concerns, leaving limited time to probe into the psycho-emotional aspects of disease. Second, "diabetes distress" is not a billable code through the International Classification of Diseases, 10th edition (ICD-10), so providers have little incentive to address this at clinic visits within the US fee-for-service model of health care. Third, few recommendations exist for how to effectively address diabetes distress, vexing management. The best evidence for ameliorating diabetes distress comes from a systematic review and meta-analysis, which found that mindfulness and cognitive-behavioral therapy interventions, particularly psychoeducation on diabetes distress, are most effective at improving symptoms (Schmidt et al. 2018). However, these types of interventions are difficult to access in the current US health-care environment in which a scarcity of mental health providers, barriers to insurance reimbursement, and a lack of interdisciplinary training restrict opportunities for care.

Quantitative measurements of diabetes distress overlook the dynamic interplay between sociopolitical context and somatization, and medical anthropologists have argued that conditions like diabetes may emerge from the embodiment of social suffering, or as a mode of resistance to it (Scheper-Hughes 1994; Krieger 1999; Rock 2003; Mendenhall et al. 2010; Mendenhall 2012). Person-centered explanatory models of diabetes among Latinx patients highlight the stress of undocumented status, family conflict, childhood trauma, and poverty as disease drivers (Mendenhall et al. 2010, 2020). By contrast, biomedical interpretations of diabetes pathogenesis in this population focus on racialized notions of genetic risk, misapplying evolutionary biology arguments like "thrifty" genotypes to a complex disease process (Neel 1962; Montesi 2014; Cerdeña, Grubbs, and Non 2022). This ontological conflict between how patients experience their disease and how clinicians interpret it manifests in frustrations with diabetes treatment on both sides of the therapeutic relationship.

IMPERATIVE RESILIENCE AND THE PHYSICAL COSTS OF SURVIVING SOCIAL ADVERSITY

"*Ay doctora*, there are so many things one has to go through," Genesis laments to Jes. "But *pa'lante*, onward." This imperative resilience has impressed Jes as she has observed how Genesis and other women have overcome hardship in their lives (Cerdeña 2023). Despite enormous personal suffering from a very young age and unabating financial and health stressors, Genesis is getting by: she rents an apartment by herself, has gathered a charming collection of porcelain trinkets, enjoys the love of her six grandchildren and the adoring attention of an affectionate new Maltese puppy named Chispita. In addition, Genesis has tucked in her medicine cabinet a few things she relies on: inhalers and metformin tablets, lidocaine patches and antidepressants, and cigarettes, her go-to source of comfort when she needs relief from her anxiety.

"I learned to be a woman by way of the hardships of my life. It's been hard because *I've* been hard. But I won't ever give up now. If you say something I don't like, I'll answer it. If you raise your hand at me, know that I'll give it right back to you."

When asked how she gets through these tough times, Genesis says she thinks of her children and, lately, her grandchildren.

"I get through it through them, through my children and my grandchildren," she reports with resolve. "If I feel that pain, that hardship, I distract myself. I put on my tablet, check Facebook or TikTok, something to clear my mind. If I have to cry, I cry. And I know that if I'm here, it's because God willed it. But I have to fix my mind because I don't want anything else to happen like what happened to my daughter."

Genesis articulates an imperative resilience by engaging cognitive avoidance, faith, and an altruistic sublimation to the needs of her offspring to cope with the traumas that defined her life of poverty, social vulnerability, and instability. In other words, despite her extraordinary suffering, she has elevated her family by pushing away her own needs in order to get by, and in many ways, thrive. Yet, she has never confronted her traumas directly in psychotherapy or with a pastor. Instead, she has had to push them into her subconscious and focus on the day-to-day tasks of preparing meals, taking medications, caring for her grandchildren, and attending medical appointments.

Genesis attests that her longstanding approach to getting by wears on the body. Her ability to stay strong for her children and grandchildren taxes her health and ability to feel unbridled joy.

"I used to be the life of the party. I was good, *happy*. I would go out and dance and drink and party, and I had all my friends I would see all the time. But now I don't go out; I don't have any interest in it. My friends will say, 'Come on, let's go out dancing,' but I just can't. I just stay home. I'm not as sociable as I was before."

When Jes asks Genesis what changed, she says, "It's because I'm *down*. I don't drink anymore because of the sugar. I'm fat now, I feel fat. And I can't afford to live downtown anymore, where I could walk everywhere. So now I'm here, without a car, cut off from everyone."

Genesis tells Jes that the addition of new diagnoses to her medical chart has changed how she views herself. She no longer looks in the mirror and finds the charming, tough *trigueñita* who could steal her sister's husband. Instead, she sees a sickly, middle-aged woman with a thick midsection and graying hair. In her view, staying strong all her life has now caught up to her: between the sacrifices she made to support her children and ultimately losing her daughter to suicide, her granite body could no longer withstand the pressure and started to crack.

THE VALUE OF COLLABORATIVE CARE

Genesis has many ideas for how medical providers can support patients like her. "I like the clinic here. You as a doctor can tell me what the problem is and how I can fix it. There are tests for everything." Genesis underscores the importance of clinicians leveraging their intellectual and cultural capital to advance the priorities of patients. In her view, if she feels something in her body, she wants to know that her physician takes her seriously and will direct the appropriate workup. This is what Genesis and Jes have done in their time together, tackling several health challenges: asthma exacerbation due to viral pneumonia, abdominal wall cellulitis resulting in a brief hospital stay, and chronic leg pain. Each occasion followed the sequence of in-office assessment, diagnostic evaluation, coordinated treatment, and follow-up.

"When I told you my leg was hurting more than usual, you got the ultrasound, and I was glad to know it wasn't a blood clot," Genesis tells me. "When I showed you that painful thing on my belly, you met with me again to check on me and then got me the antibiotics. It's good to know that I'm getting everything I need, because otherwise I get anxious."

Together, Genesis and Jes simplified Genesis's diabetes regimen, replacing frequent insulin shots with a twice-daily tablet and weekly maintenance medication. "My sugars are great now," Genesis tells Jes. "I eat lots of fruits and vegetables, and if I ever feel like it's getting too low, I know how to take care of it with some lemon water and a splash of orange juice."

Yet, each of their visits carries with it new concerns. On-and-off shoulder pain and a tingling sensation in the hands. Trouble falling asleep and frequent wakings. A tug-of-war between remitting anxiety and relapsing cigarette smoking. Even as Genesis recounts her life history, she tells Jes about all the other ways her body has betrayed her.

As her doctor, Jes never worries about Genesis not taking her medication. Some clinicians call this "noncompliance" – a stigmatizing term. Genesis diligently follows her regimen, which includes antiglycemic, antihypertensive, antidepressant, and analgesic medications. Still, her symptoms of pain, dysphoric mood, and insomnia dictate her life. When asked what would help her live her best life, Genesis says: "I need someone to *know* me. My life has been hard, and I can only tell my story in pieces. I need a person of *confianza*, of trust. I hate when I have to start new with another doctor, especially one who doesn't know any Spanish."

Together, Genesis and Jes have devised a few recommendations for improving collaborative care for patients with diabetes and its attendant distress. First, people with complex medical histories, particularly involving diabetes distress, deserve continuity in medical care. This means access to a single primary-care provider (PCP) who can foster trust (*confianza*) and partnership over time. The PCP should have integrated training in biomedical and behavioral health and be available for frequent follow-ups, ideally every six weeks and at minimum every three months.

"Why has it been so long since I've seen you?" Genesis will ask any time two months or more have passed between visits. "So much has happened!" Genesis feels confident that opportunities for regular medical check-ins are necessary for her to fully confide in her provider and ensure she stays on top of her symptoms.

Second, diabetes distress merits particular psychosocial resources, including individual and group therapy and psychoeducation. This calls for increased service provision and attention to the psychosocial dimensions of diabetes care. Whereas nutrition and lifestyle counseling for diabetes are available through many health-care institutions, including via telemedicine, and show proven health benefits (Sun et al. 2017), cognitive support for the emotional pain and traumatic histories that accompany diabetes diagnoses is lacking. This is especially true for Spanish-speaking patients who confront dramatic shortages of Spanish-speaking, structurally competent mental health providers (Kanel 2002; Espinoza-Kulick and Cerdeña 2022).

Genesis connects regularly with a Spanish-speaking psychiatrist in Jes's practice but has no access to a Spanish-speaking psychotherapist that accepts her Medicaid insurance. "I keep asking, but they say they have no one else," Genesis tells Jes during their clinical visit. Jes has contacted several providers, and the nearest clinic with availability for a Spanish-speaking therapist is almost an hour from where Genesis lives. Without a car and with no option for telehealth, Genesis declined the referral.

Strengthening of the mental health infrastructure to empower Spanish-speaking trainees across social work, psychology, and psychiatry, as well as increasing attention to the specialized needs of people living with diabetes distress and illness anxiety, can work toward meeting this need.

Third, health-care institutions should invest in integrated primary-care delivery that coordinates primary care, social services, behavioral health, and specialty care in an accessible and sustainable manner. The current fragmented U.S. health-care structure fails people like Genesis, whose elaborate needs fall through the cracks that separate insurers, primary-care providers, specialists, mental health providers, and supports for housing, transportation, and finances. Structural integration, as through patient-centered medical homes and value-based care models, optimizes patient well-being and health-care quality, promoting sustained, healing relationships that persist across time and institutions (National Academies of Sciences, Engineering, and Medicine 2021).

Finally, legislative action and public-private partnerships should expand access to health insurance, behavioral health services, housing support, and financial resources to mitigate known disparities in diabetes. Populations experiencing economic and racial oppression remain at high risk of diabetes due to lifelong stress and social adversity, which increases corticosteroid release and chronic inflammation, promotes reliance on affordable processed foods rich in government-subsidized corn and wheat, and restricts access to healthy produce due to persistent patterns of segregation (Cerdeña, Zhang, and Huang, forthcoming).

CONCLUSION

This ethnographic and biographic account elaborates the physical and psychological burdens of living well with diabetes. Favorable clinical data obscure the realities of coping with the strict medication regimens, negative self-concepts, traumatic histories, and sociostructural injustice that shape the lives of many people with diabetes, particularly Spanish-speaking migrant women. Recognizing the biosocial interplays between psychosocial adversity and glycemic control and the embodied costs of the imperative resilience required to survive amid oppression can shape how clinicians understand and relate to their patients. Health-care reforms to increase availability, integration, and sustainability of services across primary care and behavioral health can reshape the life trajectories of people like Genesis. Trusting relationships with providers who have the infrastructural capacity and structural competency to uphold patient partnerships can foster the clinical collaboration needed for people with diabetes to achieve their full potential.

REFERENCES

Beulens, Joline W. J., Maria G. M. Pinho, Taymara C. Abreu, Nicole R. den Braver, Thao M. Lam, Anke Huss, Jelle Vlaanderen, et al. 2022. "Environmental Risk Factors of Type 2 Diabetes – An Exposome Approach." *Diabetologia* 65 (2): 263–74.

Cerdeña, Jessica P. 2023. *Pressing Onward: The Imperative Resilience of Latina Migrant Mothers*. Berkeley, CA: University of California Press.

Cerdeña, Jessica P., Vanessa Grubbs, and Amy L. Non. 2022. "Genomic Supremacy: The Harm of Conflating Genetic Ancestry and Race." *Human Genomics* 16 (1): 18.

Cerdeña, Jessica P., Angela Y. Zhang, and Timothy J. Huang. Forthcoming. "Beyond the Numbers: Ending Race-Based Diabetes Screening to Address Structural Inequities." *The Lancet Regional Health – Americas*.

Csordas, Thomas J. 1990. "Embodiment as a Paradigm for Anthropology." *Ethos* 18 (1): 5–47.

Dennick, Kathryn, Jackie Sturt, and Jane Speight. 2017. "What Is Diabetes Distress and How Can We Measure It? A Narrative Review and Conceptual Model." *Journal of Diabetes and Its Complications* 31 (5): 898–911.

Espinoza-Kulick, Mario Alberto Viveros, and Jessica P. Cerdeña. 2022. "'We Need Health for All': Mental Health and Barriers to Care among Latinxs in California and Connecticut." *International Journal of Environmental Research and Public Health* 19 (19): 12817.

Geronimus, Arline T., Margaret Hicken, Danya Keene, and John Bound. 2006. "'Weathering' and Age Patterns of Allostatic Load Scores Among Blacks and Whites in the United States." *American Journal of Public Health* 96 (5): 826–33.

Gravlee, Clarence. 2009. "How Race Becomes Biology: Embodiment of Social Inequality." *American Journal of Physical Anthropology* 139 (1): 47–57.

Hermanns, Norbert, Marijke A. Bremmer, and Frank J. Snoek. 2018. "Diabetes Distress." In *Depression and Type 2 Diabetes*, edited by Khalida Ismail, Andreas Barthel, Stefan R. Bornstein, and Julio Licinio. Oxford: Oxford University Press.

Kanel, Kristi. 2002. "Mental Health Needs of Spanish-Speaking Latinos in Southern California." *Hispanic Journal of Behavioral Sciences* 24 (1): 74–91.

Krieger, Nancy. 1999. "Embodying Inequality: A Review of Concepts, Measures, and Methods for Studying Health Consequences of Discrimination." *International Journal of Health Services: Planning, Administration, Evaluation* 29 (2): 295–352.

Kuzawa, Christopher W., and Elizabeth Sweet. 2009. "Epigenetics and the Embodiment of Race: Developmental Origins of US Racial Disparities in Cardiovascular Health." *American Journal of Human Biology* 21 (1): 2–15.

Kwak, Soo Heon, and Kyong Soo Park. 2016. "Recent Progress in Genetic and Epigenetic Research on Type 2 Diabetes." *Experimental & Molecular Medicine* 48 (3): e220.

Lock, Margaret. 2017. "Recovering the Body." *Annual Review of Anthropology* 46 (1): 1–14.

Mendenhall, Emily. 2012. *Syndemic Suffering: Social Distress, Depression, and Diabetes among Mexican Immigrant Women.* 1st ed. New York, NY: Routledge.

Mendenhall, Emily, Abednego Musau, Edna Bosire, Victoria Mutiso, David Ndetei, and Melanie Rock. 2020. "What Drives Distress? Rethinking the Roles of Emotion and Diagnosis among People with Diabetes in Nairobi, Kenya." *Anthropology & Medicine* 27 (3): 252–67.

Mendenhall, Emily, Rebecca A. Seligman, Alicia Fernandez, and Elizabeth A. Jacobs. 2010. "Speaking through Diabetes: Rethinking the Significance of Lay Discourses on Diabetes." *Medical Anthropology Quarterly* 24 (2): 220–39.

Montesi, Laura. 2014. "Beyond Race and Ethnicity: How an Ethnography of Diabetes Can Contribute to a Socially Complex Approach to Hyperglycemia, Human Suffering, and Care." *Society, Biology, and Human Affairs* 78 (1): 83–104.

National Academies of Sciences, Engineering, and Medicine, Health and Medicine Division, and Committee on Implementing High-Quality Primary Care. 2021. "Integrated Primary Care Delivery." In *Implementing High-Quality Primary Care: Rebuilding the Foundation of Health Care*, edited by Sarah K. Robinson, Marc Meisnere, Jr., Robert L. Phillips, and Linda McCauley. Washington, DC: National Academies Press.

Neel, James V. 1962. "Diabetes Mellitus: A 'Thrifty' Genotype Rendered Detrimental by 'Progress'?" *American Journal of Human Genetics* 14 (4): 353–62.

Rock, Melanie. 2003. "Sweet Blood and Social Suffering: Rethinking Cause-Effect Relationships in Diabetes, Distress, and Duress." *Medical Anthropology* 22 (2): 131–74.

Scheper-Hughes, Nancy. 1994. "Embodied Knowledge: Thinking with the Body in Critical Medical Anthropology." In *Assessing Cultural Anthropology*, edited by Robert Borofsky. New York, NY: McGraw-Hill, Inc.

Scheper-Hughes, Nancy, and Margaret M. Lock. 1987. "The Mindful Body: A Prolegomenon to Future Work in Medical Anthropology." *Medical Anthropology Quarterly* 1 (1): 6–41.

Schmidt, C. B., B. J. Potter van Loon, A. C. M. Vergouwen, F. J. Snoek, and A. Honig. 2018. "Systematic Review and Meta-Analysis of Psychological Interventions in People with Diabetes and Elevated Diabetes-Distress." *Diabetic Medicine: A Journal of the British Diabetic Association,* June.

Skinner, T. C., L. Joensen, and T. Parkin. 2020. "Twenty-Five Years of Diabetes Distress Research." *Diabetic Medicine* 37 (3): 393–400.

Sun, Yu, Wen You, Fabio Almeida, Paul Estabrooks, and Brenda Davy. 2017. "The Effectiveness and Cost of Lifestyle Interventions Including Nutrition Education for Diabetes Prevention: A Systematic Review and Meta-Analysis." *Journal of the Academy of Nutrition and Dietetics* 117 (3): 404–21.e36.

Thayer, Zaneta M., and Amy L. Non. 2015. "Anthropology Meets Epigenetics: Current and Future Directions." *American Anthropologist* 117 (4): 722–35.

Worthman, Carol M., and E. Jane Costello. 2009. "Tracking Biocultural Pathways to Health Disparities: The Value of Biomarkers." *Annals of Human Biology* 36 (3): 281–97.

Epilogue

Emily Mendenhall and Jessica Hardin

In medicine and public health, the focus on *fixing* and *curing* people overlooks the ways in which life happens in the quiet moments. The foods we prepare that delight us. The people we love who support us. The places we go that comfort us. It is in these moments within our journey, or pursuit of a good life, that flourishing happens. Rarely are these moments, however, situated in medical spaces, conversations, or treatments.

Without recognizing the dynamic ways in which our lives exist well beyond the metrics and diets prescribed to define notions of health and well-being, we can become stuck in a perception of ill-health. Yet, some aspects of living well cannot be divorced from structural factors that impede well-being. Sarah Willen and colleagues' (2022) work on flourishing points to the roles that financial and material resources play in impeding one's ability to flourish. However, the collective reckoning we create with the relational opportunities afforded us can be extraordinary medicine. In this way, flourishing becomes a pursuit through which someone navigates challenges and opportunities in their life, often in the company of others.

Recognizing structures – both visible and invisible – that impede good health has long been the project of medical anthropologists. Time, money, and social support cannot be untangled from the policies that make our society tick and have a powerful role in what defines well-being. These might be policies designed far from those who bear the brunt of them, shaping what people eat, where, and how they move in the world. These policies – from what's *in* our food to how much time we must devote to each other (apart from labor in the home and at work) – are crucial for living well with and without illness. However, a condition like diabetes that requires a deep daily devotion to managing inputs and outputs makes it difficult to see beyond the metrics that define illness.

Clinical contexts also play an important role in how people think about their disease as well as their journey to wellness. This brings us back to ideas of *fixing* and *curing* because many people are interested in managing their condition amid a full life of preferred foods, activities, and interactions. Making sense of how people live well while living fully should be a clinical project. For instance, care that does not break the bank is essential, particularly when health care is expensive and, for some, hard to reach. However, holistic care means that clinical support is not only medical but also social and legal. To achieve health and well-being, many people need legal and social services to navigate their environments and allow them to spend time on what really matters. Perhaps most importantly, nutritional experts that speak the same love language as patients, so they can design healthy meals that fit their needs and preferences, are key. In this way, diabetes directives that cultivate well-being through food plans are more effective than ones that curb ill-health through food restriction.

Spaces for learning and sharing extend well beyond the clinic. Creating opportunities for people to meet and thrive together in community with others following a similar journey is imperative. Community groups. Prayer circles. Book clubs. Religious gatherings. Parties. Clubs. Alcoholics Anonymous. Whatever brings people around a shared goal and experience can foster opportunities to cultivate well-being. It's well documented that peer support and community partners can elevate people's health, particularly when they engage around the same grocers, streets, parks, and activities.

Translating how we live in the world with others is an anthropological project. And through these stories, we show how writing together with our colleagues and interlocutors emboldens how we imagine the ways people live with diabetes in the world and navigate the troubled waters of disruption – to individuals, families, and communities – brought by chronic illness. By playing with genre, from ethnography and vignette to fictional ethnography, we explore how the people we have met throughout this research may engage in ways that are less apparent in different forms of writing. Rooted in years of collective research, these stories describe how people cultivate meaning and well-being through their relationships and in doing so flourish in ways that oppose biomedical notions of good and bad, healthy and sick, and variants of *diseased*. Although medication is powerful, so are the people who care for us throughout our lives, the foods that sustain us, and the ways in which we navigate the competing layers that make up a meaningful life.

We leave you with a few questions as you think about these stories in relation to your own experiences. How might the people in your life foster good health or ill-health? How do the social relations around you influence the foods you consume, the places you visit, and the ways you perceive your health and body? How do the small everyday moments in your life contribute to your sense of well-being? How can you foster environments – whether at home or at work – that support the flourishing of others? By recognizing how we foster good health with others and flourish in the face of structural challenges – in some cases, crises – we recognize the power of being in the world together and realizing that well-being is a journey, one that ebbs and flows through many phases and dynamics in the complex lives we travel together.

Author Biographies

Tausala Aiavao is not only a nursing lecturer and keen researcher at the National University of Samoa, but also an experienced logistical coordinator for community development, research, and family events. Passionate about fostering critical thinking in her students, Tausala continues to innovate in the classroom.

Laurel Bellante is a human-environment geographer who specializes in critical food studies, food justice, and sustainable food systems in the US-Mexico Borderlands and Latin America more broadly. She is an assistant professor in the School of Geography, Development, and Environment at the University of Arizona.

Ramona Boodoosingh is an avid researcher with experience in research on gender, health, and development issues in Samoa. She is passionate about health education projects and building the capacity of researchers in resource-constrained countries. She earned her bachelor's degree in Chemistry/Management from the University of the West Indies, Trinidad and Tobago; a master's in Environmental Health from Tufts University, USA; and her PhD in Development Studies from the National University of Samoa. Her work has been published in *World Development, BMC Public Health,* and *Journal of Environmental Research and Public Health,* among others. Her work has been supported by USAID, the Australian Research Council, and the British Academy.

Edna N. Bosire has a multidisciplinary background in medical anthropology and public health. She is currently an assistant professor at the Brain and Mind Institute and Department of Population Health, Aga Khan University, East Africa. She is also the lead for the Brain and Mind Institute's Living Lab in East Africa and holds an honorary appointment as a researcher at the Developmental Pathways for Health Research Unit, University of the Witwatersrand, Johannesburg, South Africa.

Emma Nelson Bunkley is a critical medical anthropologist specializing in women's health, embodiment, and the gendered nature of chronic disease. She is an assistant professor of Health and Behavioral Sciences at the University of Colorado Denver. Her research focuses on Senegalese women's experiences with metabolic diseases to better understand embodiment, changing social networks, and kinship relationships.

D. Burnett is a medical anthropologist focused on the complex relationship between race/racism, identity formation, religion and spirituality, and inequities in health. Theoretically, her work is engaged with critical approaches to the study of indigeneity and Blackness, global public health, medical anthropology, and religion and spirituality. Burnett enjoys writing about how spiritual practices inform well-being, health, and healing. Burnett holds a PhD in sociocultural (medical) anthropology from the University of Pennsylvania, where she also concurrently pursued a Master of Public Health. Prior to this, she earned a Master of Divinity from Yale Divinity School and a BA from Hampton University.

Megan A. Carney is a feminist medical and sociocultural anthropologist specializing in critical migration and diaspora studies, the politics of care and solidarity, and critical food studies. She is associate professor of anthropology and director of the Center for Regional Food Studies at the University of Arizona.

Lindile Cele is a research associate who has conducted research in Soweto, South Africa, at the Developmental Pathways for Health Research Unit at the University of the Witwatersrand. She holds a master's degree from the University of KwaZulu-Natal in biology, focused on marine molecular ecology. She has worked on several research projects, including Helti, Soweto Syndemics, Soweto Stress, Effects of COVID on Mental Health, and Flourishing/ukuphumelela. Lindile's research interests include mental health and how it impacts healthy populations and those living with chronic illnesses.

Jessica P. Cerdeña is a family physician and medical anthropologist committed to promoting health justice. She authored *Pressing Onward: The Imperative Resilience of Latina Migrant Mothers* (University of California Press, 2023) to narrate the experiences of women who migrated from Latin America to Connecticut to build futures for their children. She is a gratis professor at the University of Connecticut Institute for Collaboration on Health Intervention and Policy (InCHIP) and is completing her family medicine residency at Middlesex Health.

Fatoumata Diagne graduated from Gaston Berger University in Saint-Louis, Senegal, with a Master of Arts in languages, literatures, and civilizations of the Anglophone world. Her research work focuses on the traumatic experiences of African American women, the manifestation of their post-traumatic stress disorder in their daily life, and their struggle to rid themselves of the ghosts of their past, relying on a powerful network of women and rituals that promote cultural reappropriation and a recovery of their full female identity. Her subject interest, the condition of women, perfectly embraces this research project on women's health in Africa and in Senegal in particular. Today, she serves as interpreter/translator at the South African Embassy in Dakar, promoting communication and mutual understanding between communities from different social, political, and cultural backgrounds through French and English languages.

James Doucet-Battle has an extensive interdisciplinary background in medical anthropology; sociology; science, technology, and society studies (ST&S); and African diaspora studies. His research contributes to a growing literature in critical studies of race and bioethics via ethnographic work analyzing health disparities and their remedial projects. A key focus of his research platform examines the translational challenges facing genomics researchers and community education outreach efforts toward recruiting individuals and communities of African descent. Doucet-Battle's work contributes integrally to the building of a new field of social scientific inquiry on race and risk, community health, and the cultural economies of science and medicine. He is the author of *Sugar in the Blood: Race, Risk, and Type 2 Diabetes* (2021).

Manuela Fuentes: I was born in San Antonio Texcala on October 10, 1977. I come from a family of three siblings, my parents were Margarita and Trinidad Fuentes. I have a family: my husband, Saúl Pacheco, and my children, Lesslie and Saúl. Here in New York, I met wonderful people and gentle beings, Father Grange and my great friend and co-author. I studied in high school in my country; here in New York I have studied English, parenting courses, nutrition, computing, mental health, and first aid. I have volunteered in community centers in my community. I like astronomy and nature; I like to read and learn new and interesting things to be able to contribute and support the people in my community. My dream is to be able to see my children fulfilled and (that all immigrants can see again the place where we grew up) to return to the place where I was born and visit my mother's grave.

Saunima'a Ma Fulu-Aiolupotea is a registered nurse, a registered midwife, and lecturer in the School of Nursing at the National University of Samoa. She also holds diplomas from the Malua Bible School and earned a post-graduate diploma in Tertiary Teaching and a certificate in Adult Teaching from the National University of Samoa. She is from Papa Sataua in Savaii and Fusi Saoluafatain in Uplou. Her parents' villages include Taua'i Fulu Lili'o and Nuufou Taua'i Fulu Lili'o. Mr Aiolupotea Fiu Kolia, her husband, was from Sili and Gataivai Savaii. His father was from Sili and Gataivai and his mother from Tufutafoe Savaii. She is seventy-four years old and the mother of five children with twelve grandchildren. Her work has been published in *Asia Pacific Viewpoint, Journal of Samoan Studies*, and the *Journal of Visual Communication in Medicine*, among others.

Alyshia Gálvez is a cultural and medical anthropologist whose research is at the intersection of food, health, and migration. She is a professor of Latin American and Latino studies at Lehman College and anthropology at the Graduate Center of the City University of New York. She is the author of several books: *Guadalupe in New York: Devotion and the*

Struggle for Citizenship Rights among Mexican Immigrants (NYU, 2009); *Patient Citizens, Immigrant Mothers: Mexican Women, Public Prenatal Care, and the Birth Weight Paradox* (Rutgers University Press, 2011); and *Eating NAFTA: Trade, Food Policies, and the Destruction of Mexico* (University of California Press, 2018).

Tine M. Gammeltoft is Professor of Anthropology at the Department of Anthropology, University of Copenhagen. Her research explores how families handle health challenges, with a particular focus on sexual/reproductive health and chronic health conditions, including diabetes. Gammeltoft has conducted collaborative ethnographic research in Vietnam for over three decades and is the author of the award-winning *Haunting Images: A Cultural Account of Selective Reproduction in Vietnam* (University of California Press, 2014). Her work on diabetes includes creative formats such as the short story "Waiting," published by the Society for Cultural Anthropology's Fieldsights section, and the award-winning photograph "Perseverance."

Emilia M. Guevara is a medical anthropologist with interests in global health, im/migration, women's health, rural health, disability, and violence, focusing on underserved and vulnerable populations in the Americas. Broadly, her research endeavors to establish and sustain relations between anthropology and medicine/public health by articulating critical health disparities on a transnational scale, providing insight into the individual and social experiences of disease and the social, economic, and political forces that shape health outcomes. Her current work considers how chronic illness, debility, and varied forms of violence influence migratory careers. Her research also illuminates the life-course trajectory of migrant women who experience the embodiment of disability as a broader household and community-wide phenomenon.

Jessica Hardin, PhD, is a medical anthropologist, Associate Professor, and Honorable Barber B. Conable Jr. Endowed Chair in Global Futures at Rochester Institute of Technology. Her work has appeared in leading journals, including *American Anthropologist, American Ethnologist,* and *Social Science & Medicine.* She is the 2022 winner of the Rudolf Virchow Award for her paper "Life before Vegetables: Nutrition, Cash and Subjunctive Health in Samoa," published in *Cultural Anthropology*. She has published several books including *Faith and the Pursuit of Health: Cardiometabolic Disorders in Samoa* (2019) and *Fat in Four Cultures: A Global Ethnography of Weight in Samoa, Paraguay, Japan and the US* (2019, co-authored with Cindi SturtzSreetharan, Alexandra Brewis, Sarah Trainer, and Amber Wutich). Her work has been supported by Fulbright, Fulbright-Hays, the National Science Foundation, the Australian Research Council, and the Wenner Gren Foundation.

Tommey Jodie (Diné) is a senior at the University of Arizona, pursuing bachelor's degrees in food studies, nutrition and food systems, and creative writing. Originally from the small community of Teesto within the Navajo Nation and raised in nearby Winslow, Arizona, she is a poet, essayist, community organizer, and Indigenous rights and climate activist. As a researcher, her work focuses on the intersections of Indigenous food sovereignty, critical food studies, and community health and well-being. Her commitment to Indigenous food sovereignty and the legitimization of Indigenous knowledge systems is deeply rooted in her lived experiences as a Diné woman. She is dedicated to the collective liberation of colonized and oppressed peoples, and she strives to facilitate the return to sacred, ancestral knowledge that has sustained Indigenous communities since time immemorial.

Pallavi Laxmikanth is a medical anthropologist and former start-up leader from Hyderabad. Her research interests span metabolic health, food systems, embodiment, and human–technology relationships. She holds a PhD from the University of Adelaide and a Master's degree from the University of Oxford. Her doctoral thesis examined the foods, technologies, and embodied practices used by middle-class Indians to "outwit" type 2 diabetes. Her interest in food and metabolic health is rooted in her previous leadership roles in Indian food-technology start-ups, where she worked across growth hacking, marketing, UX, and product design.

Tauaitala Poloie Lees is a lecturer at the School of Nursing at the National University of Samoa. She is a registered nurse and a registered midwife. Her father is from Papa Sataua in Savaii, and her mother is from Solosolo in Upolu. Her husband, Limutau Herbert Lees, is from Fa'atoia. Tauaitala has an MA from the University of Technology Sydney, a BS from Southern Cross University, and an advanced diploma in primary health care from the Department of Health of Samoa.

Uila Laifa Lima earned her MD from the Oceania University of Samoa. She serves as House Surgeon for the Ministry of Health of Samoa for two years. Before this, she was a registered nurse and lecturer in the School of Nursing at the National University of Samoa. She comes from the villages of Sasa'ai, Faletagaloa, Iva Savaii, and Vailele Uta Apia. Her work has been published in the *Asia Pacific Journal of Health, BMC Women's Health,* and the *Journal of Visual Communication in Medicine.*

Falelua Maua is Principle Nurse in the Midwifery Division (Ministry of Health) and a former senior nursing lecturer at the National University of Samoa. She brings considerable prior experience in emergency, acute, and perioperative care in the Samoan health system. Falelua was born in Savaia Lefaga to church ministers and remains grounded by family, culture, and faith.

Ndèye Aminata Mbaye is a graduate from Gaston Berger University in Saint-Louis, Senegal. She earned a master's degree in English with a specialization in linguistics. Her thesis, *Morphological Processes in English and Wolof, a Comparative Study,* examines through contrastive analysis cross-linguistic similarities and differences, not between two national languages, but between a national language and a foreign one. Ndèye Aminata's professional career started six years ago with a part-time job as translator/interpreter. Since then, she has made her way and now holds the position of receptionist at the South African Embassy in Dakar, Senegal.

Emily Mendenhall is a medical anthropologist and professor in the Edmund A. Walsh School of Foreign Service at Georgetown University. She has published widely at the boundaries of anthropology, psychology, medicine, and public health and is the author of several books, including *Syndemic Suffering: Social Distress, Depression, and Diabetes among Mexican Immigrant Women* (2012); *Rethinking Diabetes: Entanglements with Trauma, Poverty, and HIV* (2019); *Unmasked: COVID, Community, and the*

Case of Okoboji (2022); and *Invisible Illness: A History, from Hysteria to Long Covid* (2026). She was awarded the George Foster Award for Practicing Anthropology in 2017 from the Society for Medical Anthropology and a Guggenheim Fellowship in 2023 from the John Simon Guggenheim Memorial Foundation.

Laura Montesi is a CONAHCyT researcher based at the CIESAS (Centre for Research and Higher Studies in Social Anthropology) in Oaxaca, Mexico. She is a medical anthropologist specialized in the study of chronic diseases and conditions, particularly among Indigenous populations, with a focus on health disparities. She is co-editor of the books *Managing Chronicity in Unequal States: Ethnographic Perspectives on Caring* (UCL, 2021) and *Los huaves en el tecnoceno. Disputas por la naturaleza, el cuerpo y la lengua en el México contemporáneo* (INAH-Editpress, 2022).

Edward Narain is a Fijian political analyst, researcher, and writer, whose work regularly appears in the *Fiji Times* and *Fiji Sun*. Descended from Indian indentured laborers and immersed in Indigenous culture from a young age, Narain's storytelling is informed by an intimate understanding of race and class politics in Fiji. Based between Melbourne and Suva, Narain is a senior advisor with the Fiji Labour Party. His ethnographic novel, *Sugar*, co-authored with Tarryn Phillips, is forthcoming through University of Toronto Press.

Jesse Pablo (Tohono O'odham) is pursuing his bachelor's degree in agriculture, technology, and education at the University of Arizona. He has lived most of his life on the Tohono O'odham reservation located in the Sonoran Desert of southwest Arizona. As a youth, he grew fond of agriculture and how it pertains to the cultural roots of his people.

Tarryn Phillips is a medical anthropologist, writer, and socio-legal scholar at La Trobe University, Melbourne, Australia. She has conducted ethnographic research alongside Fijian communities for over a decade on issues of poverty, nutrition, and social justice. Her academic writing has been published widely in the top journals of medical anthropology, including *Social Science and Medicine, Medical Anthropology*

Quarterly, *Medical Anthropology*, and *Sociology of Health and Illness*. Her ethnographic novel, *Sugar*, co-authored with Edward Narain, is forthcoming through University of Toronto Press.

Genesis Santos (pseudonym) migrated from Arecibo, Puerto Rico, to Middlesex County, Connecticut. She was the mother of three children, including a late daughter, and a beloved Maltese. Genesis tragically and unexpectedly passed away in May 2025 due to health complications. She was surrounded by her siblings, sons, and her primary physician, Dr. Cerdeña, when she entered God's arms.

Dung Vũ is a lecturer at Thái Bình University of Medicine and Pharmacy's Faculty of Public Health. Trained as a medical doctor and public health researcher, Dung Vũ has a strong interest in health inequalities and works toward enhancing the health of disadvantaged and underserved communities. She has conducted research on type 2 diabetes and gestational diabetes in Vietnam since 2018 and has published extensively in local academic journals such as Tạp Chí Y Học Việt Nam (*Journal of Medicine in Vietnam*). Her photographs from ethnographic fieldwork in Thái Bình play significant roles in her research, and her photograph "Perseverance" was awarded First Prize in the Danish National Research Foundation's 2023 Photo Competition.

Lesley Jo Weaver is a biocultural medical anthropologist and author of the book *Sugar and Tension: Diabetes and Gender in Modern India* (Rutgers University Press, 2018). At the University of Oregon, Weaver is an associate professor of global studies and director of the Global Health program. Her research focuses, broadly, on the social production of health and illness in India, Brazil, and the USA.

Emily Yates-Doerr is an anthropologist at Oregon State University, where she works at the intersections of feminist science studies, food studies, and anthropology. Her books include *The Weight of Obesity: Hunger and Global Health in Postwar Guatemala* (UC Press, 2015) and *Mal-Nutrition: Maternal Health Science and the Reproduction of Harm* (UC Press, 2025). She is currently carrying out research on memories of nuclear weapons testing in the United States.

Index

acarajé (food, service), 61
acceptance, practice, 21
acculturation, 116; degrees, 116
action, opportunities, 182
activism, impact, 85
acute illnesses, focus, 168–9
Adams, V., 155
adulthood, nutrition-related non-communicable diseases, 152
affordances, presentation, 186
Africa, enslavement, 60
African Americans: diabetes education, 107; Great Migration, 108; interest/care/concordance, 115; meeting, 114–15
African-descent community, type 2 diabetes: incidence, 113; research, 111
African diaspora, arrivals, 114
African immigrants, diabetes risk, 116
agricultural cooperative, work (Vietnam), 89
akkara, preparation, 38
alimentary dignity, cultivation, 9
aloo pyaz, consumption, 211
alternative providers (South Africa), practice (commonness), 26

amputation: feet, 163; limb amputation, diabetes-related complications (Fiji), 51; little toe, 183; necessity, 2; partial amputation, 188; suffering, 54
ancestors: resilience, 64–5; reverence, devotion, 67; survival, fight, 128–9; teachings, reversion, 125
ancestral connection, 63
ancestral foods, structural barriers, 137–8
ancestral healing, 57; journey, work, 65; meaning, discovery, 64–5
ancestral knowledge: passage, 125; usage, 63–6
anger, feeling, 21–2
Anthropocene, decolonizing, 126
anticipative meditation, 202
anti-colonial approaches, 12
antiretroviral medication, taking (consistency), 22
antiretroviral therapy, usage, 22
Aristotle, philosophy, 185–6
Arizona (native youth disruptions), health/food (impact), 120
art, creation, 125–6
arthritis, relaxation, 19

artisanal work, patience
   (requirement), 182–3
ashwagandha, usage, 212
assimilation, resistance, 124
asthma exacerbation, viral
   pneumonia (impact), 231
attaya, preparation, 38
axé, meaning/manifestation, 59–60
Ayurvedic medication, charitable
   trust origin, 213
Ayurvedic traditional medicine
   system, usage, 212

Bailey, Merlene, 112–14;
   background, 117
baingan bharta, consumption, 196
balance, principles, 122
bananas, consumption, 205–8
banganapalli, consumption, 200;
   reaction, 200–4, *202*
barakah (blessings), 34
Bà Son, 71; confrontation
   (husband), 98; death, 94;
   depiction, 96–7; diabetes, social
   emergency, 102–3; Dung visit,
   100; ethnographic fieldwork,
   94–5; home life, *99*; life story,
   work, 94; presence, sense, 94;
   remembrance, *95*; shared lives,
   carrying, 102; wheelchair, usage,
   95–6
beadwork, 129–30; *I'm Going Home to
   Harvest, 130*
beans, usage, *148*
beauty (Three Graces component), 34
behavior, change, 12; avoidance, 23
behavioral health services, access
   (expansion), 233
benishaan, consumption, 201
Bible reading, usage, 26
biobehavioral reputation, 109
biochemical measurements,
   anthropological scholarship/
   criticism, 206

bioethical injustices, 110
biomedical advice, 37–8
biomedical care (neglect), religious
   practices (impact), 26
biomedical diabetes treatment,
   rejection (India), 219
biomedicine, tenets (differences),
   62–3
biopolitics, 143–4
biosocial facts, 106–7
biosocial interaction,
   understanding, 83
black beans: consumption,
   boredom, 164–5; usage, *148*
black churches, plaintive appeal, 113
black flesh, decipherability, 115
blood glucose elevation, 163
blood glucose levels: problems, 196;
   reconciliation, 199
blood glucose management, 166;
   improvement, 197
blood pressure: decline, 166;
   elevation, 163
blood sugar: burning, 198; daily
   measurement, problem, 92;
   elevation, 7, 195; fluctuation, 213;
   fluctuations, monitoring, 222
blood sugar levels (BSLs): control,
   195; stability, 205
blurry vision, symptom, 21
body: biochemical measurements,
   anthropological scholarship/
   criticism, 206; dysregulated
   glucose, impact, 4; exhaustion,
   57; Negro body, interrogation,
   109; nourishment, native crops
   (consumption), 133; numerical
   representations, criticism, 206;
   wearing, 230
body-mass index (BMI),
   social life, 194
"Body of Darkness," 115
botanas (snacks), consumption,
   165–6

Braiding Sweetgrass (Kimmerer), 126
Brazil: Africa, enslavement, 60; diabetes, prevalence (spread), 66; healing, promotion, 60–1; health, vulnerability, 61–2; healthy eating ("eat in community") principle, 156–7; language/culture/migration, exchange, 59–60; lunch, components, 61; *mãe-de-santo* (spiritual godmother), visit, 57; sugar, relationship (learning), 57; sugar production, 65; *terreiro* (spiritual temple), attendance, 60
Brazilians, diabetes experience (proportion), 65
bread box, diabetes medication (presence), *149*
bring and share, meeting, 24
buzios (shells), divination usage, 57, 61–2

cacahuatón tea, drinking, 189
capitalism, mechanics, 155
cardiometabolic disease, risk (improvement), 225
cardiometabolic illness clinical drug trials, 113
care: access, 18; collaborative care, 224; collaborative care, value, 231–3; connection, 161; mobilization, 52; willingness, 80
careful equivocation (research technique), 11
carpal tunnel syndrome, development, 214
Cartwright, Samuel, 108; ideological assertion, 108
cauliflower rice, consumption, 202
cell biology, discipline (revitalization), 110
Changing Woman, ceremony (performing), 122
checkups, frequency, 22
chemical conversions, scaling up, 154
chemistry, data scientist approach, 158
chicken heart (*corazón de gallina*) (soft-hearted), 75
chicken noodle soup, meal (feeding ability), *157*
childhood details, recounting (struggles), 225
children: medications, taking, 44; parental support, 8; support, 7
chili/coriander powder (*poriyals*), usage, 196
Chinese traditional medicine, usage, 93
chole bhature, consumption, 197
Christian rituals, goal, 27–8
chronic health conditions, diet (relationship), 75
chronic illnesses: connection, 161; coping/healing ability (beliefs), 27; indicators, 170–1; management, 23; migrant women/communities viewpoint, 170; presence, 33; research (Soweto), 25–6
chronic noncommunicable diseases, navigation, 68
chronic pain, fight, 225
church attendance, usage, 26
church water: healing powers, need, 25; receiving, 24–5
City Hall protest, *76*
clinical contexts, importance, 238
clinical diagnoses, interembodied experience, 37
clinical practices, shift, 18
Clinical Research Center (CRC): experts, diversification (absence), 117; team/administration demographic, 113
coffee, importance, 168
collaboration, importance, 10
collaborative care, 224; value, 231–3
collective orientation, balance, 5
colonialism: histories, addressing, 125; legacy, observations, 121

colonial subjugation, resistance, 125
colonization, influences, 127
colonized subjectivities, structural
    barriers, 137–8
comfort foods, overabundance, 132
comida chatarra (junk food),
    consumption, 165
Comité Guadalupano, meeting
    (attendance), 73
commensality, 23; diabetes usage, 19
commodity foods: distribution,
    reference, 127; government
    allocations, reliance (increase), 121
communal caring, source, 35
community (communities): care,
    129; connection, 64; fortification,
    122; scientists, entry, 127
community-run clinic, staffing, 167
comparative ethnographic project, 113
compassion, radiation, 74
complications knowledge, absence, 11
confianza (trust), need, 224, 232
Confucianism, 89
conspicuous consumption,
    demonstration, 7
continuous glucose monitor (CGM),
    205; experiment, 205–6
cooking: activity, 147; expertise,
    impact, 147; food, charges,
    147–8
coping, surveys, 28–9
co-poiesis, 98–9
corn tamales, meal (feeding ability),
    157
cost-effective rubrics, demands, 194
country marks, exchange, 107
COVID-19 pandemic: businesses,
    closure, 180; lockdown, 201
crafts, 175
craftsmanship, 187
creativity, 175, 187–90; usage, 43
critical anthropology, 72
crowdfunding campaign, 53;
    donations, scarcity, 49; race/

gender biases, disadvantage, 54;
    setup, 48–9
cultural beliefs, impact, 18
cultural practices, interplay, 144
cultural worlds, diabetes
    (reflection), 143–4
culture, loss, 133

dahi papdi, consumption, 197
daily experience (navigation),
    humor (importance), 36–7
dal, preparation, 211
dal makhani, consumption, 211
decolonial research, flourishing, 10
Decolonizing Methodologies (Tuhiwai
    Smith), 9, 126
demographic shift, 108
depression: comorbidities, experience,
    51; experience, overcoming, 63;
    handling, exhaustion, 63, 66;
    health, complications (impact),
    80; reason, 80, 81; suffering, 82;
    triggering event, 78–9
Desjarlais, R., 98
despair, handling (exhaustion), 63
determination, usage, 63
devastation, handling (exhaustion), 63
devotion, usage, 63
diabetes: adherence, goal, 228;
    awareness, 137–8; biomedical
    diagnosis, 197; burden ("years
    of lost life"), calculation, 152;
    comorbidities, experience, 51;
    control, 193–4; conversation,
    nominal site, 116–17; death,
    increase, 152; diet, relationship,
    143; disparities (mitigation),
    financial resources (access), 233;
    disruptions, 122; disruptiveness,
    23; education, 107; *el azúcar*
    (diabetes), suffering, 178–9;
    epidemic, impact, 129; "everyone
    suffers from" (*ai cũng bị*), 96;
    examination, 193; exercise/

obesity, Western medicine emphasis, 31–2; existence, creativity/relational care (usage), 43; experience, difference, 187; felt sense, reconciliation, 200; food, culprit (confusion), 37–8; gestational diabetes, experience, 74–5, 80–1; global rates, increase (WHO report), 151–2; handling, exhaustion, 63, 66; healing, 19; increase (Samoa), 3; industrialized labor, impact, 156; initiation, 91–2; intensification, 150; (inter)subjective experience, distribution, 206; issues, settling, 62; labor, energetics, 153–7; life story, 91–4; mediation, 34–5; medications, container, *149*; metaphor, 109; metrics, success, 224; migrant disease, 77; moralized sufferer, discrimination, 53–4; Native peoples, disruptions, 121; Native peoples disruption, 131; navigation, 68; negative emotional impact, 228; patients, arrival, 2; pill prescriptions, costs, 147; prescriptions, examination, *149*, 155; presence, 2, 38; prevalence, spread (Brazil), 66; prevalence (India), 199; prevention-and-control-only approach, weakness, 12; progress, unhappiness, 172; regimen, simplification, 231–2; relational aspects, 17, 18; relationality, disruption, 72; reversal, research, 196; rise, financial implications, 152; risk (African immigrants), 116; root causes, addressing, 127; shame, feelings, 23; side effect, liver failure, 148–9; social structures, relationship, 71; stories, sharing, 23; suffering/toll, 2–3; suicide increase, attempts, 179; target goals, meeting, 228; therapies, receiving (problems), 180–1; thriving, meanings, 219, 222; tragedies, 150; treatment, 68; type 2 diabetes, ethnographic research, 50; ubiquity (Vietnam), 92; uncontrolled diabetes, amputation suffering, 54; values, self experience (extension), 207

diabetes complications: productive activity (impact), 188; ravages (study), 2

diabetes diagnosis, 3–4, 25, 92; family support, 39; hiding, 23; life sentence, absence, 179; navigation, 64

diabetes distress: billable code, absence (ICD-10), 229; lived reality, 228–9; psychoeducation, impact, 229; quantitative measurements, problems, 229

diabetes management, 167, 221; attentiveness, 217; challenges, 121; enhancement/complication, 144; struggle, 212

diabetes prevention: core aspects, 122; information (abundance), 9

diabetes-related illnesses, burden, 156

diabetes research, 127; Indigenous voices/stories, integration, 127

diabetic life, social/environmental conditions (impact), 155

diabetic wounds, persistence, 4

dialysis, appointments, 80

diet: chronic health conditions, relationship, 75; diabetes, relationship, 143; education, 21; modification, struggle, 25

diet, change: avoidance, 23; struggle, 211

Diné-centric community, life (existence), 129

Diné family, diabetes epidemic (impact), 129

Diné (Navajo) girls, menstruation ceremony, 122

Diné life stages, 122

Diné tribe: birth (poem), 122; father (type 2 diabetes diagnosis), 120; forced relocation, impact, 128; girlhood (poem), 123; old age (poem), 124–5; womanhood (poem), 124

disease: epidemiological data (Mexico), 172–3; fear, 132–3; generative/creative capacities, 101–2; handling, exhaustion, 63; paradox (Sacks), 101; risk, race (link), 108; toll, 93–4

disparities, term (usage), 83

disruption, practice (development), 121

disruptive harms, Native youth resistance, 138–9

diverse blackness, embedding, 115

divination, usage, 57

divine, connection, 64

divinity, usage, 63

domestic caregiving, gendered patterns, 99–100

domestic labor, 74

domestic mood, 102

domestic work, avoidance (self-centered viewpoint), 221–2

Don Augustin: ancient custom, engagement, 181; color cones, *183*; creativity, 176–7; diabetes diagnosis, life sentence (absence), 179; diabetes improvement, hope, 181; foot, infection (entry), 183–4; informal sector, employment, 179–80; loom usage, *185*; loom work, lessons, 181–2; textile craft, inheritance, 178; wheels, *176*

doshas, mixtures, 215

doubt, handling (exhaustion), 63

drapetomania, 108

dreams, usage, 57–8

drought-resistant crops, 133

drowning, attempt/completion, 227

drugs, mistrust, 21

Du Bois, W.E.B., 108–9

Dumit, J., 157

Dung: home life, *99*; Ông Năng, conversation, *97*

eating: quality, problem, 82–3; structural conditions, impact, 3

eating together, cultural practice (ignoring), 38

ecologies, toxicity, 3

economic constraints, interplay, 144

economic dynamics, village rivalries, 178

economic marginalization, 72

economic potential, conversations, 152

economics, male-dominated field (impact), 157

ecosystem, evocation, 129

el azúcar (diabetes), suffering, 178–9

Elmina Castle, 107

embodied measuring, 195, 199–200; exemplar, 203–4; fleshy space representation, 207

emotional support, 38; social support, integration, 194

emotional well-being, discussion, 24

emotions, shaping, 102

employment benefits, concerns, 156

enslavement, histories (addressing), 125

entrepreneurialism, 54

epazote (Jesuit's tea), consumption, 166

epigenetic metabolic illness, 151

epigenetics, 65

ethical community-centered research, paradigms, 10

ethical self-formation, difficulties (overcoming), 28

ethnic art, consumption (increase), 178

ethnographic research, findings, 28–9

evidence-based interventions, demands, 194

exclusion, history, 127–8

exercises: completion, 171–2; obesity/diabetes, Western medicine relationship, 31–2

expertise, steps (diversification), 117

faith, self-reproach (blend), 6

faith healer, nerve-opening instrument, *214*; usage, 213–15

Familia CONUNIDAD, DIF Oaxaca., 175

familial ethical obligations, 102

family: breadwinner, purpose/status, 215–16; connection, 64; inheritance, increase, 178–9; obligation/support, 5; support, 39–40; trust, 29; violence, suffering, 64

fármacos, impact, 149

farm life, exit, 146

fasting blood glucose, reading, 32

father, role (playing), 80–1

fat synthesis, targeting, 154

fear: experience, 8; feeling, 21–2

feet: amputation, 163; numbness, 92–3; tissues, healing/recovery, 184

fibromyalgia: soreness, decrease, 166; suffering, 162

Figueroa, M., 173

Fiji: chronic conditions, sufferers (disadvantages), 53; diabetes, diagnosis (percentage), 51; diabetes (existence), creativity/relational care (usage), 43; gender roles, 52; *girmitiya* (indentured workers), 50–1; Indo-Fijian drivers, income supplementation, 53; Indo-Fijians/Indigenous Fijians (iTaukei), ethnic tensions, 50–1; limb amputation, diabetes-related complications, 51; migration, 50; military coups, 51; moral blame, reason, 52; poverty/type 2 diabetes, ethnographic research, 50; stroke/blindness, rates (elevation), 51; unrest (1987), 45

financial pressure, management, 7–8

firstborn daughter, value (comparison), 90

flaxseed roti, consumption, 202

flesh, wounding, 66

flor de colorín, impact, 167

flor de Jamaica (dried hibiscus flower), consumption, 166

flor de pasiflora (passion flower), consumption, 166, 167

flourishing, approach, 9–10

folk art, consumption (increase), 178

food: apartheid, conditions, 137; comfort foods, overabundance, 132; cooking, 132; eating, metabolic calculation, 153; importance, respect (expression), 5; insecurity, 137; medicine, relationship, 144; preparation, social dynamics, 144; producing/securing (economic capital), 154; scarcity, 21; sovereignty, loss, 125; structural barriers, 137–8; toxicity, 3; US weaponization, 128

foodways, loss, 83

foot-pedal looms, commonness, 177–8

footsteps, 107–10

forced relocation, impact, 125, 128

forced removal, 137

friendship: creation, 82, 181; healing powers, 85; importance, 25; themes, 74; trust, 29

"Fundraise or Die" (Fiji article), 53
Funeka, prayer group, 19
future, regaining, 131

gendered hierarchies, impact, 5
genocide, histories (addressing),
   125
genomic research trials, African-
   descent participation, 111
gestational diabetes, experience,
   74–5, 80–1; difficulty, 76–7
Gift of Corn (painting), 135
girls, mistreatment, 90
girmitiya (indentured workers), 50–1
global levels, food/diabetes
   relationship, 170–1
global West, shared metabolic
   destiny, 116
glucometer pen, usage, 197
glucometers: accuracy, questioning,
   203–4; dispensation, 31;
   installation, 32; outwitting, 207–8;
   relationship, transformation,
   206; technical problems, 203;
   technology, unavailability, 32–3;
   usage, 169, 199
glucometers, numbers: checking
   (resistance), 198; checking
   (worry), 202–3
glucose: checks, 37; chronic
   dysregulation, 4; monitor,
   continuousness, 193–4; reading,
   tension, 206
glycemic load, improvement, 224–5
glycemic regulation, racial
   discrimination (impact), 227–8
glyphosate (herbicide), impact, 155
God: divine grace, 34; faith, 6;
   healing power, trust, 27; life
   determination, 26–7; trust,
   importance, 26; will, impact, 27
Goeman, M., 126
grace: concept, history, 33–4;
   etymology, 33; gift, idea

(appearance), 34; gratitude/
   gratuity, 34; persistence, 37
grandchildren, management, 24
Great Migration, 108
grief, solution/remedy, 85
grupo de crónicos, chronic illness
   support group (rejoining), 169
Guatemala: black beans, cooking,
   147; cooking expertise, impact,
   147; death, tragic limits, 158–9;
   diabetes death rate, 152; diabetics,
   dietary advice, 156–7; life, 146–7;
   medications, access, 153; national
   hospital, free services, 149; open-
   air markets, produce sales, 146;
   pregnant people, feeding, 152
guelaguetzas (support, community
   network), 184

habits, change (difficulty), 3
hacienda, loom arrival, 177
Hardin, J., 27
harm: origin, 155; patterns,
   disruption, 121
HbA1C: level, decrease, 196; test,
   usage, 193–4
HbA1C, reduction: enablement,
   204; success, 224
healing: chemistry, 158; communal
   production, rituals (usage), 62–3;
   life changes, 62; life-long journey,
   58, 67–8; openness, requirement,
   65; possibilities, sowing, 121;
   powers, friendship (relationship),
   85; promotion, 60–1; recipes,
   usage, 145
health: complications, 80;
   considerations, 186;
   disappearance, injustice, 150–1;
   disparities, addressing, 106–7;
   education, resources (allocation),
   144; holistic understanding,
   194; impeding, visible/invisible
   structures (impact/recognition),

237–8; insurance, access (expansion), 233; migration, relationship, 77; ministry, composition, 111; patience, impact, 182–3; "playing dice," 219–20; remote monitoring, 163; social determinants, term (usage), 83; spiritual/personal/political triad, 66; vulnerability, 61–2
health-care access: absence, 9; impact, 220–1
health-care institutions, integrated primary-care delivery investment, 233
healthy eating ("eat in community"), Brazilian principle, 156–7
healthy/unhealthy habits, defining, 171
heart, matters (attendance), 102
"Heart of Darkness," 115
Heart of the Desert (painting), *136*
hegemonic epistemologies (disruption), power of youth (impact), 120–1
Helu Thaman, Konai, 10
hemoglobin A1C diagnostic tests, 112
Hierba de la Virgen (*Loeselia scariosa*), impact, 165
high blood pressure, management (Mexico), 161–2
Himayat (*Imam Pasand*): consumption, 204; mango type, 201
Hinduism, faith, 54
Historically Black Colleges and Universities (HBCUs), training, 117
HIV, control, antiretroviral therapy (usage), 22
HIV diagnosis, 21
hoja santa (Mexican pepper leaf), impact, 165
holistic health, principles, 122
holy water (tea) (*indayelo*), healing power (belief), 28

honesty, radiation, 74
hopelessness, experience, 8
hospitality, sale (absence), 148
huauzontle (Mexican broccoli), consumption, 166
humor, importance, 36–7
hunger, suffering, 64
hypertension: diagnosis, 25; presence, 38

iatrochemistry, 145, 157–9; practice, 157
iatrogenesis, 150; definition, 154–5; focus, shift, 154–5
identity cards, usage, 96–7
Illich, I., 154
illness: burden, 137; connections/ factors, 17–18; experience, 64; management, learning, 21–2; narrative, 227–8; origin, 155; premature death, 64–5; worsening, 76–7
imagination, usage, 189
imbiza tonic, serving, 22–5
I'm Going Home to Harvest (beadwork), *130*
immigrants: footsteps, 115–16; healthy immigrant effect, 115–16; women, experiences (focus), 76–7
Immortal Life of Henrietta Lacks, The (Skloot), 110–11
imperative resilience, 228, 229–31; articulation, 230
imported food, consumption (problem), 9
incommensurability, space (opening), 12
India: Ayurvedic traditional medicine system, usage, 212; biomedical diabetes treatment, rejection, 219; blood glucose measurement, importance, 200; care, access (struggle), 210; cooking, financial impact,

211–12; diabetes, prevalence, 199; diabetes, thriving (meaning), 219; diet, change (struggle), 211; domestic work, avoidance (self-centered viewpoint), 221–2; faith healer, nerve-opening instrument (usage), 213–15, *214*; family breadwinner, purpose/ status, 215–16; food, consumption (frustration), 197; health/ financial challenges, 210–11; insulin pumps, unavailability, 217–18; lower-income women, stress/health complications, 221; oral hypoglycemic drugs, taking, 212; preventative checkups, expense, 213; self-care routines, continuation, 217–18; self-sacrificing homemakers, function, 220; thriving, 210; type 2 diabetes, diagnosis (shock), 216–17; wealth disparity, 218–19
Indigenous communities: diabetes epidemic, 126; research, 127–8
Indigenous food: futurisms, 129–30; sovereignty scholars, solution, 125
Indigenous group, high-risk diabetes population, 109–10
Indigenous identities, reassertion, 121
Indigenous knowledge: contributions, 128; integration, 126
individual, mutual obligation, 5
individual behavioral change, insufficiency, 9
individualization, balance, 5
industrialized labor, impact, 156
industrialized metabolism, discussion (absence), 155–6
infected tissue, removal (necessity), 186–7
infections: presence, 2; rebelliousness, 186–7

ingenuity (*métis*), 185–6; impact, 187
inheritance, term (usage), 178–9
injectable insulin, prescribing, 195
Instituto Mexicano de Seguro Social (IMSS), 167; clinic, improvement, 168; directive, 170; instructions, following, 171–2; reporting, 167; treatment, 162
insulin: daily injection, 92; dependence, resistance, 196; dosage, increase, 218; dysregulation, 199; pumps, unavailability (India), 217–18; usage, 6, 20
insulin-based medication, transition, 224–5
insulin-measuring technologies, affordability, 51
interembodiment, 37–8
interlocking systems, structural focus, 71–2
intermittent fasting (IF), practice, 196
international research teams, power arrangement, 10–11

jaggery, consumption, 205–8
jamun extract, usage, 212
Jesus, faith, 23
jowar rotis, cooking, 201–2

kaal, consumption, 201–2
karela, usage, 212
karma, return (belief), 44
ketogenic diet, 196
Kimmerer, R.W., 126
Kinaaldá (menstruation ceremony), Diné (Navajo) girls (involvement), 122
kitchen (expertise), diabetes (impact), 150
knowledgeable practices, repetition, 187
Koumba (grace), 37–8

labor, energetics, 153–7
land: dispossession, 137;
    dispossession, histories
    (addressing), 125; reforms
    (Vietnam), 88
Landecker, Hannah, 154
languages, suppression, 125
la sombra de Doña Teresa (Doña
    Teresa's shadow), 168
Latin America, diabetes rise
    (financial implications), 152
Latinx group, high-risk diabetes
    population, 109–10
Lautua, T., 5
leadership, initiation, 117
learning, spaces (extension), 238
leg(s): Levi, amputation, 7–8;
    mother, amputation, 46; Tupua,
    amputation, 5–6
Levi: blood sugar, elevation, 7; legs,
    amputation, 7–8; meat/beer,
    enjoyment, 8–9; weight, gain, 7
LGBT community members, sexual/
    marital rights (advocacy), 100
life: chances, reduction, 137;
    changes, necessity, 62; creative
    tendency, 98; Diné life stages,
    122; farm life, exit, 146; menial
    sustenance, providing, 63;
    moral fabric, 102–3; numerical
    orientation, resentment, 199;
    path, purposefulness, 64; quality,
    improvement, 166; shared lives,
    carrying, 102; weft, weaving, 175
life cycles: Diné ceremonies, 122;
    disruptions, 122
life story: diabetes, 91–4; first-person
    voice, 94; interconnectedness, 68
literacy campaign (Vietnam), 89
liver failure, suffering, 148–9
living well (collective endeavor),
    137–9
loneliness: absence, 59; feeling,
    90–1; fight, 225

loom: colors, cones, *183*; cotton,
    threads (intervention), 186;
    diamond glyph design, *188*;
    Don Agustin usage, *185*; pedals,
    usage, *189*; thread, purchase,
    182; thread, weaving, 181; work,
    lessons, 181–2
loss, cycle, 80
love: devotion, 96; life, 94
loved one, care (difficulties), 52
lower-income women, stress/health
    complications (India), 221
lower-limb amputation, 2

Mãe Canela (spiritual godmother):
    divination, execution, 61;
    guidance, communication,
    62–3; message, hopefulness,
    62; salutation, power
    acknowledgement, 60–1; visit,
    plan, 57, 59
mãe-de-santo (spiritual godmother),
    visit/experience, 57, 66
male-oriented kinship system
    (Vietnam), 98
mangoes, *202*; body, attunement,
    204; types, 201
Mann, Robert, 112
marital issues, worsening, 226
*Mark My Words: Native Women Mapping
    Our Nations* (Goeman), 126
massage, pain, 214
maternal nutrition investments,
    importance, 152
meal, feeding ability, *157*
measuring body, impact, 207
mechanical social obligation, 102
medical anthropology,
    contribution, 18
medical care (finding), worries, 164
medical theory, adaptation, 187
medications: access, affordability,
    153; avoidance, noncompliance,
    232; skipping, 153

médico particular (private physician),
  charges, 163
meditation, practice, 162
memelas (picaditas), making, 77
mental health providers, shortages,
  233
meso-level thinking, 12
mestizaje logics, 173
metabolic disorders: constraints,
  36–7; impacts, 33; navigation, 40
metabolic illnesses: epigenetic
  aspect, 151; production, 154
metabolic modernity, 107–8
metabolism, calculable exchange,
  153
metformin: absence, impact, 22;
  usage, 20
metrics: meaning, 194; social life,
  194
Mexico: care, establishment,
  163; coffee, importance, 168;
  comida chatarra (junk food),
  consumption, 165; community,
  importance, 161; community-run
  clinic, staffing, 167; COVID-19
  pandemic, businesses (closure),
  180; diabetes, impact, 162–3; diet,
  166; dietary nutrition, increase,
  166; disease, epidemiological
  data, 172–3; economic dynamics,
  village rivalries, 178; employment,
  loss, 181; *grupo de crónicos*, chronic
  illness support group (rejoining),
  169; healthy/unhealthy habits,
  defining, 171; high blood
  pressure, management, 161–2;
  home, sanctuary, 168; Indigenous
  languages/Spanish dialects,
  speaking, 180; insecurity, 161;
  Instituto Mexicano de Seguro
  Social (IMSS) treatment, 162;
  life, quality (improvement),
  166; medical care (finding),
  worries, 164; *médico particular*
  (private physician), charges,
  163; online intake form, medical
  examination, 164; rural health,
  161; rural zones, diabetes (rise),
  178–9; skill, impact, 184–7;
  tamale business, understanding,
  167; tourist sector, consolidation,
  178; type 2 diabetes, management,
  161–2; type 2 diabetes mellitus,
  death cause, 172; unhealthy
  lifestyles, correction, 172–3; work
  (loss), injury (impact), 162–3
migrants: community, good (force),
  84; diabetes/disease, 77, 84;
  families, interaction, 84–5
migration: health, relationship, 77;
  nodes, disparateness, 114
milk tea (*trà sữa*), presence, 96
Minas Gerais (Brazil), 64
minimum salary, concerns, 156
minor indulgences, guilt, 195
mirth (Three Graces component), 34
Mission and Removal Period, 128
money: finiteness, 153;
  management, 24
moral blame, reason, 52
moral duty, 102
moral orientations, shaping, 102
morena (dark-skinned Mexican), 161
Morning Dawn, representation, 122
mother: leg, amputation, 46; role,
  playing, 80–1; separation, 78–9;
  suffering, 79–80
mothering, attention, 152–3
muscles, relaxation, 167

national ethical obligations, 102
Native communities: diet-sensitive
  health problems, 137; symbolic
  violence, contribution, 138
Native foods, reintroduction, 138
Native peoples: assimilation/
  reeducation, 133; cultural
  restoration/health, 129; culture,

loss, 133; diabetes, disruption, 131; diabetes, presence, 121; losses, 131–6; realities/aspirations, 138–9; US government-subsidized food assistance, 137
native *pueblo*, 177
Native schools, youth (interaction), 132
Native tribes, commodity foods (distribution), 127
Native youth, resistance, 138–9
native youth disruptions, health/ food (impact), 120
natural history, witness, 12
nausea, generation, 187
necrosis, diagnosis, 93
necrotic tissue, removal, 183
neem leaves, usage, 212
negative health outcomes, 137
Negro body, interrogation, 109
Negro population, increase, 115
Nestle, M. (message), 144
networks: connection, 64; support, 18
New York City: fact-finding missions, 79; public health-care system, navigation, 76
nimbu pani, consumption, 216
noncompliance (medication avoidance), 232
Nopal (cactus paddles), consumption, 165
nutrition, importance, 167
nutrition-related non-communicable diseases, 152

obesity, 133; cause, 194; consequence, 152; exercise/ diabetes, Western medicine emphasis, 31–2
omama bomthandazo (mothers/ women of prayer), impact, 28
Ông Năng, 71; alcohol, brewing, 94; altar placement, 94–5; Dung, conversation, *97*; identity cards,

study, 96; moral indebtedness, 102; wife, death, 98
online intake form, medical examination, 164
open-air markets, produce (sale), 146
open-heart surgery, 162
openness, requirement, 65
optimism, maintenance, 52, 54
oral hypoglycemic drugs, taking, 212
oral medications, success, 187
organisms, environments (mutual relationship), 182
orixás, divination, 62

Pacific research methodologies, development, 10
pain: absence, 79; cycle, 80; endurance, 82; healing, 73; increase, 158–9; intensity, 151; physical somatization, 80; presence, 65; relief, 75–6; witness, 84–5
painting: *Gift of Corn, 135*; *Heart of the Desert, 136*; *Squash Mother, 134*
paneer, consumption, 211
paneer butter masal, consumption, 196
paquetero (informal courier), job, 79
paracetamol, usage, 164
parenting, difficulty, 81
pastors, trust, 29
patchwork, 177
patience, requirement, 175, 182–4
patient behavior, compliance, 190
patient-physician partnerships, value, 224
Penda (grace), 39–40
people, fixing/curing (focus), 237
physical therapy, 163
physiological indicators, self-tracking, 206
poems, creation, 125–6
poiesis-on-behalf-of-another, 98–9
Poor People's Campaign, 154

poverty: comorbidities, experience,
    51; ethnographic research, 50;
    suffering, 64
prayer: diabetes usage, 19; group,
    attendance, 19–20; group,
    hosting, 22; importance, 26
preemptive refusals, encounter, 106
pregnancy, 91; difficulty, 74–5;
    USAID energy, targeting, 152
preventative health-care programs,
    treatment, 151
prevention-and-control-only
    approach, weakness, 12
prevention knowledge, availability, 11
prudence (*phrónesis*), 185–6
psychosocial support, prayer
    (importance), 26
psychosocial trauma, 227–8

quelites (edible leaves/stems/
    flowers), consumption, 166

Rabinbach, A., 153
rabri, consumption, 197
race, disease risk (link), 108
race/gender biases, disadvantage, 54
racial capitalism, impact, 72
racial categories, reinforcement,
    109–10
racial categorization, 109–10
racial discrimination, 227–8
racialized experiences, 116
racial labor, 114
racial risk, 109
rasam, consumption, 196
rebozo, weaving, 186
reciprocity, importance, 40
Red River Delta: house, description,
    94; patriarchy, 100
relational care, usage, 43
relationality, importance, 4–5
religious practices: description, 26;
    negative impact, 26

research: decolonization, 10–11;
    Indigenous knowledge,
    integration, 126
residential patterns, commonness, 74
rice farming, income source
    (Vietnam), 96
Richards, Margaret, 112
Ridaq, taking, 20
risk: co-management, 173; factors,
    term (usage), 83
Robbins, J., 27–8
romerito (seepweed), consumption,
    166
rooibos, drinking, 21
roti: consumption, 211; flaxseed roti,
    consumption, 202; preparation,
    212

Sacks, O., 101
sadness: endurance, 82; insanity,
    81–2; period, entry, 80
Salvador da Bahia (Brazil),
    anthropology, 60–1
sambar, consumption, 196
Samoa: diabetes prevention,
    information (abundance), 9;
    multigenerational settings,
    5; primary care, limitations
    (sharing), 11; systemic
    problem, 4
Samoan Pentecostals, healing
    (everyday activity), 27
saving, calculus, 151–3
scarcity, driver, 154
Schwittek, David, 84
Seguridad y Solidaridad Social
    (Security and Social Solidarity),
    168–9
self-care: frame, 173; importance,
    teaching, 4; routines, continuation,
    217–18; source, 35
self-medication, 81
self-prayer, usage, 26

self-sacrificing homemakers,
function (India), 220
Senegal: childcare, trade, 33;
education, 35; life, 31; Three
Graces version, diabetes
context, 34
settler colonialism: disruptive
harm, 121; manifestations, 128;
struggles, 127; type 2 diabetes,
pathology, 137
Seventh-day Adventist Church:
brothers, assistance, 184; network,
181
severity (mitigation), humor
(usage), 36–7
shared responsibility, 173
sharing, spaces (extension), 238
shells. *See buzios*
shift work, concerns, 156
sickle cell disease, 109
sickness: description, 58; spirituality,
exploration, 66
side effects, unbearability, 187
Simmons, D., 154
Sirah (grace), 35–7
skill (*téchne*), 185–6
skilled practices, repetition, 187
skills, learning, 188
Skloot, R., 110
slavery: afflicted slave, diagnosis,
108; Africa, enslavement,
60; durée, 108; existence,
225–6; slaves, subsistence-level
deprivations, 109
Slave Voyages (website), 107–8
sleep schedules, concerns, 156
sobadores (healers of muscle pain and
sprains), impact, 166–7
*Sobrepeso, Obesidad y Diabetes: Hacía
Una Vida Saludable y en Armonia
(Overweight, Obesity, and Diabetes:
Towards a Healthy, Harmonious
Life)*, 169–70

social adversity, survival (physical
costs), 230–2
social contexts, 116; risk levels,
creation, 71–2
social inequalities, impact, 18
social networks, web (intricacy), 33
social relations, impact, 239
social relationships: interplay, 144;
networks, combination, 184
social science, approaches, 194
social structures, diabetes
(relationship), 71
social support, emotional support
(integration), 194
social upheaval (Vietnam), 88
social wave, 111
social worlds, diabetes (reflection),
143–4
socioeconomic status: elevation,
health results, 221; impact, 220–1
socio-somatic generativity, 88
solidarity, issues, 11–12
somatic issues, anthropological
characterizations, 227–8
Soteropolitanos, healing, 60–1
Soweto: chronic illness, research,
25–6; HIV, presence, 23
space, creation, 1
spirit, compassion/honesty
radiation, 74
spiritual godmother. *See* Mãe Canela
spiritual inheritance, 65
spirituality, description, 125
Squash Mother (beadwork), *134*
states of being, embodiment, 38
STEMM disciplines, challenges, 117
stoicism, 43
story, creation, 125–6
storytellers, 125; observations, 121
storytelling, approach (creative/
collaborative method), 120–1
strategic thinking, requirement,
116–17

strength (*fuerza*), 189
stress, surveys, 28–9
stretching, practice, 162
stroke, suffering, 94
stroke/blindness, Fiji rates
    (elevation), 51
structural conditions: observation,
    4–5; reality, 4
struggles (capture), creative
    expressions (usage), 126
subsidy system (Vietnam), 93–4
subsistence-level deprivations
    (slaves), 109
sugar: avoidance, 48; blood sugar,
    elevation, 7; catalyst, problem,
    109; control, *imbiza* (drinking),
    22–3; diabetes, entanglement,
    65–6; imbalance, 21; increase,
    77–8; management, 193–4;
    plantation industrial complex,
    profit, 114; racial project
    metaphor, 107; relationship,
    learning (Brazil), 57;
    transformative power, 66
sugar-industrial complex, demands/
    profits, 108
suicidal ideation, demonstration,
    179
suicide, increase (attempts), 179
support, importance, 39–40
sustainable foods, production, 138
sweetness, conversion, 58
symbolic violence, contribution, 138
sympathy entrepreneurs, 53
syndemics: term, usage, 83; violence,
    immigration, diabetes, depression,
    and abuse (VIDDA syndemic), 83
systemic problem, 4

tai chi, practice, 162
tamale business, understanding, 167
taxi driving, gendered/racialized
    affordance, 52–3
telemedicine, usage, 233

terreiro (spiritual temple),
    attendance, 60
Theoharis, L., 154
thieboudienne, fish (preparation), 36
Three Graces (mirth/beauty/
    youth), 34–5
thriving, discussion, 2
tinkering, 43; care, metaphor
    (development), 51–2
tissue: death, diabetes (cause),
    93; infected tissue, removal
    (necessity), 186–7
titanium mechanical heart-valve
    replacement, chronic illness
    (appearance), 162
Tohono O'odham people: foods,
    presence, 132; Sonoran Desert,
    existence, 133; traditional crops,
    growing, 133–6
tortillas, consumption (boredom),
    164–5
traditional food: Native people
    definition, 132; sustainability, 138
trauma: haunting, fighting, 225;
    pain, healing, 73; pain (physical
    effects), simple solution
    (absence), 85; psychosocial
    trauma, 227–8; release, 65
tribal relations, structural barriers,
    137–8
trigueñita (light brown skin
    coloring), 226
Trostle, J., 189–90
Tuck, E., 11
Tuhiwai Smith, L., 9–10, 126
Tupua: diabetes medication,
    avoidance (reasons), 6; food,
    availability (change), 6; imported
    food, consumption (problem),
    6; leg, amputation, 5–6; sickness,
    prolongation, 6–7
Tuskegee Syphilis Study, 113
type 2 diabetes, 106–7, 110;
    diagnosis, shock, 216–17;

ethnographic research, 50; management (Mexico), 161–2; pathology, 137; racial biology, unmooring, 111; redounding, 109; research focus, reprioritization, 111

type 2 diabetes mellitus, death cause (Mexico), 172

type 3 diabetes, 111–12

uncontrolled diabetes, amputation suffering, 54

unhealthy lifestyles, correction (Mexico), 172–3

United States, migration, 73–4

University of Arizona, youth storytelling project, 120

usos y costumbres, 178

vascular tension, impact, 227–8

vatapá (paste, service), 61

vendors, search, 146

Vietnam: agricultural cooperative, work, 89; diabetes, ubiquity, 92; domestic mood, 102; ethnographic fieldwork, 94–5; family, building, 89–91; feet, numbness, 92–3; girls, mistreatment, 90; highly processed foods, presence, 96; ID cards, *101*; identity cards, usage, 96–7; land reforms, 88; LGBT community members, sexual/ marital rights (advocacy), 100; literacy campaign, 89; loneliness, feeling, 90–1; male-oriented kinship system, 98; marriage, women resistance, 99–100; milk tea (*trà sữa*), presence, 96; patrilineal/patrilocal kinship system, 97–8; post-war starvation, 90; rice farming, income source, 96; social organization, 97–8; social upheaval, 88–9; socio-

somatic generativity, 88; subsidy system, 93–4; tea, invitation, 95–6; traditional medicine, 93

violence, immigration, diabetes, depression, and abuse (VIDDA syndemic), 83

Virgen morena, 178

vitamins: transfer, 154; usage, absence, 83

waist size, importance, 170–1

water, toxicity, 3

water walking, practice, 162

Wayne Yang, K., 11

weight: gain, 7; management, 166

well-being: emotional well-being, discussion, 24; impacts, 32; impeding, 237; sense, contributions, 239

wellness, 38

Western knowledge, contributions, 128

Western knowledge production, challenge, 10

Western medicine, harshness, 92

wheelchair: donation, 49; need, 46–7

wheels (Don Agustín creation), *176*

Whyte, K., 126

willpower, impact, 3

wives, grace, 31

women: abuse, story, 225–7; interviews, 36–7; learning, 230; lower-income women, stress/ health complications (India), 221; mobility, limitation, 171; resources, sharing, 40; support, importance, 39–40

wool: natural dyes, preparation, 182; thread, weaving, 177

work: domestic work, avoidance (self-centered viewpoint), 221–2; loss, injury (impact), 162–3; skill, 184–7; value, 181

work-based health care, qualification
    (absence) (Mexico), 172
wounds: gangrenous impact,
    163; healing, slowness, 2;
    improvement, absence, 48

Xaagá: community identification,
    178; entrance, *179*

Yaets-Doerr, E., 11
yoga, practice, 162

Yoonu Njub ("way of righteousness"),
    31; organizers, activity, 31–2
youth (Three Graces component),
    34
youth storytelling project, 120

Zarate, Gustavo, 84, *84*
Zárate, López de, 177–8
Zion Christian Church (ZCC),
    attendance (growth), 28
Zionist church, joining, 22